How to Write the Thesis and Thesis Protocol

A Primer for Medical, Dental, and Nursing Courses

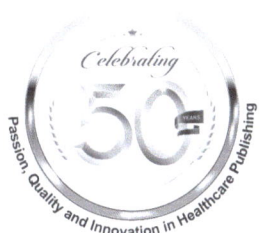

How to Write the Thesis and Thesis Protocol

A Primer for Medical, Dental, and Nursing Courses

Editors

Piyush Gupta MD FIAP FNNF FAMS
Professor and Head
Department of Pediatrics
University College of Medical Sciences
and Guru Teg Bahadur Hospital
New Delhi, India

Dheeraj Shah MD FIAP MNAMS
Professor
Department of Pediatrics
University College of Medical Sciences
and Guru Teg Bahadur Hospital
New Delhi, India

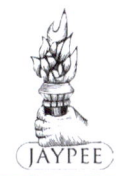

JAYPEE BROTHERS MEDICAL PUBLISHERS
The Health Sciences Publisher
New Delhi | London

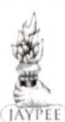
Jaypee Brothers Medical Publishers (P) Ltd

Headquarter

Jaypee Brothers Medical Publishers (P) Ltd
4838/24, Ansari Road, Daryaganj
New Delhi 110 002, India
Phone: +91-11-43574357
Fax: +91-11-43574314
Email: jaypee@jaypeebrothers.com

Overseas Office

J.P. Medical Ltd
83 Victoria Street, London
SW1H 0HW (UK)
Phone: +44 20 3170 8910
Fax: +44 (0)20 3008 6180
Email: info@jpmedpub.com

Website: www.jaypeebrothers.com
Website: www.jaypeedigital.com

© 2021, Piyush Gupta

The views and opinions expressed in this book are solely those of the original contributor(s)/author(s) and do not necessarily represent those of editor(s) of the book.

All rights reserved. No part of this publication may be reproduced, stored or transmitted in any form or by any means, electronic, mechanical, photocopying, recording or otherwise, without the prior permission in writing of the publishers.

All brand names and product names used in this book are trade names, service marks, trademarks or registered trademarks of their respective owners. The publisher is not associated with any product or vendor mentioned in this book.

Medical knowledge and practice change constantly. This book is designed to provide accurate, authoritative information about the subject matter in question. However, readers are advised to check the most current information available on procedures included and check information from the manufacturer of each product to be administered, to verify the recommended dose, formula, method and duration of administration, adverse effects and contraindications. It is the responsibility of the practitioner to take all appropriate safety precautions. Neither the publisher nor the author(s)/editor(s) assume any liability for any injury and/or damage to persons or property arising from or related to use of material in this book.

This book is sold on the understanding that the publisher is not engaged in providing professional medical services. If such advice or services are required, the services of a competent medical professional should be sought.

Every effort has been made where necessary to contact holders of copyright to obtain permission to reproduce copyright material. If any have been inadvertently overlooked, the publisher will be pleased to make the necessary arrangements at the first opportunity. The **CD/DVD-ROM** (if any) provided in the sealed envelope with this book is complimentary and free of cost. **Not meant for sale.**

Inquiries for bulk sales may be solicited at: jaypee@jaypeebrothers.com

How to Write the Thesis and Thesis Protocol:
A Primer for Medical, Dental, and Nursing Courses / *Piyush Gupta, Dheeraj Shah*

First Edition: 2014

Second Edition: **2021**

Reprint: 2024

ISBN: 978-93-90020-71-3

Printed at Repro India Limited

Contributors

Aashima Dabas MD
Associate Professor
Department of Pediatrics, Maulana Azad Medical College and Lok Nayak Hospital
New Delhi, India
Email: dr.aashimagupta@gmail.com

Alpana Raizada MD FICP
Associate Professor
Department of Medicine
University College of Medical Sciences and Guru Teg Bahadur Hospital
New Delhi, India
Email: alpanaraizada@yahoo.com

Amir Maroof Khan MD FAIMER (CMCL)
Associate Professor
Department of Community Medicine
University College of Medical Sciences
New Delhi, India
Email: khanamirmaroof@yahoo.com

Bhupendra Kumar Jain MS FAMS FAIS FCLS
Former Director Professor and Head
Department of Surgery and Medical Superintendent, University College of Medical Sciences, and Guru Teg Bahadur Hospital
New Delhi, India
Email: bhupendrakjain@gmail.com

Devendra Mishra MD FIAP
Professor
Departments of Pediatrics and Medical Education
Maulana Azad Medical College
New Delhi, India
Email: drdmishra@gmail.com

Dheeraj Shah MD FIAP MNAMS
Professor
Department of Pediatrics
University College of Medical Sciences and Guru Teg Bahadur Hospital
New Delhi, India
Email: shahdheeraj@hotmail.com

Jaya Shankar Kaushik MD
Professor
Department of Pediatrics
Pt B D Sharma Postgraduate Institute of Medical Sciences
Rohtak, Haryana, India
Email: jayashankarkaushik@gmail.com

Kirtisudha Mishra MD DNB FIPNA FISPN
Associate Professor
Department of Pediatrics
Chacha Nehru Bal Chikitsalaya
New Delhi, India
Email: kirtisen@gmail.com

Naveen Sharma MS
Professor
Department of General Surgery
All India Institute of Medical Sciences
Jodhpur, India
Email: drnsemail@gmail.com

Navjeevan Singh MD
Former Director-Professor
Department of Pathology, and Co-ordinator of
the Medical Education Unit
University College of Medical Sciences
New Delhi, India
Email: navjeevansingh@hotmail.com

Nidhi Bedi MD
Associate Professor
Hamdard Institute of Medical Sciences
New Delhi, India
Email: drnidhibedi@gmail.com

Nitin Agarwal MS MNAMS FIAGES
Professor
Transplant Unit
Department of Surgery
ABVIMS and RML Hospital
New Delhi, India
Email: drnitinagarwal76@gmail.com

OP Kalra MD DM FICP FACP
Vice Chancellor
Pt B D Sharma University of Health Sciences
Rohtak, Haryana, India
Email: opkalra1@yahoo.com

Pankaj Kumar Garg MS MCh FACS FRCS
Additional Professor
Department of Surgical Oncology
All India Institute of Medical Sciences
Rishikesh, India
Email: dr.pankajgarg@gmail.com

Piyush Gupta MD FAMS FNNF FIAP
Professor and Head
Department of Pediatrics
University College of Medical Sciences
and Guru Teg Bahadur Hospital
New Delhi, India
Email: prof.piyush.gupta@gmail.com

Pooja Dewan MD FIAP
Professor
Department of Pediatrics
University College of Medical Sciences
and Guru Teg Bahadur Hospital
New Delhi, India
Email: poojadewan@hotmail.com

Rehan Ul Haq MS MAMS
Professor and Head
Department of Orthopaedics
All India Institute of Medical Sciences
Bhopal, India
Email: docrehan1975@gmail.com

Romit Saxena MD IFPCCM EPIC Dip
Assistant Professor
Department of Pediatrics
Maulana Azad Medical College
New Delhi, India
Email: drromit@gmail.com

Sahiba Kukreja MD
Professor and Head
Department of Biochemistry, Dean (UG)
Director (Biomedical Research)
Sri Guru Ram Das University of
Health Sciences
Amritsar, Punjab, India
Email: drsahibakukreja@gmail.com

Sanjay Gupta MS FRCS
Director Professor and Head
Department of Surgery
University College of Medical Sciences
and Guru Teg Bahadur Hospital
New Delhi, India
Email: drsanjaygupta1@gmail.com

Sharmila Banerjee Mukherjee MD
Professor
Department of Pediatrics
Lady Hardinge Medical College and
Associated Hospitals
New Delhi, India
Email: theshormi@gmail.com

Siddarth Ramji MD
Director-Professor
Department of Neonatology
Maulana Azad Medical College
New Delhi, India
Email: siddarthramji@gmail.com

Somashekhar Nimbalkar MD
Associate Dean (Research), Head
Department of Pediatrics
Pramukhswami Medical College
Karamsad, Gujarat, India
Email: somu.somu@gmail.com

SV Madhu MD DM (Endocrinology)
Director-Professor and Head
Department of Endocrinology
University College of Medical Sciences
and Guru Teg Bahadur Hospital
New Delhi, India
Email: drsvmadhu@gmail.com

Tejinder Singh MD DNB MHPE Dip Human Resource Management
Professor of Pediatrics and Medical Education
SGRD Institute of Medical Sciences and Research
Amritsar, Punjab, India

Upreet Dhaliwal MS CMCL-FAIMER Fellow
Former Director-Professor
Department of Ophthalmology
University College of Medical Sciences
and Guru Teg Bahadur Hospital
New Delhi, India
Email: upreetdhaliwal@gmail.com

Foreword

I am delighted to learn that you are going ahead with the second edition of your highly in demand, an absolute must for all budding postgraduates and even their teachers and guides, the very apt book on "How to Write Thesis." You have done a commendable job and this new edition with additional inputs will be liked even more by all postgraduate students and teachers in various Medical, Paramedical, Nursing, Biomedical, Biotechnical, and Pharmaceutical Institutions involved in conduct of research. In today's world of competence and competition, good research is a core issue.

Thesis writing is an integral part of postgraduate training. With increasing pool of trainees being admitted into various medical postgraduate courses every year, it is extremely important to impart them knowledge and skills related to thesis writing and the related intricacies of the process of research. With over 500 medical colleges running postgraduate training programs in various specialties and even higher number of institutions conducting Diplomate of National Board (DNB) postgraduate teaching, it is also imperative to create a large pool of faculty who can supervise and mentor these young postgraduate students.

This multiauthored book is very well planned with 28 chapters covering all aspects of protocol and thesis writing. Starting from explaining the rationale and planning of research and thesis writing, this treatise provides reader a smooth ride to various intricacies of thesis writing. Taking care of affective domain, the book provides excellent information about mentor-mentee relationship, and ethical principles in carrying out research and related publications. The book is written in a simple and instructional language and is replete with simple and understandable examples.

This book is so well written and is almost like a Bible. I am confident, it will be so much liked that it would be in possession of all postgraduates and PhD scholars of medical and allied sciences and their institutions. I heartily appreciate the enormous efforts put in by the editors and the acclaimed authors.

With best compliments and regards.

Professor (Mrs) S Chooramani Gopal
MS MCh (AIIMS) FAMS
Padmashree Awardee
DR BC ROY Awardee
Distinguished Professor (Pediatric Surgery)
President, National Academy of Medical Sciences
Former Vice-Chancellor, K.G. Medical University, Lucknow
Former President, All India Association of Pediatric Surgeons

Foreword

Conducting Medical Research is essential for the understanding of the problems that affect individuals, communities, or health systems. It allows for a systemic and scientific assessment of the problem and provides knowledge that allows for instituting a change in the practice of clinical medicine.

A thesis is seen as the culmination of research conducted as a postgraduate and is submitted as the final end product. Making the thesis submission mandatory for postgraduates need not be viewed as a statutory requirement for acquisition of postgraduate medical degree alone, but an opportunity to get exposure to conduct research. Such an opportunity encourages postgraduates to not only convert this thesis research into a publication in a scientific journal but also opens pathways in selecting future career and related research areas.

Each thesis is a unique piece of research, with an intent to extend the academic information in the area of specialization. The structure of the thesis explains the purpose, the previous research literature related to the topic of the study, the methods used, and the findings of the study conducted. The most difficult elements of writing a thesis include framing a research question and hypothesis, identifying appropriate material and relevant methods, collating the scientific literature, and using appropriate statistical tools for interpretation of data.

Currently, there is a void in the scope of medical literature which provides guidance to the postgraduate students regarding conducting a good quality research and about writing the thesis. Students are usually scared from the idea of thesis and teachers are left scratching their heads for want of innovative or meaningful research topics.

This book fills this gap and provides useful tools to improve thesis writing. It covers the basic information about conducting a good quality research and converting it into a quality thesis. There are chapters on each and every aspect of thesis with emphasis on important areas like protocol, elements of thesis headings including research designs, estimation of sample size, statistical analysis, and a separate chapter on references.

I congratulate Professor Piyush Gupta for bringing out the second edition of this book after the success of the first edition. I also compliment Dr Dheeraj Shah and all other authors for their contribution for the release of the second edition. This edition finds addition of new chapters namely *"Converting Thesis into a Scientific Paper"* and *"Manuscript-based Thesis: A New Paradigm"* I am sure that this book shall also encourage the young medical researchers to convert their thesis into scientific papers in national and international acclaimed journals.

Professor Pawanindra Lal
MS DNB FIMSA FCLS FRCSEd
FRCS (Glasg) FRCS (Eng) FACS FAMS
Executive Director, National Board of Examinations
Director Professor of Surgery, MAMC
New Delhi, India

Preface to the Second Edition

While the first edition of this book was inspired by a series of workshops on thesis writing organized for postgraduate students by our team, in this thoroughly revised second edition, we have attempted to accommodate the additional perceived needs and demands of students participating in workshops conducted by us since the publication of first edition. To achieve this, we provided a set of objectives and the desired content and flow to the author of each chapter, simultaneously providing them liberty to incorporate new ideas and examples. This process mandated inclusion of illustrious authors who are the best in the fields of medical education and research in the country. Though this revised edition essentially maintains the sequence of chapters as per the events in engaging with a thesis, each chapter is thoroughly revised with inclusion of plenty of examples from various medical and nonmedical subjects for easy understanding. We have included two new chapters—"*Converting Thesis into a Scientific Paper*" and "*Manuscript-based Thesis: A New Paradigm*"—in order to further stimulate the readers to culminate this process of thesis writing in form of a scientific paper in a reputed journal. We have tried to keep the language simple and conversational so as to achieve a better connect with the readers. An updated list of references for further reading is provided for readers to explore more details of the processes of research and thesis writing. A pleasing two-color format and inclusion of Key Messages and Concluding Paragraph with every chapter will result in better visual appeal and understanding. We hope that this book will continue to serve not only the needs of novice researchers such as undergraduate/postgraduate medical/nursing students and PhD students, but also of their supervisors and young research scientists who have to consolidate their research knowledge and skills for further dissemination and implementation.

Piyush Gupta
Dheeraj Shah

Preface to the First Edition

This book has evolved from a series of workshops organized for postgraduate students by the Medical Education Unit of the University College of Medical Sciences. The objective of the workshops was to introduce them to the basics of biomedical research as a prelude to writing a protocol for a thesis, and subsequently, to writing the thesis itself. As the number of postgraduate admissions increased exponentially in 2009, the three-day "thesis writing workshop" was split into two one-and-a-half day workshops; the first a protocol writing workshop at the beginning of first year of residency, and the second a thesis writing workshop, some three months prior to thesis submission.

To maintain the true character of a hands-on workshop, with more time for group exercises than for didactic lectures/presentations, each workshop was conducted for batches of only up to 35 participants. Four identical workshops in sequence over a week, gave us the opportunity to groom more workshop faculty, the result of which is visible in the depth of academic talent in the list of authors in this book. Today our institution can boast of at least three independent teams capable of conducting these workshops.

As word of our workshops spread, we began receiving requests from other institutions to conduct them for their students; however, it quickly became clear that we could not possibly do justice to too many each year. At the same time, there appeared to be a dearth of resources dealing with thesis writing—material that could serve as self-help tools for the beginner. In this setting, it appeared rational to write this book. As with our workshops, this book is written for the novice desirous of entering the research arena: for whom a thesis is mandatory, undergraduate students wishing to venture into research by way of summer projects and working with supportive faculty, and, in fact, any beginner in research. It can be used as a bench manual—to be referred to at every stage of working on a thesis. It may also be useful to thesis supervisors, and institutions wishing to design and administer their own training workshops similar to ours.

The text is organized into 26 chapters which follow the sequence of events in engaging with a thesis. A unique feature is the numerous examples in each chapter illustrating what to do, and often, what not to do. The language is simple, the style conversational, and we hope, easy to follow. A bibliography is provided at the end of each chapter for those wishing to delve further into the intricacies of biomedical research.

We hope the readers will find answers to many of their questions related to the thesis; that the book arouses their curiosity, propelling them to further their reading, and continues to be a useful reference whenever they contemplate research.

Piyush Gupta
Navjeevan Singh

Contents

1. **Rationale for Thesis and Research in Postgraduate Courses** — 1
   Siddarth Ramji

2. **Dealing with the Supervisor: Mentor–Mentee Relationship** — 5
   Sahiba Kukreja, Tejinder Singh

3. **Process of Thesis Writing: Plan it Well** — 10
   Alpana Raizada, OP Kalra

4. **Thesis: The Essential Elements** — 18
   Nitin Agarwal

5. **Formulating a Research Question/Hypothesis: The First Step** — 26
   Bhupendra Kumar Jain

6. **How to Select the Study Design** — 33
   Aashima Dabas, Devendra Mishra

7. **Framing a Suitable Title** — 45
   Piyush Gupta

8. **Electronic Search of the Literature** — 51
   Romit Saxena, Jaya Shankar Kaushik

9. **Writing Aim and Objectives: Getting Clarity** — 60
   Upreet Dhaliwal

10. **Writing the Introduction: Justifying Your Research** — 66
    Naveen Sharma

11. **Review of Literature: Recalling the Past** — 69
    Sanjay Gupta

12. **Material and Methods: How will I do it?** — 76
    Dheeraj Shah

13. **Sample Size Estimation** — 85
    Amir Maroof Khan

14. **Ethical Issues in Thesis and Conducting Research** — 97
    Kirtisudha Mishra

15.	**Preparing a Case Record Form: Get, Set, and Go** *Pankaj Kumar Garg*	106
16.	**Planning the Statistical Analysis** *Pankaj Kumar Garg*	109
17.	**Results: Fruits of the Labor** *Rehan Ul Haq*	124
18.	**Converting Results to Text, Tables, and Graphs: Represent the Findings** *Amir Maroof Khan*	131
19.	**Discussion: The Most Read Part of the Thesis** *SV Madhu, Dheeraj Shah*	138
20.	**Writing the Conclusion: Bringing Down the Curtains in Style** *Nidhi Bedi, Pooja Dewan*	143
21.	**Summary: The Essence of Thesis** *Pooja Dewan, Nidhi Bedi*	148
22.	**Writing References** *Piyush Gupta, Amir Maroof Khan*	154
23.	**Publication Misconduct and How to Avoid it** *Sharmila Banerjee Mukherjee*	165
24.	**Elements of Writing Better English** *Navjeevan Singh*	175
25.	**Showcasing Thesis through an Effective PowerPoint Presentation** *Pooja Dewan, Piyush Gupta*	185
26.	**Writing the Thesis Protocol** *Dheeraj Shah, Navjeevan Singh*	197
27.	**Converting Thesis into a Scientific Paper** *Dheeraj Shah*	202
28.	**Manuscript-based Thesis: A New Paradigm** *Somashekhar Nimbalkar*	208
	Annexure: Case-Record Form	212
	Index	213

CHAPTER 1

Rationale for Thesis and Research in Postgraduate Courses

Siddarth Ramji

INTRODUCTION

As a medical practitioner we would always have to query ourselves about the *whys, hows, whats,* and *whens* related to problems people present with or situations that arise as part of the discharge of our professional responsibilities. How does one get answers to these concerns and queries? The easiest way is search for published material on the subject (which nowadays is just a few taps away in this digitalized world). If we do manage to find a solution, we feel happy and get on with our lives. But, how many of us pause for a moment and give a thought to the quality of evidence for this solution; most of us take the information obtained as the "gospel truth." Decisions based on low-quality evidence could have the potential to adversely impact the outcome—either by not improving the person's condition or hurtling him/her down the abyss of death or disability—though both being the result of a decision that was unintentional on the part of the medical practitioner.

IMPORTANCE OF RESEARCH IN MEDICINE

There are several reasons for the need of research in medical sciences; the most salient ones are outlined below.

For the Practicing Physician

Imagine a physician deciding to use prophylactic daily aspirin therapy to prevent myocardial infarction (MI) in a 50-year-old postmenopausal woman because her father had history of MI at 60 years, based on the result of a single randomized control study.
- If with this treatment, the woman does not develop MI, can one conclude that the physician's decision validates the study results?
- On the other hand, if the woman was to develop MI, would it refute the study results?
- Or if she was to develop serious gastrointestinal bleeding without developing MI, would it mean aspirin therapy is unsafe for use for prevention of MI in postmenopausal women?

These and many similar questions require an understanding of how to evaluate the strength of evidence available to be able to translate the findings into clinical practice. Understanding of research principles and methods facilitates the physician to adopt evidence-based results into their medical practice, which would not only make it more scientific but also more ethical.

For Problem-solving

Research is also needed to find a way forward to handle health problems afflicting humankind, which either have no solution, or a solution with low-moderate efficacy, or prevent the occurrence of such health maladies. The Coronavirus (COVID-19) epidemic which had its origins in China in the late part of 2019 is a case in point, where neither a vaccine for its prevention nor a drug for its treatment was available when the epidemic began. However, the attempts to characterize the virus genome and consequent efforts at vaccine development are good examples of how research is being used to address human health problems.

For Professional Qualifications and Academics

Research work is an integral part of any academic *milieu*, be it for award of a professional degree/qualification or for those who aspire to become part of the academic fraternity and grow within these academic institutions. The consequent academic recognition brings name and fame to the individual.

■ DEFINING RESEARCH

We have outlined the importance of research in medicine but for different people it probably means different things. While there are many ways of defining research, a useful way to define it is to say that *it is a systematic inquiry into a particular concern or problem*. The systematic inquiry process is essentially the research methodology. Understanding research methodology process is the key to one's successful journey as a practicing physician, researcher, or an academician.

The outputs of this systematic inquiry process are the thesis or dissertation. What do these terms mean?

Thesis and Dissertation

The word thesis has its origin from the Greek word "thesis" meaning "something put forth," while the word dissertation has its origins from the Latin word "dissertare" meaning "continue to discuss." Thesis or dissertation is a document of research findings in support of one's candidature for award of an academic degree/professional qualification. The terms have generally been used interchangeably for both award of a Masters' degree and a doctoral degree.

The quantum and quality of research and the duration needed to complete the thesis/dissertation vary with country and university. However, there are those who wish to distinguish the two from one another. A thesis maybe understood as a tool to test the students' understanding of their field of study/work wherein they formulate a proposition based on work done by others in the field and analyze it. In a dissertation, the student is expected to focus on an original research question and prove or disprove the hypothesis by doing the research work. A thesis submitted for postgraduate courses in medicine or nursing probably includes both the elements.

■ RESEARCH OPPORTUNITIES FOR MEDICAL TRAINEES

As stated earlier, key to translating evidence to practice lies in comprehending research methodology. Classroom or workshop exposure at best sensitizes the learner to the principles of research and its process, but being able to understand it sufficiently well to look at published evidence for translating into clinical practice requires one to engage in some actual research work, even though for a brief period.

Unlike overseas, where students have several opportunities for research exposure and experiences even during their graduate medical training period, these opportunities are limited in India. The Short Term Studentship (STS) offered by the Indian Council of Medical Research is probably the only opportunity that an undergraduate student has to carry out research projects under the supervision of a mentor in their own medical college without disrupting their ongoing medical training. However, not all undergraduate students get selected for the Studentship. The primary opportunity for medical graduates to experience research work in India is therefore during the pursuance of their postgraduate courses wherein the thesis related research work is an obligatory requirement for the award of their postgraduate degree.

ROLE OF THESIS IN POSTGRADUATE COURSES

The aim of postgraduate training is not restricted to ensuring the acquisition of clinical skills to work as specialist/consultant in the concerned specialty. The objectives are manifold. The thesis should empower the postgraduate student as follows:
- Enable them to critically evaluate and synthesize evidence available in published medical literature.
- To be able to translate available evidence into clinical practice.
- To be able to ask probing questions to solve clinical problems.
- To be able to enthuse some of the postgraduate students to enter the academia or research pathways.

The experience of thesis work hones the students' skills to search medical literature systematically, synthesize available evidence, identify unanswered queries, plan a study for gathering appropriate data, get to know how to analyze their data, and finally present their work as a written document.

The thesis, eventually, will form the launching pad for those who may choose to spend a greater part of their career contributing to the growing body of medical literature by writing and publishing. The thesis also exposes them to the ethics of healthcare, which is often a neglected area in one's daily practice of clinical medicine.

How did my thesis affect me?

It improved my critical thinking, ability to look at data and its analysis, and infused a passion for academics and research and eventually launched me on that trajectory. My mentor (research guide) was an important factor in my transformation. I was also fortunate to have trained in a department which fostered and supported academic excellence, publication and research, and encouraged its postgraduate students to present papers in local and national conferences. It activated the dormant "competitive" spirit in us.

Advantage and Disadvantage of Thesis

Working on a thesis bestows several advantages to the student. It improves critical thinking of the students, helps in problem solving, would facilitate adoption of evidence-based medical practice, and improves their medical writing skills. The only disadvantage that one may put forth is time spent on thesis is relatively large and could have been put to better use for acquiring their core subject specific skills. However, in the tradeoff between the pros and cons, the advantages outweigh the disadvantages.

TRANSLATING THESIS INTO VALUABLE RESEARCH

One needs to understand the fate of the thesis after its completion. An important question is whether it should be viewed only as a passport to award of degree with the thesis left forgotten in the institutional archives? The answer to this is a definite "No." Few theses get translated into a publication as they are not necessarily pursued any further thereafter. But there are examples wherein the thesis has become the beacon for ongoing research in the field which eventually changed practice and policy. The following experience of the author is an illustration of how thesis can translate into long-term research impacting practice and policy.

My first thesis as a mentor attempted to answer the question as to "whether room air could be used for resuscitation of newborns at birth instead of 100% oxygen", which was driven by the observation that mouth to mouth resuscitation was being practiced successfully by primary health workers to revive asphyxiated newborns without supplemental oxygen. The question was relevant and novel but challenged by the ethical concerns of lack of any experimental or clinical data to support the proposed hypothesis. The search for this tenacious evidence to support the hypothesis led me to meet up with a researcher in another part of the world, who was independently attempting to unravel the answer to the same question in porcine models which was driven by the observation that use of excessive oxygen following hypoxia could be detrimental to the newborn due to its ability to generate free radicals. This thesis research effort was published (Ramji S et al. 1993) and translated into a journey of international collaborative research spanning three and half decades which eventually changed both practice and policy globally.

- The existing practice at that time was to use 100% oxygen to resuscitate newborns at birth.
- The thesis concluded that room air could be as effective as 100% oxygen for neonatal resuscitation, a finding that was confirmed by several clinical trials thereafter.
- Today the current policy is to initiate resuscitation in newborns with room air.

There are also other examples wherein thesis work has contributed to ongoing research and change in policy. Some of the examples include delayed cord clamping at birth to improve iron stores in infancy, use of zinc in diarrhea, lack of maternal protection against rotavirus infection in newborns, iron supplementation in exclusively breastfed infants, and serum antigliadin antibody for diagnosis of celiac disease in tropical countries.

CONCLUSION

Postgraduate students must view the thesis as an educational tool to enhance their skills to practice medicine rationally. They must enjoy this learning experience which could launch them into a successful career. To make this a stimulating experience and rather than a drudgery of doing a thesis, teachers and institutions must strive to create a conducive ambience for learning and doing.

KEY MESSAGES

- It enables the physician to evaluate evidence systematically and scientifically for practice.
- Individuals gain recognition through their research and publications by way of awards/honors and academic recognition.
- The research work done by way of thesis may eventually contribute to change in practice and policy.

FURTHER READING

1. Cheung BMY. Medical student research: is it necessary and beneficial? Postgrad Med J. 2018;94(1112):317.
2. Dzirasa K, Krishnan RR, Williams RS. Incubating the research independence of a medical scientist training program graduate: a case study. Acad Med. 2015;90(2):176-9.
3. Garg R, Goyal S, Singh K. Lack of research amongst undergraduate medical students in India: It's time to act and act now. Indian Pediatr. 2017;54(5):357-60.
4. Morbitzer KA, Rao KV, Rhoney DH, Pappas AL, Durr EA, Sultan SM, et al. Implementation of the flipped residency research model to enhance residency research training. Am J Health Syst Pharm. 2019;76(9):608-12.
5. O'Brien JM. Conceptualizing the research culture in postgraduate medical education: Implications for Leading Culture Change. J Med Humanit. 2015;36(4):291-307.
6. Personett HA, Hammond DA, Frazee EN, Skrupky LP, Johnson TJ, Schramm GE. Road map for research training in the residency learning experience. J Pharm Pract. 2018;31(5):489-96.
7. Ramji S, Ahuja S, Thirupuram S, Rootwelt T, Rooth G, Saugstad OD. Resuscitation of asphyxic newborn infants with room air or 100% oxygen. Pediatr Res. 1993;34:809-12.
8. Tullu MS, Karande S. Quality research in Indian medical colleges and teaching institutions: the need of the hour. J Postgrad Med. 2016;62(4):213-5.

CHAPTER 2

Dealing with the Supervisor: Mentor–Mentee Relationship

Sahiba Kukreja, Tejinder Singh

■ INTRODUCTION

Preparing a thesis is one of the major stressors of a student's life. We all have experienced it during our studies. How we wished that the supervisor showed us the path to tread rather than just shoving the papers back to us and saying, "write it again."

Fortunately, things are changing. There is a growing realization that "children must be taught how to think, not what to think." It can be achieved through mentoring program, rightly described as "a brain to pick, an ear to listen, and a push in the right direction" by John Crosby. The intellectual, trusted, highly regarded, and an experienced individual who has the ability to guide is referred to as a **Mentor**, while the person who is being guided is referred as the **Mentee**.

■ ORIGIN OF MENTORSHIP

The origination of mentorship program has historical roots. Mentor was mentioned in the Greek mythology as a person who taught the son of Odysseus after he left for the Trojan War. The way he taught was later conceptualized and modified to give rise to the mentorship program.

Mentorship program was once a part of the earlier Indian education system of *gurukuls*. This system of education included a *Guru*, who acted as the mentor for the budding *Shishya* or the mentees. This system helped the mentees rise to become an individual with utmost achievements. Let us try to extrapolate some concepts of this relationship to the supervisor-supervisee relationship.

■ MENTORSHIP IN POSTGRADUATE COURSES IN MEDICINE

Mentorship program is important in almost all the educational fields, besides medical education. There are several issues faced by individuals enrolled in medical education. Some of these issues are difficult education system, difficulty in handling patients, and issues in further career advancements. Though both undergraduates and postgraduates in medical education require comprehensive mentorship program, the requirement is more crucial for the postgraduate students. Mentoring postgraduates is usually a completely different task, in contrast to the undergraduates. Let us look more closely at it.

THESIS SUPERVISOR AND SUPERVISEE (CANDIDATE)

The success of postgraduate students hangs on a thin thread balanced by an exemplary supervisor. Unfortunately, this relationship has deteriorated over time due to rising competition, increased expectations, and lack of trust. Strong and directional efforts are necessary for ensuring a fruitful relationship. The supervisor is expected to provide personal and administrative support to the student. Studies have shown that a balance is necessary between the role of supervisor and expectations from a student. Stok-Koch et al. pointed toward the importance of practicing with the student and being a role model for developing a lifelong relationship.

Dobbs et al. focused on the expectations of supervisee from their supervisors. The study highlighted that the supervisor is expected to be approachable, ethical, assertive, willing to walk the extra mile, knowledgeable, experienced, helpful, available, and resourceful. Another study by Woolhouse concluded the expectations of a supervisor from their supervisee. The supervisee, in general, is expected to show motivation and to take initiative in research and to carry out independent research. The student is expected to be committed, thoughtful, focused, honest, and realistic. **Table 2.1** lists the expectations from a supervisor and a supervisee (student). Many problems between supervisor and supervisee arise when either or both tend to fall short of the expectations.

Supervisor as a Mentor

The need of the hour is to convert the supervisor–student relationship to mentor–mentee relationship. The scholarly review by Mellon and Murdoch-Eaton highlights the key factors necessary for the supervisor to transform into a mentor. The supervisor is required to discuss the career ideas of the student, help the student in exploring possible options, challenge the current assumptions, providing new information source, encouraging commitment, review progress, treat the student as a peer, support and promote the mentee, act as a friend, and help in pushing the mentee to achieve new heights and face new challenges.

Mentees often refrain themselves while discussing with the mentor. The most common topics discussed among mentor and mentee are often limited to education, future career, role as a doctor, and balancing work with personal life. It is important to understand that topics regarding professional and private issues faced by the mentees are discussed less.

> *Mentoring* is a brain to pick, an ear to listen, and a push in the right direction.

Relationship and Challenges

Supervising a postgraduate student is a colossal task teeming with several lacunae. A report by Wadesango and Machingambi highlighted that both students and supervisors often face several issues while working with each other. The students often feel that their supervisor is unable to provide ample quality time. The feedback provided by the supervisor is often considered conflicting, infrequent, and lacking in depth. The level of commitment and interest shown by the supervisor are considered unfulfilling. The cosupervisors of thesis often have conflicting perspectives, thus building tension among them. The most common problem faced by the students is poor communication and disagreement regarding

TABLE 2.1: Expectations from a supervisor and student.

Supervisor	Student
Approachable	Motivated
Ethical	Take initiative
Assertive	Show commitment
Knowledgeable	Be focused
Experienced	Honest
Helpful	Realistic
Available	Thoughtful
Willing to walk that extra mile	Knowledgeable

the research. Other issues of the students are selfishness, disrespectful nature, and lack of knowledge about expertise of the supervisor.

It is important to understand that issues are also faced by the supervisors. Some of the common issues have been described in literature by Mafa et al. They reported that students pose challenge related to thesis work. They underestimate the importance of research in their career. The students tend to follow unethical measures in their research work such as plagiarism and stealing data from others. They feel that the students lack knowledge, are unwilling to gain new knowledge, and lack research experience and the competency to achieve it.

Do's and Don'ts of Relationship

Mentor plays a crucial role of giving advice to the assigned mentee. There are several important qualities that are required in a true and able mentor. A mentor has to be enthusiast for working with the mentee. A mentor is considered as unfitting if he/she is selfish in providing time, lacks in mentoring skills, and wishes for all the glory without providing any acknowledgement to the mentee. A mentor must never exploit the mentee, and instead promote the academic and personal development of the mentee. The individual personalities of the mentee have to be nurtured, without influencing it with personal bias (**Table 2.2**).

■ ADVANTAGES TO MENTEE AND MENTOR

Both mentor and mentee can be positively benefited from this relationship.

Advantages to Mentee

The mentee may receive someone who can act as a role model and boost the confidence and self-esteem of the individual. The mentor can provide the mentee a shoulder to lean on during stressful situations. Open communication and fruitful discussions can improve the personal and professional life of the mentee. The career aspect is also improved due to quality publications, research, and improving teaching skills of the mentee.

Mentor is considered as an individual who would be supportive and will provide new and improved knowledge to the mentee. Mentees feel that mentor provides emotional support to them, besides guidance. Majority of students feel that the mentorship helped in improving their knowledge and critical thinking.

Advantages to Mentor

Mentorship program is often considered as a "give and give" relationship where mentor provides knowledge and guidance to the mentee, and nothing is being offered to the mentor in return. However, this is not entirely true. Mentorship program is a great initiative for reinforcing the current knowledge. It is important to understand that we can teach others only when we have thorough knowledge regarding the concept. It provides rejuvenation to the concepts and knowledge of the mentor. Mentor gains new perspectives while dealing with their mentee. Mentor develops the skills of empathy and sensitivity toward other individuals. The professional relationships and contacts are further enhanced when the mentee enters the profession. And the biggest reward for the mentor is when the mentee excels in life and career and gains recognition.

TABLE 2.2: Making most of mentoring.

Mentor	Mentee
Have a clear understanding of your motivation to mentor	Have a clear understanding of your motivation to be mentored
Agree to be a mentor based on a realistic assessment of your skills and experience	Use the relationship on a pre-established criterion relevant to your career goals

EXPECTATIONS OF SUPERVISOR AND SUPERVISEE

The relationship between supervisor and a student is crucial for any academic success. A positive relationship between the two can benefit the institution they work in. In order to understand the relationship between the supervisor and a supervisee, an investigation was conducted that involved interviewing supervisors and supervisee. During the interview, the participants were asked to elaborate on the expectations that they have from each other in the working environment. **Box 2.1** summarizes what not to expect from the mentorship program.

Expectations of a Student from the Supervisor

Here are the view of two students:
Student 1:
- I expect my supervisor to show some positive and a cooperative attitude toward me. I wish my supervisor can be more aware regarding his professional duties.
- My supervisor should communicate and guide me in such a way that the necessary information reaches well to me.
- I would like my supervisor to be open for discussions and to listen to my perspectives patiently.
- I wish my supervisor could understand that the negative imposing attitude can undermine my performance and credibility.
- I would like my supervisor to provide a comfortable and safe environment to me so that I feel safe enough to talk about my personal issues when necessary and not take advantage of it.

Student 2:
- I wish my supervisor could provide me safe affection and trust as a parent rather than a boss. An environment of mutual trust creates a comfortable situation for me and I will be able to focus more on my work.
- I feel that my communications with my supervisor must be kept confidential and the information must not be shared with any other members of the group.
- I would like to receive a positive feedback and appreciation for my efforts from my supervisor.
- I also feel that moral support from my supervisor would encourage me to work hard and be productive.

Expectations of the Supervisor from Student

Here are the views of a Supervisor:
- I expect my postgraduate students to select a topic that is within the area of interest so that the student can be responsive and focused.
- I believe that positive interest from my student would boost my own enthusiasm toward them.
- I wish my students could come up with novel ideas and to reach at certain findings on their own rather than waiting for me to spoon-feed the same.
- I would like the student to submit their written material on time without any reminders.
- I wish my students could approach me freely without any apprehensions in mind. I believe that if the students could come to me during the early stage of postgraduate studies, it would build a stronger bond with me.
- I would like the student to give at least three presentations during the research, in the beginning, middle, and the in end, so that the track of their progress can be ensured.

> **Box 2.1: What mentoring does not mean.**
> **Mentoring is not:**
> - A guarantee of advancement
> - An unlimited tap on resources
> - A means of bypassing seniors
> - A mechanism for taking unfair advantage
> - A way of working outside the system

CHANGING TRENDS

There have been many changes in the recent times regarding the roles of mentors and mentees. While the traditional view was for the mentor to initiate the process, the contemporary view is that mentee should initiate the process. The interactions should be specific goal-oriented rather than being of a general nature. What it means practically is that mentee should not always wait for the supervisor to call him for thesis related work rather he should himself take the initiative. Please do not forget that ultimately it is mentee's career that is going to be affected.

Interest is also being generated in the concept of peer mentoring, where students can help each other for many things, rather than depending on one supervisor only. This is especially true for issues such as literature search, data entry, and statistical methods.

CONCLUSION

Mentorship program is more or less like a roller coaster ride with several ups and downs during its course. But once the individuals involved in this process get a hang of it, the ride becomes much more fun and beneficial as well. This program is in continuation with the traditional concepts of education system. Mentorship provides professional and personal support to both of them. It opens new realms of learning where newer concepts and skills are learnt.

KEY MESSAGES

- Mentoring offers benefits which go beyond the traditional academic exchange.
- Both mentor and mentee have defined roles and responsibilities.
- Mentor can only show the path: To walk therein is the responsibility of the mentee.
- Mentoring is not a means to work outside the system rules and regulations.
- Mentoring relations are beneficial for both the mentor and the mentee.

FURTHER READING

1. Anderson EM, Shannon AL. Toward a conceptualization of mentoring. J Teach Educ. 1988;39(1):38-42.
2. Brand M. Breaking down the walls: Partnerships and progress in higher education. J High Educ Outreach Engagem. 2010;8:14-25.
3. Dobbs A, McKervey H, Roti E, Stewart R, Baker BM. Supervisees' expectations of supervisor characteristics: Preclinical fellowship year versus postclinical fellowship year. Contemp Issues Commun Sci Disord. 2006;33:113-9.
4. Jacobi M. Mentoring and undergraduate academic success: A literature review. Rev Educ Res. 1991;61(4):505-32.
5. Ludwig S, Stein RE. Anatomy of mentoring. J Pediatr. 2008;152(2):151-2.
6. Mafa O, Mapolisa T. Supervisors' experiences in supervising postgraduate education students' dissertations and theses at the Zimbabwe Open University (ZOU). Int J Asian Soc Sci. 2011;2:1685-97.
7. Mellon A, Murdoch-Eaton D. Supervisor or mentor: is there a difference? Implications for paediatric practice. Arch Dis Child. 2015;100(9):873-8.
8. Moberg DJ. Mentoring for protégé character development. Mentoring & Tutoring. 2008;16(1):91-103.
9. Nachimuthu P. Mentors in Indian mythology. Manag Labour Stud. 2006;31(2):137-51.
10. Smith L, Herry Y, Levesque D, Marshall D. On Becoming a Teacher: A Longitudinal Tracking Study. Toronto: Queen's Printer for Ontario; 1993.
11. Stok-Koch L, Bolhuis S, Koopmans RT. Identifying factors that influence workplace learning in postgraduate medical education. Educ Health. 2007;20(1):8.
12. TCTMD (Cardiovascular Research Foundation). On mentoring: a brain to pick, an ear to listen, and a push in the right direction. [online] Available from https://www.tctmd.com/news/mentoring-brain-pick-ear-listen-and-push-right-direction. [Last accessed July, 2020].
13. Tobin MJ. Mentoring: seven roles and some specifics. Am J Respir Crit Care Med. 2004;170(2):114-7.
14. Wadesango N, Machingambi S. Postgraduate students' experiences with research supervisors. J Sociology Soc Anth. 2011;2(1):31-7.
15. Woolhouse M. Supervising dissertation projects: Expectations of supervisors and students. Innov Educ Teach Int. 2002;39(2):137-44.

CHAPTER 3

Process of Thesis Writing: Plan it Well

Alpana Raizada, OP Kalra

■ INTRODUCTION

The prospect of penning a brief guide to the process of thesis writing took us back to our own postgraduate days where we distinctly remember being told by our seniors that thesis writing was a grueling, futile task with no immediate- or long-term gains. A substantial majority of first-year postgraduates may voice the same opinion and if given an option, many would choose not to write a thesis.

Years later, we have realized that it was a process worth undertaking as it laid the foundation of our career as a teacher and a researcher.

■ THESIS WRITING: THE PROCESS
Why should a Thesis be Written?

A thesis is not just a mandatory requirement for an academic degree but is an opportunity to apply systematic scientific methods to questions in medicine. For most, it serves as the first exposure to the process and practice of research.

Above all, it may serve to be the means of communication to a larger audience.

Step 1: Need for a Plan, a Roadmap

Though it may be viewed as an unpleasant obligation on the way to acquiring a degree, the spirit of scientific enquiry and the drill of scientific writing, induced by thesis writing process, have long-term benefits.

Feel convinced that writing a thesis is a task worth undertaking and start planning for it. Planning is the most important part of the formula called "time management." A plan is a roadmap for achieving an objective which in your case happens to be the timely submission of a thesis of an appropriate standard and format.

"If I had 60 minutes to cut down a tree, I would spend 40 minutes sharpening the axe and 20 minutes cutting it down."
— Abraham Lincoln

A medical postgraduate must master the art of juggling time between patient care, academic expectations, personal issues, and of course, the inevitable task of conducting research and writing a thesis. Absence of a robust plan and the commitment to stick to the plan can lead to mental agony and have significant repercussions.

Step 2: Find the Supervisor

For most theses, the next logical step is finding a supervisor. As against a PhD thesis where finding an available, approachable, committed supervisor is probably one of the biggest hurdles in thesis writing, this is not the case with a medical postgraduate. In most departments, random allocation or systematic randomization of candidates to potential supervisors or *vice versa* is the norm. The medical postgraduate has no option but to accept his destiny. Therefore, a word of advice is to spend a little time understanding the characteristics of your supervisor and to adapt and modify your own working style to optimize time and effort.

Step 3: Select Topic and Research Design

Selecting the thesis topic and the research design may be the biggest hurdle you would face. You have got to write the thesis, but if you choose the wrong topic, you may not even get started. You shall undergo following three stages:

1. *Selecting an area to study*: In a medical thesis, often the supervisor has a specific area of interest and the student is advised to work in the same area. Rarely, the student suggests various areas and the supervisor chooses an appropriate one. In either case, the first task is to select an area that you are going to study. Zero-in on a broad area in the first or second meeting. If you are keen on pursuing your area of interest, then be prepared to indulge in a good amount of labor before your first contact with your appointed supervisor. There is no virtue in being passive at the time of topic allocation and then actively cribbing once you start executing the research process. Try to bring some of your own individuality and interests to bear on the choice. Since you will be spending more than half of the duration of the total length of your postgraduate course for studying a single subject in depth, very often you develop deep interest in the area. This may even guide your future decision for choosing an area for super specialization.

2. *Formulating the research problem*: Once a general area has been selected, the next task is to select the specific problem within this area. This involves two processes: reading and discussion. The reading might already have been done by your supervisor or you may be entrusted the task of skimming all relevant research articles on the area under contemplation from the library and e-sources. The goal for you at this stage is not mastery of the area but is an attempt to gain a "feel for the area." Once you are aware of the relevant literature, then embark upon discussions with your supervisor to identify the lacunae or gaps in knowledge in the existing medical literature. Remember most of the best research ideas are generated from discussions and divergent thinking.

   If you fail to find a specific research question, then replicate a good recent study which may not be original but will serve to extend the generality of the finding you are replicating. During this process, you could propose some changes to make it relevant to the needs of our society. Alternatively, you can modify so that it adds something new to the existing study.

3. *Designing the study*: Selection of the research question must be accompanied by selection of a design which can answer the question. *The type of question is less important than ensuring that a design is available which is capable of answering the question.*

Once you have accomplished all of the above, ask yourself the following questions before you finally nod in affirmation:

- Is my institution's infrastructure conducive to my thesis topic?
- Shall I be able to recruit subjects with ease?
- Is my thesis a financial burden to me or to my subjects?
- Do I need to rely on several people and multiple investigations?

- Is my thesis topic too ambitious?
- Is this topic something I can speak about with enthusiasm and insight?
- Shall I be able to offer a fresh perspective on this topic?

If in doubt, confide in your supervisor and clarify your doubts. Problems are more likely when more people and things are relied upon. So, keep your thesis simple. The four basic attributes of a good thesis are as follows:

1. Feasibility
2. Precision
3. Arguability
4. Originality/replication with a modification.

Reminder for the supervisor: The aim of thesis writing is not to produce a number of research papers. Too broad and ambitious topics are invariably watered down, uninformative, and dull.

Step 4: Drawing a Timetable

Pilson's law: "It always takes longer"
No matter how disciplined and efficient you are, you might still underestimate the amount of time that is needed to put a good piece of work together. So,

- Structure your time
- Enlist intermediate targets
- Assign dates for completion of intermediate targets
- Convert your timetable into a chart
- Check off items as you finish them.

This will provide you with a lot of mental peace and will keep you focused on future targets. Remember, the plan has to be realistic and should adjust for all anticipated and some of surprise hurdles too.

Start Writing: What is Not Started will Never Get Finished

The four integral components of scientific writing as per Barrass are to think, to plan, to write, and to revise. Translate thoughts into plans and plans into words. Do not postpone writing because it is easier to improve upon what has been written previously. But how and where from to make the beginning? You may start writing your thesis inside out. Start with what you are most comfortable with, like the material and methods section which is usually straightforward and without ambiguity. Writing is a cyclic process and not a linear one. What appears first in the thesis may be written last using the unified perspective which becomes available after certain other sections have been dealt with.

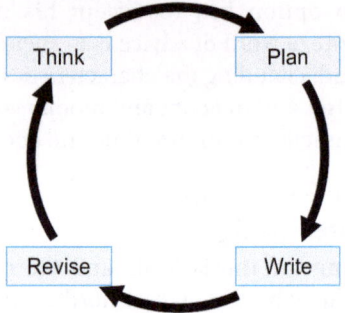

Regularly keep submitting drafts of sections written to your supervisor and take a positive attitude to all the scribbles which decorate your text. The process of writing the thesis is like a course in scientific writing where each chapter is like an assignment in which you are taught, but not assessed. Remember, only the final draft is assessed.

Step 5: Writing a Thesis Proposal/Protocol

What is a thesis proposal? It is a means to:
- introduce the research topic;
- briefly outline the relevant literature;
- specify the problem and objectives; and
- describe methodology to achieve the objective (s).

It is to convince the committee (departmental/institutional) that the research is worth undertaking and serves as a guide to elaborate the thesis upon. The components of a thesis protocol are the same as that of a thesis *sans* Results, Discussion, Conclusion, and Acknowledgments.

THESIS WRITING: THE SCIENTIFIC CONTENT

Writing a Thesis

Scientific writing is embodied by the three S's which are as follows:
1. Structure
2. Substance
3. Style.

The structure of a thesis is invariably a logical and fixed sequence of sections and is irrespective of the subject. The substance varies with subject, and its quality is determined by the knowledge and acumen of the student. Style is influenced by language and layout.

The thesis is constituted by several sections. We are summarizing here the salient points of each of these sections that you need to keep in mind while writing. Detailed description of each section will follow in the subsequent chapters in this book.

Introduction

This section introduces the topic and explains reasons to choose this topic. It very briefly reviews relevant literature and answers:
- *What is known*: Quote pertinent studies
- *What is not known*: Controversies/lacunae in the literature
- *Why this study*: Briefly state what you plan to do and why.

It can be written best once the other sections of the thesis have already been written. So, do revisit this section again after you are done with writing all other sections.

Avoid the Following

- Use of the first person ("I") unless it is intentionally included for emphasis
- Being too critical of previous research
- Referring to your proposed study in each paragraph of the introduction (other than in the first paragraph)
- Avoiding your supervisor lest you might miss some critical issues

Review of Literature

The literature review portion of the master's thesis is designed to:
- Familiarize you with essential background on your topic
- Familiarize the reader of your thesis with what has already been written on the topic

Tips for Writing a Review

- Do not write literature review as a series of disjointed paragraphs, each summarizing a different article or book.
- Do not simply list the literature you identify but read, summarize, discuss, synthesize, and analyze it.
- Do not rely on only one method for identifying relevant literature.
- Read the cross-references from articles and books.
- Reference all identified literature.
- Acknowledge the source of table/figure at the bottom of the same or mention as "adapted from" if modified.

Aim and Objectives

Aim and objectives are not synonymous. At the onset, you have to be clear that Aim = intention or what you hope to achieve, whereas Objective is a step taken to achieve the aim. Thus, *Aim* is usually written in broad terms, whereas *Objectives* are specific statements. Each aim should be matched with specific objectives. Objectives should be *SMART*, *i.e.* they should be:
- *Specific*: Denote precisely what you are going to do.
- *Measureable*: You will know when you have reached your goal.
- *Achievable*: As per the available timeframe and not very ambitious.
- *Realistic*: Match the available resources.
- *Time constrained*: Determine when each stage needs to be completed with allowance for unexpected delays.

There are two types of objectives. Principal or *primary objective* is the one that dictates the research design and methods of your study. *Secondary objectives* are other objectives of interest, which can be achieved with same study design.

Reminder for supervisors: Good work done and well in time is better than shabby work done or not in time. So, keep the thesis simple. Have only one or two specific objectives in the study.

Material and Methods

- This section should be written with precision to enable reproducibility by any other competent researcher.
- You can initiate writing your thesis with this chapter as it is one of the easiest chapters to write.
- Use past tense in this section.

The components of this section depending on the type of thesis are as follows:

- Study design and setting
- Study period
- Study subjects with inclusion and exclusion criteria
- Sample size:
  o Do not forget to mention the basis for calculating sample size.
  o Correct for estimated dropouts, if any, during study
- Method of recruitment
- Randomization, if applicable
- Blinding/masking
- Intervention, if any, discuss in detail
- Follow-up of the study participants
- Method of measurement of outcome of interest
- Study questionnaire and formats (to be placed in Annexure)
- Data collection methods
- Data management and statistical analysis
  o Describe procedure to enter data
  o Software to be used for data entry and statistical analysis.

Tips for Material and Methods

- Be simple and precise.
- Always use international standard units of measurement, with the correct abbreviations. Nonstandard abbreviations must be listed in an "Abbreviations" section at the front of your thesis.
- Use the correct Greek letters such as α, ß, and μ rather than incorrect Latin letters such as a, b, or u.
- Do not capitalize the names of chemicals; for example, Sodium Chloride and Sodium chloride are incorrect, sodium chloride is correct.
- When writing formulae, be careful always to use the appropriate subscripts and superscripts, for example: H_2O and not H2O.
- Use the correct word to describe actions. For example, do not use the word "spin" if you mean "centrifuge".
- Learn about the conventions of notation in your field. For example:
  o Human gene names should be written in italicized capital letters (*CTBP2* and *VCP*).
  o By convention when writing names of organisms, these are written in italics, with a capitalized genus name and a species name that begins with a small letter, for example, *Escherichia coli*.
- Mention the name, model number, and manufacturer of the piece of equipment you used, because this may also affect your results.
- Reference computer programs, databases, and websites.
- Use figures and tables to convey bulky and/or detailed information.

Results

This section summarizes the data collected and their statistical treatment. It consists of the observations and measurements recorded while conducting the procedures described in the methods section. Figures (graphs and diagrams) and tables present the complete findings in numerical, visual, or graphical terms, while the accompanying text helps the reader to focus on the most important aspect of the results.

- Do not present an overwhelming amount of detail, or an exhaustive compilation of every analysis you conducted. Instead, present the important findings so that your reader does not lose focus.
- Break up your results into logical segments by using subheadings. Start with making the reader comfortable with your measures and your sample, then present your main findings relevant to the purpose of the study and finally present any additional analyses you feel are of importance.
- Mention negative as well as positive results.
- Quarantine observations from interpretations.
- Provide a clear description of the magnitude of a response or difference. It is more effective to use percentage of change rather than exact data.
- Frame clear sentences to highlight key results; such as "X had significant positive relationship with Y ($P < 0.01$)" rather than a less informative statement like "There is a significant relationship between X and Y".

Discussion

This is by far the most difficult section to write. Keep it simple and structured. This section is a "Discussion of your results" and not a recap of review of literature. Start this section with a crisp brief on the most important results. Follow it with subsections each dedicated to answering the following questions:

- What are the major patterns in the observations? What are the relationships, trends, and generalizations among the results?
- What are the exceptions to these patterns or generalizations?
- What are the likely causes underlying these patterns?
- Is there similarity or conflict with previous work?
- What are the strengths and limitations of your work?
- What are the new findings in the present work?
- What are the significance and practical implications of the present results?

Finally, believe your findings and avoid being too critical of your work.

Conclusions

This section should usually be reasonably short. It should:
- Summarize major findings
- Present implications
- Suggest directions for future research.

"Conclusions" should give a word of finality to your thesis. It should present a unified perspective to all the work done and should not leave the reader with remorse.

Acknowledgments

Acknowledge all who have assisted:
- Intellectually
- Technically
- Financially

References

The purpose of writing proper references is that the reader should be able to retrieve the referred document without difficulty.
- Note down the citation as soon as you obtain data from any source.
- Follow the same citation style throughout the thesis (preferably the Vancouver/ICMJE style).
- Do not quote a reference that you have not read, because reading the abstract alone is not sufficient. As far as possible, quote the reference from the original article rather than from a cross reference cited in another article.
- If you have read other supporting articles that have helped in the research, but you have not cited them in the thesis, place them in a separate "Bibliography" section.
- Double check all references with their position in text as any sloppiness reflects very poorly on your abilities.

Annexure and Appendices

Following are to be included in this section:
- Reference data/materials not easily available (theses are used as a resource by the department and other students).
- List of equipment used for an experiment or details of complicated procedures.
- Questionnaires/measurement tools/elaborate classification systems which have been mentioned in review of literature.
- Patient/parent information sheet and consent form: Both in English and local languages.
- Competing interest, if any. Disclose source of funding, association, etc.
- Master chart depicting raw data about various clinical parameters and laboratory investigations of the entire study population, which may need to be referred to at a later stage.

■ THESIS WRITING: FINAL STEPS

Work done may not be necessarily "well done". Good editing will save you from embarrassment. Some useful tips to follow:
- Proofread your thesis a few times.
- Do the final spell check by eye for spell checkers are useful for initial checking, but fail to catch homonyms (e.g., there and their).
- Use complete sentences.
- Check your grammar.
- Do not use double negatives.
- Avoid qualitative adjectives when describing concepts that are quantifiable ("most of the subjects had severe anemia" vs. "90% subjects had hemoglobin <8%").
- Do not use unexplained acronyms and abbreviations. Spell out all acronyms the first time that you use them.
- Ask colleagues to read and comment.
- Write for brevity rather than length but do not sacrifice accuracy for the sake of brevity.

Research is:
1. To know;
2. To know what to do;
3. To do it; and
4. To make it known.

■ MAKING A SCIENTIFIC PAPER OUT OF THESIS

By the time you submit your thesis, you are already in the last lap of your master's course. Most of you would focus on reading for university examination rather than on writing a thesis paper. If you are already not too sick of your thesis, then making a paper out of your thesis should be the most logical and final step in this scholarly journey of yours. Since you have already invested so much time and energy into your thesis, our advice is to attempt taking this one final leap because science which is not communicated should not have been done in the first place. So, keep reading, start writing, and keep trying till your paper reaches its desired destination. In addition, scientific communication is likely to help in the growth of your career.

■ CONCLUSION

Thesis writing is an opportunity to understand the process and practice of research. The integral components of writing a thesis are thinking, planning, writing, and revision. A good thesis is one where a suitable scientific enquiry is substantiated by structure, substance, and style. Meticulous planning and time-bound, disciplined approach to research are sure to result in timely submission of a thesis of an appropriate standard and format.

> **KEY MESSAGES**
>
> *The steps to plan the thesis are as follows*:
> - Step 1: Need for a plan, a roadmap
> - Step 2: Find the supervisor
> - Step 3: Select topic and research design
> - Step 4: Drawing a timetable—plot a feasible timeline along a systematic, approved plan
> - Step 5: Writing a thesis proposal/protocol
>
> *Contents of the thesis*:
> - Introduction
> - Review of literature
> - Aim and objectives
> - Material and methods
> - Results
> - Discussion
> - Conclusions
> - Summary
> - References
> - Annexures
>
> Keep your thesis simple, feasible, and achievable.

FURTHER READING

1. Barrass R. Scientists Must Write: A Guide to Better Writing for Scientists, Engineers, and Students. 2nd edition. Abingdon: Routledge; 2002.
2. Chandrasekhar R. How to write a thesis: A working guide. [online] Available from http://ciips.ee.uwa.edu.au/pub/HowToWriteAThesis.pdf. [Last accessed April 30, 2020].
3. Jamieson J. Thesis survival guide. [online] Available from http://flash.lakeheadu.ca/~jjamies/guide.html. [Last accessed April 30, 2020].
4. Kastens K, Pfirman S, Stute M, Hahn B, Abbott D, Scholz C. How to Write a Thesis? [online] Available from http://www.ldeo.columbia.edu/~martins/sen_sem/thesis_org.html. [Last accessed on April 30, 2020].
5. Lindsay D. Scientific writing = thinking in words. Australia: CSIRO Publishing; 2011.
6. Murray R. How to Write a Thesis, 3rd edition. New York: McGraw-Hill; 2011.
7. Wolfe J. How to write a PhD thesis? [online] Available from http://www.phys.unsw.edu.au/jw/thesis.html. [Last accessed April 30, 2020].

CHAPTER 4

Thesis: The Essential Elements

Nitin Agarwal

■ INTRODUCTION

Every university has a set format for writing a thesis with predefined number of components. As per the ordinance of the University of Delhi for postgraduate students pursuing the degree of doctor of medicine/surgery, the thesis must be arranged to include the following 10 components in the order specified below:
1. Cover page
2. Title page
3. Declaration by the candidate
4. Certificate from the institution
5. Acknowledgments (optional)
6. Presentation of thesis results to scientific forums and publications in scientific journals, if any
7. Table of contents
8. Glossary of abbreviations
9. Core of the thesis:
    a. Introduction/background
    b. Review of literature
    c. Objectives of research
    d. Patients/Subjects/Material and Methods
    e. Results
    f. Discussion
    g. Conclusions and recommendations
    h. Summary/Abstract
    i. Index of references: Vancouver system of references
10. Appendices: Consent form (local language and English), case record form, samples of any questionnaires used, data sheet, and certificate of approval from institutional ethics committee.

■ THE 10 ESSENTIAL COMPONENTS OF THESIS

While you may devote most of your time and effort on writing the introduction, review of literature, aim and objectives, material and methods, results, discussion, and conclusions of your thesis, which do constitute the bulk of your thesis, there are certain sections such as Title page, Acknowledgments, Declaration, Certificate, Table of contents, Glossary of abbreviations, Case record form, Data sheet, Ethics certificate, and Consent, which need to be included before a thesis can be officially certified as complete. In this chapter, we will highlight how to present these parts of the thesis in a standard format. Subsequent chapters in this book are devoted to the individual components of text of thesis.

Cover Page

Remember the saying, "Don't judge a book by its cover." This is something which is difficult to avoid, as the visual cortex constitutes about 30% of our brain's cortex. Hence, you need to take utmost care in designing the cover of your thesis which must conform to the standards set by the respective university. In most instances, the cover page is a replica of the "*first page of your thesis.*" The title of the thesis work should appear at the top of the first page and must be centered. Further down the page (middle of the page), the phrase "Thesis submitted to the Faculty of Medical Sciences, XYZ University, for partial fulfillment of the degree of Doctor of Medicine/Surgery (Discipline)" should appear. At the bottom of the cover page, your name (the name of the student), right aligned and the English month and year of thesis submission, left aligned, should appear in a single line. Generally, the title of the thesis, student's name and month of submission must appear in "ALL CAPS" font and look must be "official." Some universities may prefer to include its official logo on the title page. **Figure 4.1** illustrates a sample cover page.

Title Page

The second page of your thesis (not numbered) is designated as the Title Page. It should mention the topic of the thesis, degree (with discipline) for which the thesis is being submitted, name and educational qualifications of the candidate (you), supervisor and co-supervisor(s) and their affiliations, name of the institution where the thesis has been undertaken, and the duration of the course. Generally, the title is mentioned in ALL CAPS font and centered. The page must have appropriate margins, font must be 12, with proper spacing. See sample shown in **Figure 4.2**.

Declaration by the Candidate

You must submit a signed declaration that the thesis is your original work which has been carried out by you under the supervision of your supervisor/co-supervisors, and that the work has not been submitted earlier in candidature for any degree. A signed written consent is needed from your side for permitting the

---

INHALED IPRATROPIUM BROMIDE FOR BRONCHIOLITIS IN CHILDREN: A RANDOMIZED CONTROLLED TRIAL

Thesis submitted to the
Faculty of Medical Science, University of Delhi, towards the partial fulfillment of the degree of Doctor of Medicine
(Pediatrics)

April, 2020　　　　　　　　Dr. Samira Arora

Fig. 4.1: Sample for cover design of thesis.
(*Disclaimer*: Names and affiliations used are fictitious)

INHALED IPRATROPIUM BROMIDE FOR BRONCHIOLITIS IN CHILDREN: A RANDOMIZED CONTROLLED TRIAL

Thesis submitted to the Faculty of Medical Science, university of Delhi, towards the partial fulfillment of the degree of Doctor of Medicine
(Pediatrics)
(Batch: 2018–2021)

By
Dr. Samira Arora
Postgraduate student

Supervisor:
Dr. Prabha Kumar, Professor
Department of Pediatrics
UCMS and GTB Hospital, Delhi

Co-supervisors:
Dr. Rekha Sharma, Assistant Professor
Department of Pediatrics
UCMS and GTB Hospital, Delhi

Dr Niranjan Das, Assistant Professor
Department of Pharmacology
UCMS and GTB Hospital, Delhi

Institution
University College of Medical Sciences and Guru Teg Bahadur Hospital, Delhi

Fig. 4.2: Sample of the "Title Page" of a thesis.
(*Disclaimer*: Names and affiliations used are fictitious)

> I, Dr. Samira Arora, hereby declare that the work embodied in the thesis entitled "*Inhaled Ipratropium Bromide for Bronchiolitis in Children: A Randomized Controlled Trial*" is an original work carried out by me under the guidance of my supervisor Dr. Prabha Kumar and Co-supervisor Dr Rekha Sharma and Dr. Niranjan Das in the Departments of Pediatrics and Pharmacology University College of Medical Sciences and Guru Teg Bahadur Hospital, Delhi.
>
> I certify that the contents of this thesis have not been submitted earlier for the candidature for any degree. I hereby give my consent for the availability of the thesis for photocopying and interlibrary loan to other institutions.
>
> ———————————
> **Dr. Samira Arora**
> Postgraduate student (II year)
> Department of Pediatrics
> University College of Medical Sciences and
> Guru Teg Bahadur Delhi

Fig. 4.3: Sample of the "Declaration" by the student.
(*Disclaimer*: Names and affiliations used are fictitious)

availability of the thesis for photocopying and interlibrary loan to other academic institutions. This declaration will appear on the third page of your thesis (not numbered). See sample shown in **Figure 4.3**.

Certificate

Your thesis should be accompanied by a certificate (on fourth page, not numbered) issued to you by your supervisor and co-supervisors, certifying that you have undertaken the thesis work in the department under their direct guidance and that the thesis fulfills all the requirements stipulated by your university. The certificate must bear the complete name, designation, and affiliation of your supervisor and all co-supervisors and it must be signed by all of them. See sample shown in **Figure 4.4**.

Acknowledgments

You may (this page is not compulsory) dedicate the fifth page (not numbered) of the thesis to your family, teachers, supervisors/co-

> **Department of Pediatrics**
> **University College of Medical Sciences and**
> **Guru Teg Bahadur Hospital,**
> **Delhi**
>
> **CERTIFICATE**
>
> This is to certify that the thesis work entitled "*Inhaled Ipratropium Bromide for Bronchiolitis in Children: A Randomized Controlled Trial*" is a bonafide work of Dr. Samira Arora conducted in the Department of Pediatrics and Pharmacology, University College of Medical Sciences and Guru Teg Bahadur Hospital, Delhi, under our direct supervision and guidance.
>
> Supervisor:
> ———————————
> **Dr. Prabha Kumar**,
> Professor
> Department of Pediatrics
> UCMS and GTB Hospital,
> Delhi
>
> Co-supervisors:
>
> ———————————   ———————————
> **Dr. Rekha Sharma**   **Dr Niranjan Das**
> Assistant Professor   Assistant Professor
> Department of Pediatrics   Department of Pharmacology
> UCMS and GTB Hospital,   UCMS and GTB Hospital,
> Delhi   Delhi

Fig. 4.4: Sample of the "Certificate" issued to the student.
(*Disclaimer*: Names and affiliations used are fictitious)

supervisors, colleagues, patients, technical staff, etc. acknowledging their guidance, support, etc. Certainly, you must acknowledge all funding sources used to support the research that is reported, including university grants and external grants, if any.

Writing an acknowledgment is one of the possible loose ends to tie after the thesis is finished. Difficulty arises in ensuring that everyone is thanked or recognized appropriately, concisely, in correct order, and without sounding repetitive. *Permission needs to be taken from all those being acknowledged.*

Some Useful Tips

- Be judicious in the number of people you thank. Thank only those who have actually helped you with thesis writing.

- Classify people whom you wish to thank into groups. This will ensure that you do not leave out people and simultaneously you would not sound repetitive.
- Acknowledgment by definition is personal and meant to be written less formally than the rest of the thesis but refrain from being too strongly emotive.
- Make sure you spell names correctly. It is ironic to misspell the name of someone who means so much to you. So pay a lot of attention to spelling names correctly.

Table of Contents (Index)

Provide an "Index" or a "Table of Contents" showing a list of all the chapters/section titles and the page numbers on which they begin. The purpose is to enable the reader to search for relevant sections of the thesis. Each chapter/section must commence on a new page. The list commences from Introduction and is followed by the Review of literature, Aim and Objectives, Material and Methods, Observations and Results, Discussion, Conclusions and Recommendations, Summary, References, and Appendices/Annexure, providing page numbers in Arabic numerals (1, 2, 3,....... etc.) alongside the relevant chapter/section. See sample shown in **Figure 4.5**.

S. No.	Title	Page No.
1.	Introduction	1
2.	Review of Literature	5
3.	Aim and Methods	43
4.	Material and Methods	45
5.	Observation and Results	52
6.	Discussion	72
7.	Summary and Conclusions	81
8.	References	88
9.	Annexures:	
	• Consent form	89
	• Patient information sheet	91
	• Case record form	92
	• Master chart	95
	• Institutional ethics certificate	100

Fig. 4.5: Sample of the "Table of Contents."

Glossary of Abbreviations

You should include a glossary explaining/expanding the abbreviations or technical terminology used in your thesis on a separate page. The abbreviations/words/phrases should be arranged alphabetically, with the definitions/expanded forms formatted as a hanging indent if they are longer than a single line. Many of these are standard, e.g., HIV—Human Immunodeficiency Virus and WHO—World Health Organization.

- Do not invent abbreviations of your own (e.g., AB: antibiotic).
- Avoid using nonstandard abbreviations, as it can confuse the reader (ARF: Is it acute rheumatic fever or acute renal failure?).
- The first time that you use an abbreviation in the main text, you must expand it, e.g., "stool was cultured on xylose lysine deoxycholate (XLD) agar". The next time you can simply use the abbreviation, e.g., "organisms isolated from XLD agar were subjected to detailed biochemical analysis".
- Once you have defined an abbreviation, you should always use the same abbreviation and not revert to the original words.

Core Text of Thesis

The core of the thesis is constituted by the nine chapters listed in **Figure 4.5**. Each of these chapters needs to have certain elements which have been summarized in the previous chapter. Each one of them is described in depth in subsequent chapters in this book. You need to ensure that these chapters are written in the style (font, word limit or length, etc.) as per the norms of the university.

Appendices

Material that may be useful or related to the text, but is inappropriate for inclusion within the core text, may be placed at the end of the thesis as Appendix. You may include an Appendix or Appendices, following the list of references.

Each Appendix should begin on a separate page with the word APPENDIX (numbered) typed in upper case (capitals) and centered on the page. All appendices must be numbered consecutively. The various appendices that you may have to attach include the following:
- *Case record form*: A sample case record form used by you for recording the study parameters on each study subject during your study should be provided. The case record form should indicate the baseline and any follow-up parameters. This section is usually a replica of the case record form submitted by you to the university as a part of your thesis protocol.
- *Patient information sheet*: A sample of the patient information sheet in local language and English, as used in your study should also be attached as an appendix.
- *Consent forms*: A separate consent form in local language and English should be attached. Again, these can be replicated from those used in your protocol submitted to the university.
- *Questionnaire/Scoring/Measurement tools used*: Attach samples of every questionnaire, if such is planned to be used as the basis for collecting data. In addition, if your thesis is based on use of a standard scoring system, e.g., Glasgow Coma Scale and New Ballard Score, it may be provided as an Appendix.
- *Institutional ethics approval*: Attach the approval of the ethics committee obtained by you from your institution.
- *Copyright permissions*: Attach any permission for use of copyrighted material/tools in your study.
- *Data sheet/Master Chart*: A complete data sheet of all your subjects including the patient identification (serial number, randomization number, age, sex, etc.), clinical profile, outcome parameters, and characteristics defined in your study needs to be appended as an Appendix. Provide a footnote explaining all codes used by you in the data sheet.

The final version of the work must be printed and bound in the customary manner as described below.

■ COVER DESIGN AND BINDING

The cover design is a replica of the first page, albeit embossed using silver/golden color on a hard-bound cover (buckram covering a cardboard). A blue/black/red buckram cover is usually preferred. Avoid using covers in green, yellow, brown, pink, and white.

The paper quality of the thesis should be of sufficient weight and thickness [≥70 g per square meter (GSM)] to ensure a good keeping quality. This paper is generally called "Thesis Paper" or "Exceptional Business Paper" and it often has a watermark. Use of erasable, glossy, or colored paper is not prohibited; however, restrict its use to the figures and photographs in your thesis. These may be reproduced on glossy art paper and covered by a thin microfilm or transparency. Figures/maps/graphs should be positioned in the text as close to the first reference to the item as possible.

The *spine* of the thesis should show the short title of the thesis, the degree (with discipline) for which the thesis is being submitted, and the duration of the course (**Fig. 4.6**).

■ TYPING AND FORMATTING

Most universities have specific norms about the length of a thesis, which could vary according to the degree (PhD or MPhil or MD) and also according to the subject (Physics or Sociology or English or Medicine). A PhD thesis may have a word limit of 80,000 words (excluding bibliography or references) while an MPhil thesis may have permissible limit of only 40,000 words. Sometimes the length of the thesis may be specified in terms of typed pages. As

| Inhaled ipratropium bromide for bronchiolitis | MD (Pediatrics) | 2018–2021 |

Fig. 4.6: Spine of a thesis.

per the norms of the University of Delhi, the thesis for MD/MS degree should not exceed 100 pages. It is very important that you comply with the maximum word limit stipulated by your university. If your thesis is likely to exceed this, take appropriate steps to curtail it to the prescribed limit.

The text of thesis should be printed in English language, using 12-point font size letters, preferably using Times New Roman font (if Times New Roman font is not used, you may use another typeface such as Arial or Courier), using black ink, on both sides of A4 size paper in double space, and justification on both sides. University of Delhi advises to print on both sides of the paper, while few other universities insist on printing on a single side, leaving the reverse side blank.

- Footnotes, references, table and figure captions, and the data within tables are all single-spaced. Appendices can also be single-spaced.
- A 3 cm margin is preferred on the left to enable trimming, stitching, and binding of thesis. Keep a 2.5 cm margin on the right side.

HEADINGS AND SUBHEADINGS

You should use headings and subheadings throughout the text. Headings should represent the major division and subdivision of the thesis. You should be consistent with the heading styles (fonts, bolds) throughout the document.

Headings for Major Divisions

Each major division (Introduction, Methods, Results, Appendix, References, and Index) should begin on a new page with the heading at the top margin. Titles and headings of major divisions should be typed in bold font, and centered on the page. If a title exceeds 5½ inches in typed length, it should be divided into two or more lines with each successive line of the title being shorter than the preceding line. Multiple-line titles for major divisions of the text should be double-spaced; multiple-line titles for subdivisions should be single-spaced. Do not use any punctuation at the end of the thesis title or the heading of a chapter.

Subheadings

Use a standardized format for capitalization, placement, italics, and/or use of bold face to indicate various levels of subheadings which must be consistent throughout your text.

PAGINATION

You should number consecutive pages of your thesis beginning from the main text, i.e., Introduction and continue till the end of all appendices, using Arabic numbers. All inserted maps, diagrams, tables, and illustrations should be included in this numbered sequence. The Cover page, Title page, Declaration, Certificate, Acknowledgments, and Glossary of abbreviations, are usually not numbered, though these pages are counted. If at all you wish to number them, these preliminary pages should be numbered with small Roman numerals (i.e., i, ii, iii...). Be consistent with the placement of all page numbers; by convention place the number at the center bottom, one double space below the last line of type, or at the top right corner. The pages are numbered consecutively using Arabic numerals.

PREPARING FINAL COPIES OF THE THESIS

You will have to submit a specified number of hard copies (four for University of Delhi) and one electronic/soft copy (the proposal must be saved in a file named using your name and student's ID number on a compact diskette) of the thesis to your university toward the partial fulfillment for the award of degree of doctor of medicine/surgery, in the standard format described earlier. In addition, you need to get hard copies of your thesis for your supervisor, co-supervisors (if any), your own copy, and institutional/departmental library. You must ensure that all thesis copies have a dark, clear, and straight print on the pages. If possible, a laser printer should be used to produce the text for all copies. In case photocopies are used, you must ensure an acceptable (dark and clear) copy. You must keep in mind that most printing and photocopy centers require at least 1–2 days for printing thesis copies. So plan accordingly and never leave the printing and binding for the last day.

Note: At least a week prior to the date of your thesis submission, present an unbound copy of your thesis to your supervisor to allow him/her to proofread and suggest necessary changes and corrections in time. Get your official copies only after approval from your supervisor.

TIME GUIDELINES FOR THESIS SUBMISSION

You will have to submit your thesis for examination (after being approved by your supervisor and co-supervisors) within the maximum period of candidature or such date as stipulated by the university. As per the norms of the University of Delhi, thesis submission date for MD/MS/MDS courses is 30th April (at the end of 2nd year of the course) or 1st week of October in the second year of the course for students who have already done Diploma in the same subject. The deadline for super-specialty courses (where applicable) is 30th November (at the beginning of 3rd year of the course) as per the norms of the University of Delhi. Usually, no extension of time is granted for submitting the thesis beyond the last date. As per the guidance of the Medical Council of India, thesis needs to be submitted at least 6 months prior to the theory and practical examination. A candidate is permitted to appear for the examination only after the acceptance of the thesis by the examiners.

In case, you fail to submit your thesis within 6 months of the last date of stipulated time frame, your registration for the postgraduate course may be annulled by the university on recommendations of the Board of Research Studies.

OPTIONAL THESIS

Some universities may not mandate thesis for super-specialty courses (DM/MCh) as a part of curriculum. In lieu of a thesis, the student is expected to publish two research papers (as first/second author) during his tenure in reputed journals indexed with Medline, to enable the student to appear in the theory and practical examinations. The student is expected to submit proofs of publication like a reprint or photocopy of the papers/letter of acceptance from the editor of the journal, *in lieu* of the thesis, to the university. Diploma courses usually do not mandate thesis submission as a part of curriculum.

RECTIFICATION IN A THESIS

Every thesis is assessed by a set of external examiners and a referee and must be passed by all the examiners to enable you to appear for the examination. Hence, you must check your thesis thoroughly for any possible errors prior to submission. On a rare occasion, a gross error may be noticed by you after submission. Alternately, your thesis assessor (examiner) may advise you changes, or seek clarification regarding your thesis. This will warrant you to revise your thesis and also draft a point-wise reply to the assessor explaining the modifications done by you within a stipulated time frame. Resubmitted thesis would then be evaluated by the original set of examiners/referee unless the original examiner(s) refuses, or is unavailable. At the time of re-evaluation of the modified thesis, another examiner may substitute the examiner who had initially rejected the thesis. The thesis is allowed to be resubmitted on one occasion. A resubmitted thesis, if not accepted by all the examiners/referee, is taken as "Rejected."

CONCLUSION

While you may spend most of the time in writing the core components of your thesis namely Introduction, Review of literature, Objectives Materials and Methods, Results, Discussion,

Conclusions and recommendations, Summary, and References, you must take cognizance of that your thesis includes all the elements deemed essential by your university. These would generally also include a cover page, a title page, declaration by the candidate, certificate from the institution, acknowledgments, presentation of thesis results to scientific forums and publications in scientific journals, table of contents, glossary of abbreviations, and appendices, which must be presented in an order prescribed by the university. Ensure correct typesetting, fonts, word count, and pagination. Stick to the timelines for thesis submission. Remember that you will be eligible to appear for the university examination, only if your thesis is approved/passed by examiners appointed by the university.

KEY MESSAGES

- Always refer to the guidelines for thesis submission while preparing your thesis.
- In addition to the core elements of your thesis, certain other components must be included in your thesis to certify it as complete.
- Ensure that your protocol and thesis are synchronous.
- Adhere to the timeline and format prescribed by your university to avoid rejection of thesis.

FURTHER READING

1. Faculty of Medical Sciences, University of Delhi. Bulletin of Information. [online] Available from https://www.fmsc.ac.in/notices/pg-notice-2019/Bulletin%20of%20Information.pdf. [Last accessed April 30, 2020].
2. Faculty of Medical Sciences, University of Delhi. Postgraduate (Degree/Diploma) Post-Doctoral Courses. [online] Available from http://www.fmsc.ac.in/pg-ordinance.pdf. [Last accessed April 30, 2020].
3. Medical Council of India Postgraduate Medical Education Regulations, 2000. [online] Available from https://www.mciindia.org/documents/rulesAndRegulations/Postgraduate-Medical-Education-Regulations-2000.pdf. [Last accessed April 30, 2020].
4. Smith JU, Murrell G, Ellis H, Huang C (Editors). Research in Medicine. Planning A Project: Writing A Thesis, 3rd edition. New York: Cambridge University Press; 2010. p. 129.
5. University of Delhi. Amendment to Appendix II to Ordinance V(2) & VII of the Ordinances of the University regarding Examination relating to M.S., M.D.,D.M., M.CH (effective from the academic session 2005-2006), (Page 350 of the University Calendar, Volume II, 1989)/(E.C. 1.4.2005). [online] Available from http://www.du.ac.in/du/uploads/Rules_Policies_Ordinances/Acts/pages/ordinanceamendments.pdf. [Last accessed April 30, 2020].
6. University of Leeds. Submitting your thesis for examination. [online] Available from https://students.leeds.ac.uk/info/10125/assessment/773/submitting_your_thesis. [Last accessed April 30, 2020].

CHAPTER 5

Formulating a Research Question/Hypothesis: The First Step

Bhupendra Kumar Jain

■ INTRODUCTION

Selecting a research topic for your thesis is the first important step toward thesis writing. For a postgraduate student, who has joined the course only a few weeks back, it may be an unfamiliar and onerous task. Stimulus for conducting research on a particular topic may stem from your own experience or observations, perceived gaps in knowledge, cues from previous studies, hot topics under discussion, brainstorming, curiosity about something being covered by the media, passion for a specific field, need to solve a problem, and/or pressure to become involved in research. You must exploit all these opportunities for finding a suitable topic for your thesis.

■ TYPES OF RESEARCH

At the onset, you must familiarize yourself with certain terms used to categorize the research (**Table 5.1**).

- *Basic research* is the research driven by the curiosity or interest of a scientist in a particular subject. The main purpose of this exercise is to study the fundamental aspect of phenomena and to expand the existing pool of knowledge. There may not be any obvious/immediate commercial value of the outcome of basic research.
- *Applied research,* on the other hand, is designed to solve some practical problem or to improve prevailing conditions.

The research can also be categorized according to the nature of the problem and level of current understanding about the problem.

- *Quantitative research* is an inquiry into an identified problem, usually based on testing a hypothesis, measured with numbers, and analyzed using statistical methods. Quantitative research is conclusive in nature.
- *Qualitative research* is exploratory in nature and it is used when we do not know what to expect. It is commonly used for understanding human knowledge, attitude, behavior, feelings, values and opinions, etc. Qualitative research is conducted in a natural setting. The qualitative research may generate ideas or hypotheses for exploring the subject further through quantitative research.

As a beginner, you must explore the domain of quantitative research for your thesis work. The quantitative research is the basic building block of the research process.

TABLE 5.1: **Examples of various types of research.**

Research category	Examples
Basic research	• Do black-colored items absorb more heat than white-colored items? • What is the mechanism of infection by human immunodeficiency virus (HIV)? • What is the genetic code for humans?
Applied research	• Is black- or white-colored umbrella more suitable for protection from heat on a sunny day? • How can one cure HIV infection? • How to alter genetic code to detect and cure disease?
Quantitative research (What? When?)	• Did boys or girls perform better in CBSE class 12 examinations in the year 2020? • What is the prevalence of tobacco smoking in medical students? • What is the demographic profile of men seeking no-scalpel vasectomy for family planning in Delhi?
Qualitative research (How? Why?)	• How can parents' attitude help a student to cope up with poor results in examinations? • Why do medical students smoke? • Why is no-scalpel vasectomy poorly accepted by eligible men in Delhi?

FIELDS OF RESEARCH

A large number of fields are available from which you can choose a topic. These are summarized below. Awareness of the list would be of great help to you in selecting a topic relevant to your discipline.

- Intracellular and biological processes, genetic studies, studies on properties of drugs, and animal experiments
- Distribution of diseases and/or health-related characteristics in the population
- Profile of cases of a specific disease
- Risk factors and their contribution to a condition
- *Efficacy of treatment*: Drugs and procedures
- Efficacy of diagnostic tests
- Health economics and cost-effectiveness
- Health policy, health systems, and health services
- Quality of healthcare and quality of life
- Reviews and meta-analysis

RESEARCH QUESTION AND HYPOTHESIS

Research Question

It is the question that you are trying to answer when you do research on a topic. At times, the question may not be very specific in the beginning due to the lack of available research on the topic of your interest. You can frame more than one research question on a topic. However, in a postgraduate thesis, it is desirable that the number of research questions should be restricted. Large number of questions makes your task more complex.

The research question can be of different levels: Descriptive or Inferential.

Descriptive Research Question

Descriptive research question seeks description of a phenomenon. It usually covers only one variable.

Examples

- What is the prevalence of scabies in primary school children in village "X"?
- What is the socioeconomic status of patients presenting with scabies at dermatology outpatient department (OPD) of Guru Teg Bahadur (GTB) Hospital?

Inferential Research Question

Inferential research question aims at drawing inference from a sample of the population. It involves a minimum of two variables—independent and dependent.

Examples

- What is the relationship between socioeconomic status and occurrence of scabies among the students of primary school in village "X"?
- Is drug "A" better than drug "B" for curing scabies in children?

Hypothesis

Hypothesis is a statement that makes a prediction about the result of an experiment. It is an educated guess based on existing knowledge. You would be trying to test the hypothesis by applying research methods.

- A hypothesis is very specific and it is based on previous empirical research. Hypothesis is used in quantitative research.
- Hypothesis can be framed in different forms: *null hypothesis* or *alternate hypothesis*.
    - *Null hypothesis* predicts that no relationship or significant difference exists between the groups in respect of a variable.
    - The alternate hypothesis, on the other hand, predicts that there exists a significant difference between the study groups. *Alternate hypothesis* can be stated as either a nondirectional hypothesis or as a directional hypothesis (**Box 5.1**).

A null hypothesis (abbreviated as H_0) is a hypothesis to be disproved. When a null hypothesis is rejected, alternate hypothesis is accepted—at least for the time being.

You may use either research question or hypothesis for your thesis. However, it is desirable that you generate a hypothesis after gathering all available information on the subject. It is preferable to state the hypothesis as null hypothesis, as clinical trial can be justified ethically only if an honest uncertainty exists in respect of the results under investigation.

> **Box 5.1: Examples of different types of hypotheses.**
>
> **Null hypothesis**
> - There is no difference between day-scholars and hostellers in respect of proportion of students who abuse drugs
>
> **Alternate—non-directional/two-sided hypothesis**
> - There is a difference between day-scholars and hostellers in respect of proportion of students who abuse drugs
>
> **Alternate—directional/one-sided hypothesis**
> - The proportion of students who abuse drugs is greater among hostellers as compared to day-scholars
>
>   OR
> - The proportion of students who abuse drugs is greater among day-scholars as compared to hostellers

PICO: Essential Elements of Research Question/Hypothesis

While transforming your research topic into the research question/hypothesis, you should make efforts to incorporate certain elements in your research question/hypothesis to make the research focused and feasible, for example, the population/problem, independent variables, and the dependent variables.

In practice, well-built research questions usually contain four elements represented by *PICO*—an acronym which stands for:

- *Patient, Population, or Problem*
- *Intervention*

- Comparator
- Outcome

The intervention and comparator represent independent variables, while the outcome represents the dependent variable.

Example

Suppose you want to find out *"Efficacy of a specific operative procedure on the outcome of the treatment of anal fistula,"* you may use the PICO format to translate the clinical problem into a structured research question which identifies specific key concepts (**Table 5.2**).

Application of PICO strategy results in a clear, specific, focused, and achievable research question, e.g., *How does fistulotomy compare with fistulectomy in terms of the postoperative pain and wound healing in the management of patients with simple anal fistula?*

This research question can also be stated as "null hypothesis": We hypothesize that there is no difference in postoperative pain and wound healing following fistulotomy and fistulectomy in patients with simple anal fistula.

The elements of the research question/hypothesis should be operationally defined to remove any scope for ambiguity in interpretation. In the above-mentioned example, postoperative pain and wound healing need further elaboration: postoperative pain as measured with visual analog scale; and wound healing as measured in terms of median wound healing time.

It may not be practical to identify/define all the four PICO elements in each and every research plan. It is more applicable to analytic and experimental studies. However, awareness of PICO format helps you improve your research question irrespective of the type of study you choose to undertake.

■ FRAMING A RESEARCH QUESTION/HYPOTHESIS

It would be a good strategy for you to first choose an interesting broad topic. You must jot down what you already know and what you would like to know about the topic. You must further expand your knowledge about the topic by studying coursework, journals, and information available on internet. Nonavailability of enough studies, inconclusive studies, and studies conducted with inappropriate designs justify further exploration of the topic. Patients' hospital records can provide valuable material for clinical topics. You must consult peers, advisors, and research workers interested in the topic to get useful information and guidance.

Once you have enough information, you should narrow down the topic to suit your and the research community's interest. A pilot study can provide you with an insight regarding the feasibility of the proposed study and the difficulties likely to be faced by you. You should work on a few topics in this manner, and then select the most appropriate topic in consultation with your supervisor.

TABLE 5.2: PICO format for translating clinical problem into a research question.

		Tips for formulating	Example
P	Patient/population/problem	What is the study population?	Patients with simple anal fistula
I	Intervention/cause/prognostic factor/treatment	Which main intervention is considered?	Specific/new operation: fistulotomy
C	Comparison (alternate to that above)	What is the main alternative for comparison?	Alternate/standard operation: fistulectomy
O	Outcome	What could this intervention really affect?	Postoperative pain and wound healing

Depending upon whether the topic chosen by you is suitable for qualitative or quantitative research, you must transform the research topic to a well-defined research question or a hypothesis.

The success of your thesis project and the degree of its contribution to your career development will depend on the goodness of your research question/hypothesis. Seven important characteristics of a good research question/hypothesis are shown in **Box 5.2**. You must evaluate your research question/hypothesis on goodness parameters before finalizing it.

> **Box 5.2: The seven characteristics of a good research question.**
> 1. *Novel*: Addresses a defined gap in knowledge.
> 2. *Relevant*: Applicable to day-to-day practice, and significant enough.
> 3. *Clear*: Well-defined and focused.
> 4. *Appropriately complex*: Neither very ambitious nor very simple, well suited to caliber/commitment of student and supervisor
> 5. *Ethically sound*: Research process is acceptable to the study population, and it causes no potential harm to them.
> 6. *Interesting*: Interesting enough to engage the student, the supervisor, and the research community.
> 7. *Feasible*: Must be answerable. Feasibility of completion of the study using available resources: time, subjects/materials, tools, etc.

Good and Bad Research Questions/Hypotheses

Carefully study the research questions printed below to understand the difference between a good and a bad research question/hypothesis.

Example

Unclear: Do the patients suffering from carcinoma of lung smoke more?

Clear: Is the frequency and quantum of smoking—in terms of pack years—greater among patients diagnosed as carcinoma of lung by biopsy, as compared to the controls?

The unclear version of this research question does not specify or define carcinoma of lung, the comparator, and the measurement for smoking. Clear version provides the definitions of various elements that are necessary to conduct the research.

Example

Unfocused: What is the effect of television viewing on students?

Focused: Does increase in the duration of television viewing adversely affect the sleep pattern of the primary school students?

The unfocused research question may cover the academic, psychosocial, and lifestyle characteristics of students—too broad a topic for postgraduate thesis. The independent variable (duration of television viewing), dependent variable (sleep pattern), and study population (primary school students) have also not been defined in the unfocused version.

Example

Too simple: What measures are being taken to prevent postoperative wound infection at XYZ hospital?

Appropriately complex: What are the risk factors associated with deep surgical site infection following laparotomy for acute perforation peritonitis in patients presenting at XYZ hospital?

The simple version of this question can be answered in a few sentences. There is no scope for analysis. The more complex form of this research question requires observation, systematic data collection, analysis, and evaluation by you.

Example

Novel, focused, and relevant: What is the effect of yoga therapy on "Perceived Stress Score" in low-risk pregnancy?

The question is novel and focused. It is relevant to holistic management of pregnancy. You may need to involve a yoga expert to identify the appropriate yoga exercises and to train the patients.

Example

Clear and relevant but incomplete: There is no difference between treatment with centchroman and tamoxifen for relief of symptoms of mastalgia.

Complete: There is no difference between treatment with centchroman and tamoxifen for relief of symptoms of mastalgia in women of childbearing age.

The hypothesis may be improved by including "population under consideration": Ethical concerns regarding the use of these drugs, if any, will need to be addressed.

Exercise

A few more research questions are listed below for you to brainstorm. Please spend a few minutes on each question to discover if it is good for postgraduate thesis according to the seven goodness criteria mentioned in **Box 5.2**. You would find some of the deficiencies of the questions printed below the questions.

- *What is the difference between hypertonic saline (7.5%) and Ringer's lactate resuscitation on the mortality following burns?*
  Procurement of hypertonic saline for clinical use may be a challenge and its availability is to be verified. Patient population has not been defined: age group/severity of burns.
- *What is the frequency and the site of local recurrence following conservative breast surgery for carcinoma of breast?*
  The usual 18-month study period would be insufficient for studying local recurrence.
- *What are histopathologic changes seen in trucut liver biopsy specimen in patients undergoing cholecystectomy?*
  Performing trucut biopsy to obtain liver tissue for the study in patients undergoing cholecystectomy involves ethical issues—the procedure has the risk of complications. The relevance of performing this study is also questionable.
- *What is the role of iron deficiency in the formation of gallstones?*
  The topic lacks clarity and is probably too ambitious for a postgraduate thesis.
- *What are the incidence and pattern of various neoplastic thyroid swellings with particular reference to surgical management?*
  The topic is not clear and not focused. It has a few terms such as "incidence, pattern, and neoplastic thyroid swellings" which need to be defined. Would it be a hospital-based or population-based study? The study lacks novelty.

Once you assess your research question/hypothesis on the seven goodness parameters and identify deficiencies, you can improve upon your proposal or drop it in favor of a more suitable one. A simple scheme for developing a research question/hypothesis is depicted in **Flowchart 5.1**.

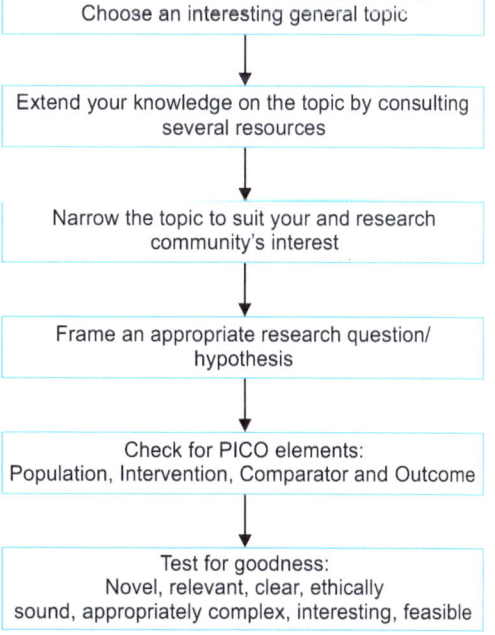

Flowchart 5.1: Path for developing a research question/hypothesis.

CONCLUSION

You must exercise due diligence for selecting a good research topic and framing the research question/hypothesis for your thesis. Reflection on all the currently available information on the proposed topic is vital. Consultation with peers, advisers, and experts is rewarding. Finally, you must evaluate your research question/hypothesis for the application of PICO strategy and compliance of goodness criteria.

KEY MESSAGES

- The research can be categorized as quantitative and qualitative. Quantitative research is based on testing a hypothesis, measured with numbers, and analyzed using statistical methods. Qualitative research is exploratory and used for understanding human knowledge, attitude, behavior, feelings, values and opinions, etc.
- The research question can be descriptive or inferential.
- Well-built research questions usually contain four elements represented by PICO—an acronym which stands for: Patient, Population, or Problem; Intervention; Comparator; and Outcome.
- Follow the acronym FINER for a good research question, i.e., the research question should be Feasible, Interesting, Novel, Ethical, and Relevant.

FURTHER READING

1. Creswell JW. Chapter seven. Research questions and hypotheses. In: Research design: qualitative, quantitative, and mixed methods approaches, 3rd edition. California: Sage Publications, Inc.; 2009.
2. De D, Singh S. Basic Understanding of study types and formulating research question for a clinical trial. Indian Dermatol Online J. 2019;10(3):351-3.
3. Dhadwal DS, Mazta SR, Gupta A. Judicious selection of MD thesis topic: Role of faculty in improving research in public health. Indian J Community Med. 2013;38(3):184-5.
4. Duke T. How to do a postgraduate research project and write a minor thesis. Arch Dis Child. 2018;103(9):820-7.
5. Durbin Jr CG. How to come up with a good research question: framing the hypothesis. Respir Care. 2004;49(10):1195-8.
6. Fandino W. Formulating a good research question: Pearls and pitfalls. Indian J Anaesth. 2019;63(8):611-6.
7. Farrugia P, Petrisor BA, Farrokhyar F, Bhandari M. Research questions, hypotheses and objectives. Can J Surg. 2010;53(4):278-81.
8. Joob B, Wiwanitkit V. Formulation of research question. J Indian Assoc Pediatr Surg. 2020;25(1):62.
9. Macfarlane MD, Kisely S, Loi S, Looi JC, Merry S, Parker S, et al. Getting started in research: research questions, supervisors and literature reviews. Australas Psychiatry. 2015;23(1):8-11.
10. Meadows KA. So you want to do research? 2: developing research question. Br J Community Nurs. 2003;8(9):397-403.
11. Ratan SK, Anand T, Ratan J. Formulation of research question–stepwise approach. J Indian Assoc Pediatr Surg. 2019;24(1):15-20.

CHAPTER 6

How to Select the Study Design

Aashima Dabas, Devendra Mishra

▪ INTRODUCTION

Selection of the Study Design is the most critical component of the research cycle. It is essential to plan how, where, and when will the study commence; who will participate; and how the study participants will be selected. The Study Design provides a direction and plan of recruitment, and helps you to collect and analyze the generated data with credibility and validity. In this section, you will learn about the different types of study designs and how to choose the most appropriate design for a research question.

▪ QUALITATIVE VERSUS QUANTITATIVE STUDY DESIGNS

While answering a research question, data collection can be *qualitative* or *quantitative*.

Qualitative Studies

Qualitative study designs record data which may not be totally convertible into numbers for statistical analysis such as data of experiences after injection administration, reasons for a particular behavior, and problems with a new intervention. The data generated are usually heterogenous but may give us vital information about an event/problem, and frequently serve as the basis of further quantitative studies or community-based interventions.

For example, a researcher wants to find out the reasons why students avoid attending clinical postings. This research question can be answered in a purely qualitative study design by just asking the possible reasons, using one-to-one interviews or focused group discussions. The results are presented based on themes that emerged, rather than numbers/proportions. These studies are not limited by sample size.

Quantitative Studies

Quantitative studies are the most common type of study for thesis and dissertations. The study variables can be presented in the form of numerical values. A quantitative study can be further planned to be *observational* or *experimental* (**Flowchart 6.1**).

- *Observational studies* are the ones where the researcher decides to make observations about various events, without interfering with the process (in a way that it changes the outcome). Observational study designs can be further classified into *descriptive* where data of only one group is being "described,"

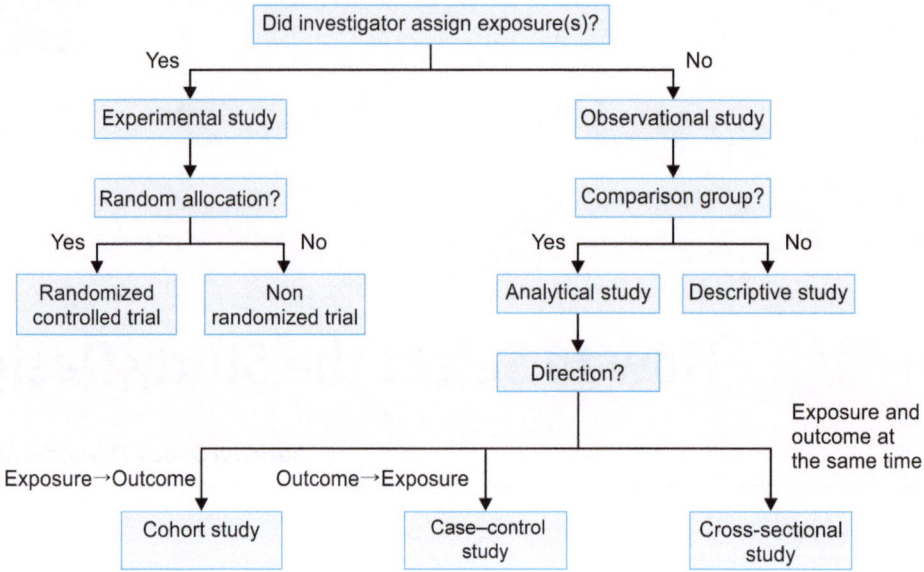

Flowchart 6.1: Outline of study designs.

or *analytical* where data generated are being "analyzed by comparing" these between two or more study groups.
- *Experimental studies* are those where the researcher carries out an intervention in one group of subjects, which is likely to affect the outcome in them, and compare it to another group/s not receiving that intervention/receiving a different intervention.

Details are discussed later in this chapter.

■ CHOOSING THE STUDY DESIGN

Identify the most suitable study design based on the research hypothesis and considerations such as disease, logistics, and time. Spell out the flow of the study right from preparation of the protocol to recruitment process, study methods, and data collection.

You should be able to judiciously decide which study design is most feasible for a given research question in your specific situation. The following factors need to be considered during selection of a study design:
- *Disease characteristics*: Descriptive studies may be the earliest evidence to report something new about an event. The rarity of exposure and outcome can further determine which type of analytical study will be suitable. In diseases with long natural course such as cancers, case–control study would be more appropriate where the researcher divides the population on the basis of outcome and evaluates the likely past exposure(s). A cohort study can assess for multiple exposures and more reliably establish their association with the outcomes than case–control studies.
- *Resources, feasibility, and time*: Cross-sectional and case–control studies are easier to perform than cohort studies which need long follow-up, implying need for human resources, finances, and logistics. Similarly, an experimental design needs finances, logistics and human resource, and are not easy to conduct.

For example, in previously discussed study of use of public transport and time to arrival in college, an experimental design would be most ambitious and scientifically strong. However, it will be difficult to execute and conduct, and thus may not be the best option for a thesis.

- *Type of research question*: The efficacy/safety of a drug/intervention can be observed in controlled settings such as an experimental study design. A diagnostic study where a new method/innovation about a diagnostic testing is being explored can be done in a cross-sectional study design. Similarly, cross-sectional studies can estimate prevalence of a disease in the population. Study for risk factors of a disease can be done as case–control or cohort keeping in mind few salient features (**Table 6.1**).
- *Ethical consideration*: A new molecule being tested on humans/human tissues should first be found safe in animal studies. Randomized trials have added ethical concerns as intervention group is more likely to be benefited or be exposed to side effects of an intervention than the control group. Therefore, it becomes important to plan the intervention in a way that it abides by the ethical standards.

OBSERVATIONAL STUDIES

Descriptive Studies

These studies merely record observations or data without any comparison groups. Examples of descriptive observational studies are: Case reports and case series, risk/disease profile of a group of persons, or description of a study population. Such data are important as they provide initial clues/understanding about the problem or disease. Descriptive studies are usually done to assess the burden of disease or report findings of a disease. All surveys, questionnaire-based studies, and clinicoetiological profile studies are primarily descriptive studies.

For example, a study on hand washing practices in ICU will report quantitative data on use of soap and hand-rub and knowledge about hand hygiene. Similarly, outcomes of a new surgical procedure (already in use) may be done in a descriptive study (as there is no need of a comparison group). Another example

TABLE 6.1: Comparison of case–control and cohort studies.

	Case–control	Cohort
Direction	Outcomes under study have already occurred and are known in the study population. Researcher traces back data on likely associated exposures	Exposures are already known. Participants are followed up for likely outcomes
Feasibility and timeliness	Can be done quickly and easily. Feasible for rare disorders and those with long incubation period	Need time period of observation. Not feasible for diseases with long incubation period
Multiplicity of factors	Multiple risk factors can be studied for one outcome	Multiple outcomes can be studied for one exposure (risk factor)
Controls	Controls may have unidentified confounders	Better control over selection of controls as likely confounders can be adjusted
Causality estimation	Establishes only an association between exposure and outcome	Establishes link between exposure and outcome
Strength of association	Expressed as odds ratio	Expressed as risk ratio
Bias	Recall bias among participants, selection bias among researchers	Matching of controls may introduce selection bias

could be a study reporting on CT chest findings in patients of COVID-19.

Analytical Studies

Analytical study designs are those where there is analysis or comparison of different risk factors or outcomes within two groups selected from the study population. These two groups are predecided at the time of stating the research question or hypothesis—otherwise, even in a descriptive study, you would report differences within subgroups, e.g., urban–rural and male–female. The statistical tests of significance are applicable for analytical studies. A hypothesis statement should be written before planning an analytical study as shown in example below.

As evident in example above, the mere mention of reasons for coming late gives us only some information regarding the problem but does not suffice to decipher whether they are actually responsible for the outcome or are associated by chance. For the above-mentioned example, the researcher decided to better comprehend the risk factors of arriving late to college and modified the research question as "whether the use of public transport is associated with first-year college students reaching late to the college?" Therefore, a null hypothesis for this would read "use of public transport does not affect the arrival timings of first year college students for 8 AM lecture." A comparison of the usage of public transports between students coming in-time and late will help decipher whether public transport (exposure) is a risk factor. The different ways of conducting this analysis is discussed below in analytical study designs.

Analytical studies are further divided into *Cohort*, where the participants are enrolled before the occurrence of study outcomes (on the basis of presence or absence of the risk factor being studied); *Case-control*, where the outcomes have already occurred and the participants are being enrolled on the basis of presence or absence of outcome; and *Cross-sectional*, where both exposure/risk factor and the outcome are measured simultaneously at the time of enrollment, and it may be difficult to decide what came first. The classic example for a cohort study is comparison of smokers and nonsmokers (presence or absence of risk factor) for occurrence of lung cancer (outcome). For case–control study, the example is comparison of lung cancer patients and healthy persons (presence or absence of outcome) for history of smoking (risk factor). The groups in Cohort studies are decided based on the exposure/risk factors, whereas in Case–Control studies, they are decided based on the outcome.

- A *cohort* means a group of people with common characteristics. A cohort study analyzes the likely outcomes by monitoring different exposures over a period of time in a group of participants. The direction of study thus "looks forward" from exposure to outcome (**Fig. 6.1**). For example, antenatal nutrition (exposure) and occurrence of low birth weight in neonates (outcome); prophylactic antibiotics (exposure) and postoperative infection (outcome); and hygiene (exposure) and occurrence of diarrhea (outcome).

  Multiple outcomes can be simultaneously evaluated in a cohort study. For example, antenatal malnutrition (exposure) and occurrence of low birth weight in neonates (outcome). In the same study, effect of antenatal malnutrition (exposure) can also be assessed on preterm birth (outcome), birth asphyxia (outcome), and congenital malformations (outcome).

- In a *case-control* study, the outcome has occurred to define the study population into two groups. For example, cancer survivors and deceased, graft failure and graft uptake, diarrhea and no diarrhea, and malignant and benign. The risk factors or variables under study in these two groups are now examined by "looking back" at their salient features (**Fig. 6.2**). Thus, the direction (of collecting data) in a case-control study is from outcome to exposure. In the first example, the researcher goes back and asks the use of public transport (exposure)

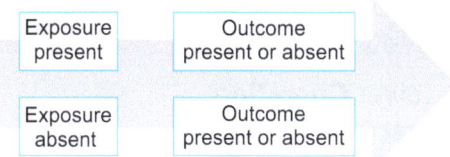

Fig. 6.1: Cohort study.

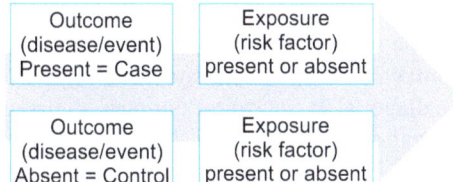

Fig. 6.2: Case–control study.

between those who arrived on time and those who were late (outcome).

- In a *cross-sectional study*, the exposures and outcomes have occurred and are analyzed at one point of time. For example, hygiene practices and diarrhea, consumption of sweetened beverages and obesity, preoperative antibiotics with postoperative infection, use of public transport, and arrival timing of students. A pictorial description with the previously discussed example is shown in **Figure 6.3**, where four possible permutations of exposure and outcome exist. The researcher thus records the observations/outcomes and analyzes them as difference between these four groups to establish an association between exposure and outcome. The researcher contacts each participant only at one point of time to collect data.

- *Selection of controls*: A control is identified as a participant for comparison of the risk factor in a cohort study, and presence of an outcome in a case–control study. In a cohort study, the controls should be free from the risk factor under investigation and free of likely confounders associated with the risk factor. The researcher selects a control by *matching* them for certain features with the cases. Caution should be exercised for matching for likely confounders, which are defined as variables or factors which can independently affect the outcome and exposure and can result in misinterpretation of an association. In a case–control study, the control should be free from the outcome being studied.

- *Example of a confounder*: In a study on risk of obesity (outcome) with intake of high calorie fast foods (exposure), increased television viewing is a confounder as it can be independently associated with both obesity and intake of high calorie fast foods. It should be matched/controlled during the selection of controls (preferred method) or should be adjusted during the analysis of results.

As evident from few of these examples, the same research question can be addressed by different types of analytical study designs. The salient features of case–control and cohort studies are mentioned in **Table 6.1**.

Studies of Diagnostic Accuracy

Diagnostic studies are a form of observational studies that are done to test the performance

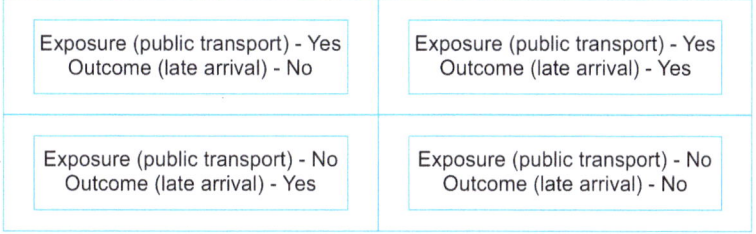

Fig. 6.3: Snapshot of a cross-sectional study.

of a diagnostic test. As they are usually done to look for some test variable that is present when the disease is also present, these are primarily cross-sectional study designs, unless they are being done for markers of risk of disease or prognosis.

These can be of two types, you are either comparing a new test (Index test) against a gold standard (Standard test) or you are comparing two tests. In the former case, you are able to use measures of diagnostic accuracy such as sensitivity and specificity, whereas, in the latter, you can just calculate the degree of agreement between the two tests.

For the former, it is essential to choose a valid gold standard against which the test under study will be compared. For example, researcher "A" wants to test the performance of a new biochemical test in predicting a complication in a disease. The patients will undergo investigation with the new test (Index test) and the traditional test (Standard test) and results from both will be compared as shown in **Table 6.2**. This table can help us deduce the sensitivity and specificity to understand the performance of a diagnostic test. Remember, that both sensitivity and specificity are characteristics of the test under study. An ideal screening test should be able to suspect more patients with the disease or complication (true positives) and hence should have better sensitivity than specificity. On the contrary, a confirmatory test should be specific for the disease/complication under question and should be able to filter true negatives better, implying need for higher specificity than sensitivity.

Receiver Operating Characteristic Curve

A receiver operating characteristic (ROC) curve is a useful statistical tool that helps to determine the best cut off value for a diagnostic test under question. It is constructed by plotting the true positive rate on *y-axis* against the false positive rate on *x-axis* as shown in **Figure 6.4**. The diagonal in the center denotes occurrence by chance or as random. As clarified in the discussion for a diagnostic test, the new test under question will be compared with a gold standard to establish true and false positivity. ROC curve is also known as the curve between sensitivity (true positive rate) and 1-specificity (false positive rate). The researcher can also calculate the area under the curve (AUC) for that diagnostic test (ranges from 0 to 1), a higher AUC implying a better performance or accuracy of a diagnostic test. This means AUC of 1 is perfect while of 0.5 means no diagnostic ability.

For example, a researcher aims to check whether the serum levels of "X" are useful to diagnose sepsis. The gold standard for the diagnosis of sepsis is positive blood culture. The researcher now checks the sensitivity and specificity at different values of new test, such as $x1, x2, x3,$ and $x4$, which will also calculate true positive and false positive for each set of cutoffs. Thus, different curves can be made representing the different cutoffs as in

TABLE 6.2: 2 × 2 table for diagnostic test.

	Standard test positive (Disease positive)	Standard test negative (Disease negative)
Index test positive	True positive	False positive
Index test negative	False negative	True negative

Notes:
Sensitivity = True positives/(True Positives + False negatives)
Specificity = True negatives/(True Negatives + False positives)
Positive predictive value = True positives/(True positives + False positives)
Negative predictive value = True negatives/(True negatives + False negatives)

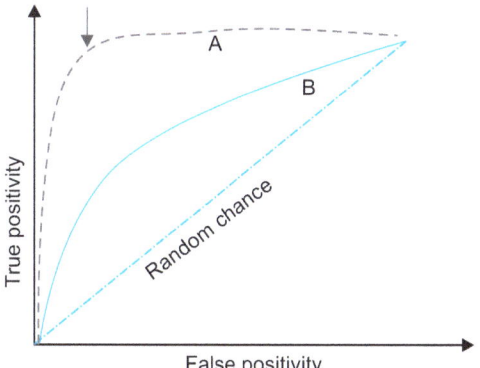

Fig. 6.4: Receiver operating curve for two tests—A and B. Better cut offs with curve A (best at tip of arrow) with higher true positivity rate than curve B.

Figure 6.4. The test is a good diagnostic test if the curve lies in the upper left quadrant of the graph A (arrow), i.e., a cut off value which gives maximum true positivity and minimum false positivity or type I error rate.

■ EXPERIMENTAL STUDY DESIGN

Experimental study design is where the researcher decides or dictates the occurrence of an event, such as treatment or therapy, in a group of participants. These study designs will also record observations about exposure and outcome, but these observations would not have occurred if the researcher had not intervened. In an experimental study, the exposure and the outcomes both have NOT occurred. The researcher controls assignment of the exposure to different groups and then measures the impact of this exposure on the outcome. Experimental study designs can be randomized or nonrandomized depending on how the researcher chooses who will receive intervention and who will not.

Nonrandomized Study

In nonrandomized studies, the researcher allots the intervention but in a nonrandom manner. It could be by consecutive numbers, odd-even numbers, or based on presentation on certain days of a week.

A researcher chooses to ask first 10 patients to use public transport and next 10 patients to use own vehicle. Students with the first 10 roll numbers therefore have no chance of coming in own vehicle for the study making this a nonrandom selection.

Randomized Study

In a randomized study, each participant has an equal chance of being selected for the study intervention. This selection can be made through various methods of randomization such as simple lottery, stratified, block, or cluster randomization. Thus, a participant gets "randomized" to an intervention or control arm.

The researcher can study the use of public transport as a risk factor for reaching late to college. He can make two groups in the class and decide the exposure, where one group will strictly use self-vehicles (control), while the other group will strictly use public transport (case).

Each student gets equal chance of being chosen into the own vehicle or the public transport group by a process called randomization, which may be either by generating random numbers using a software, through the web, or random number tables.

Randomization can be done by the following methods:
- *Simple randomization*: This can be done by lottery methods as simple as flipping the coin or choosing between two colored balls from a bag where one choice is randomized to receive group A and the other choice gets group B. More commonly, a random sequence of numbers is generated through a computer or random number table where participants will be randomized into group A or B as per the sequence.
- *Stratified randomization* helps to divide the participants into different strata to ensure equal enrollment from each strata. Example: Randomization for vitamin D therapy in children with fractures—here limb of fracture (upper or lower limb) or

gender (boy or girl) can be used to stratify the participants.
- *Block randomization*: Here, participants are divided in different blocks at one time which are multiple of intervention arms. For example, for a two-limb randomization, blocks can be of sizes 2, 4, 6, and 8 and of three-limb study, block sizes can be 6 and 9. If we take block size of four for a two-limb study, the randomization sequence shall read as AABB or ABAB or ABBA or BABA or BAAB or BBAA till the entire sample size gets covered. Thus, at any given point, a block of chosen size will contain equal number of participants of both groups for analysis. However, the investigator will be able to guess the group for the fourth participant in a block. To avoid this bias, blocks of varying sizes can be used to generate the randomization sequence.
- *Cluster randomization*: This form of randomization is used in large epidemiological studies where the population is divided into clusters based on their natural properties such as geographical location. Each cluster so identified is then sampled further for the study.

A randomized study is said to be a randomized controlled trial (RCT) as the researcher has control on who receives what intervention. The researcher may choose to create a parallel or crossover design. In the parallel study design, the participants get randomized into either of two groups and continue to receive the respective interventions till the study is completed. In a cross-over design, the respective interventions get interchanged between the study groups after a period of observation. The study participants thus act as controls for themselves. Most RCTs are parallel group studies with two groups. The research question and the type of intervention usually determine whether a crossover design is needed. The comparator group in an RCT emerges after randomization. These subjects are expected to have (*and almost always have*) similar baseline characteristics as the test group.

Blinding

The procedure by which the researcher now deidentifies the control and test groups is called blinding or masking. This is done to reduce the researcher's bias in interpreting data. For example, a researcher wishes to compare the efficacy of a new drug A versus drug B for hypertension in adult males. He selects a group of 50 newly diagnosed hypertensive adult males and randomizes them to groups A and B for respective drug administration. He compares the mean blood pressure in both groups after 4 weeks. The study design can be made single-blinded when the patients do not know which drug they have received—drug A or drug B. For an unbiased measurement of outcome, the researcher should also be blinded to which group the patients belong, known as double blinding. The design is sometimes labeled as triple-blinded when the person analyzing the mean difference in blood pressure also does not know the drugs belonging to codes A and B. However, these terms are not very well-defined, and it is always better to clarify in your methodology who all were blinded/masked.

Blinding is helpful as it reduces the bias in the study. There are various methods to introduce blinding such as packaging drugs in similar form, color, and taste. This prevents the participant and the researcher from knowing the likely study group of the patient during follow-up and analysis. However, not all interventions can be blinded, e.g., comparison between an exercise program and a drug for reduction in blood pressure, or performance of an open versus laparoscopic surgical technique.

Allocation Concealment

It is different from blinding and is an essential part of an RCT. It literally means concealing the likely group allocation of a participant to be enrolled in the trial. For example, in efficacy study of drug A versus B, the researcher may keep the complete randomization list with him and allot to participants consecutively.

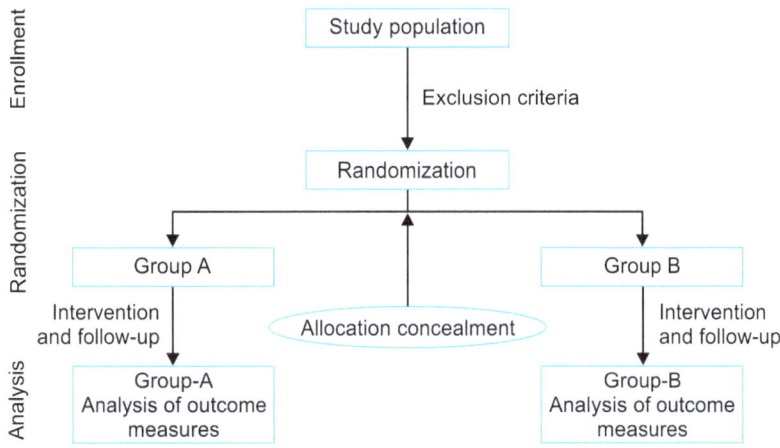

Flowchart 6.2: Randomized controlled trial—parallel group.

However, he may be tempted not to treat a sicker or less sick or one's relative with the newer drug than conventional drug and the allocation of randomized group may be interchanged with the next number. To reduce this selection bias, allocation order should be concealed which is known as allocation concealment. This can be done by keeping all randomized codes sealed in envelopes which can be opened one per participant, or the randomization codes can be generated real-time through a server and accordingly allotted from the main randomization sequence.

The flow of a parallel group randomized controlled trial is shown in **Flowchart 6.2**. Other RCT designs include factorial and cluster randomization which will not be discussed here.

ADDITIONAL STUDY DESIGNS

Systematic Reviews and Meta-analysis

These studies *per se* are studies on already collected data, or secondary data. It summarizes the pooled estimate from available evidence for a study hypothesis or problem. These form the highest level of evidence as data from multiple sources are being analyzed and summarized by using appropriate statistical tests. A systematic review can address a problem related to epidemiology, etiology, diagnosis, management, or prognosis of a disease. Systematic indicates that the process of collection and compilation of secondary data is done systematically and in a sequential manner. This usually includes the following steps:

- Identify a research question.
- Outline a search strategy and select libraries or online databases where the search string will be run.
- Identify inclusion and exclusion criteria of selecting studies for data retrieval.
- Check the quality and risk of bias of shortlisted studies.
- Pool or tabulate data for analysis—assess how important were the findings/risk associations/odds ratio/effect size for each respective study in comparison to the others.

Meta-analysis is the statistical process of combining results in a systematic review of randomized controlled trial or observational studies. Cochrane collaboration (*www.cochranelibrary.com*) publishes systematic review of highest possible quality to generate the best evidence for a particular topic. A meta-analysis performs the tabulation of results in a quantitative manner to generate a statistical plot called as a Forest plot. The forest plot shows the magnitude of the main outcome measure of each study represented by squares and the overall pooled result is shown as a diamond in the end.

Nested Case–control

This is a type of case–control study within a predefined group or a cohort. The outcomes of interest have occurred at the point of beginning the study but the exposures are studied within a well-defined population. Thus, a random sample of cases and controls emerges from a defined group instead of a large population making it a convenient design for studying a different outcome within a cohort study.

Crossover Study Design

This is a type of randomized controlled study design with two arms where each arm is allocated as specific intervention. After a minimum period of intervention and follow-up, the participant groups can be interchanged with each other to see the effect of the other intervention of the groups. There is usually a period of wash-off or waiting which is meant for the effect of the first intervention to wane or disappear. For example, to see the effect of two drugs A and B on blood pressure, groups I and II are randomized to drugs A and B for 4 weeks. After a drug-free period of 2 weeks, the groups get interchanged such that groups I and II receive drugs B and A, respectively. A crossover design requires a lesser sample size than parallel group design. However, it is sometimes difficult to conduct, wash-out period may not be possible or ethically correct in few instances, and there may be higher chances of attrition.

Mixed-methods Study

These studies use both qualitative and quantitative research methods in the same or related populations. For example, in a study on unintentional childhood injuries, the authors may note the prevalence of child injuries (quantitative part) and also try to study the opinion of stakeholders (older children, parents, community leaders, and public health engineering experts) by various methods (qualitative part).

■ LEVELS OF EVIDENCE

A random search of medical information available today is frequently fraught with risk of it not being reliable, valid, and applicable in the current situation. To ease the process of weighing information available through research, levels of evidence were proposed to stratify the validity and strength of information. An experimental study design is graded superior over observational study design as it removes bias and helps in the analysis of results in a controlled manner. Systematic review and meta-analysis of RCTs are considered superior to results from an individual RCT. Evidence from case reports, anecdotal experiences, and cross-sectional studies is considered as a weaker evidence. The hierarchy of levels of evidence is shown in **Figure 6.5**.

The levels of evidence thus help us interpret information available through different studies/pooled analysis. RCTs may not exist for few research questions where conducting a RCT was illogical or not feasible. In such cases, data from a well-conducted systematic review of cohort studies or a large cohort study are informative.

The readers should also be wary that the above pyramid is only an outline of the levels of evidence, not degree of recommendations for a given question. The researcher may find more relevant and valid data in a cohort study than a meta-analysis on a similar topic. Sample size and effect size of different studies should also be taken into consideration. For example, a cohort study on a large sample size is more powerful than a RCT on a handful of patients. Other measures which decide the quality of the study such as study methods, data handling, and

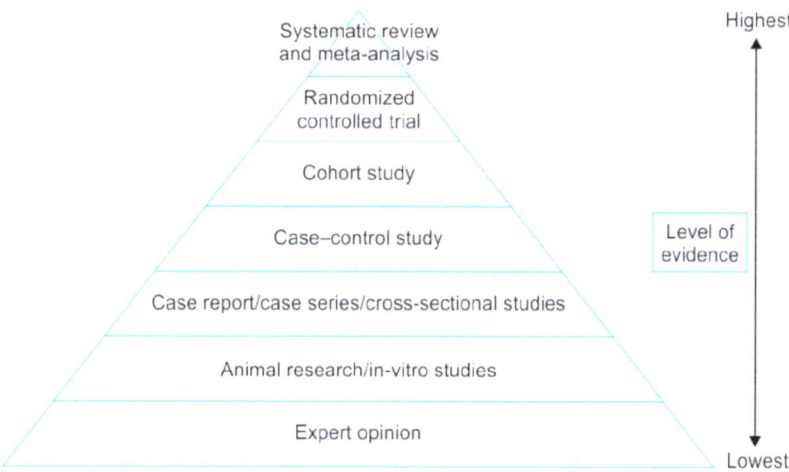

Fig. 6.5: Hierarchy of level of evidence in scientific research.

TABLE 6.3: Levels of evidence for different research questions.

Type of study/research question	Best type of level of evidence	Other suitable levels of evidence
Prevalence study	Locally relevant cross-sectional studies and surveys	Systematic reviews of cross-sectional data
Diagnostic study	Systematic review of cross-sectional studies with consistently applied reference standard and blinding	Cross-sectional studies with consistently applied reference standard and blinding
Prognosis of therapy/disease	Systematic review of cohort studies with large sample size	Inception cohort studies
Efficacy studies	Systematic review of RCTs or systematic review of high-quality cohort studies	Individual RCTs or cohort study with large sample size or high effect size*

*Effect size is the measure of outcome seen after exposure which can be compared between the study groups calculated statistically.

quality assurance in the study should also be regarded. **Table 6.3** shows how different levels of evidence can be used for different research questions (The Oxford 2011 Levels of Evidence. *http://www.cebm.net/index.aspx?o=5653*).

Reporting Guidelines

Reporting guidelines are standard guidelines (with checklists) for reporting of a specific type of study design. These provide details of different components of research study and methods and can be used to validate whether your study plan has all the necessary components. There are different guidelines for different study designs, e.g., STARD (Standards for Reporting Diagnostic Accuracy Studies) for diagnostic studies, STROBE (Strengthening the Reporting of Observational studies in Epidemiology) for observational studies, and CONSORT (Consolidated Standards of Reporting Trials) for randomized control trials. Details guidelines in a checklist form can be accessed at *https://www.equator-network.org/*.

■ CONCLUSION

It is important to develop a robust plan before commencing on any research idea. Study design is an integral component of a research protocol and should be used in compliance with standard guidelines in the relevant context regarding disease characteristics and logistic issues. **Table 6.4** summarizes the salient features of common study designs.

TABLE 6.4: Strengths and limitations of study designs.

Study design	Strengths	Limitation
Case studies	No logistics required, easy to report, and first clue of an event in literature	Biased reporting and lacks analysis
Cross-sectional	Prevalence analysis, hypothesis generation, and easy to conduct in terms of logistics and time	No temporal relationship and cannot determine causality
Case–control	Quick, easier logistics, and can analyze multiple risk factors	Recall bias, matching may be improper, and difficult due to confounders
Cohort	Cause and effect relationship, can analyze multiple outcomes	Time consuming, costly, and attrition of study participants may affect analysis
Experimental	Causality and robust scientific evidence	Expensive, ethical concerns, difficult, and attrition depending upon the time of study

KEY MESSAGES

- The study design guides the methodology, sample size calculation, and also the statistical analysis.
- When the researcher observes the effects of an exposure occurring naturally, it is an observational study.
- Two types of observational studies are descriptive (describing a single group) and analytical (comparing ≥2 groups).
- Interventional studies (trials) are characterized by the researcher deciding who receives the exposure, and then comparing outcomes.
- Studies evaluating performance or diagnostic tests are called diagnostic accuracy studies.

■ FURTHER READING

1. Anglemyer A, Horvath HT, Bero L. Healthcare outcomes assessed with observational study designs compared with those assessed in randomized trials. Cochrane Database Syst Rev. 2014:MR000034.
2. Ioannidis JP, Greenland S, Hlatky MA, Khoury MJ, Macleod MR, Moher D, et al. Increasing value and reducing waste in research design, conduct, and analysis. Lancet. 2014;383(9912):166-75.
3. Khan AM, Gupta P, Mishra D. The 3-Question approach: A simplified framework for selecting study designs. Indian Pediatr. 2019;56(8):669-72.
4. Melamed A, Robinson JN. A study design to identify associations: Study design: observational cohort studies. BJOG. 2018;125(13):1776.
5. OCEBM. (2016). The Oxford 2011 Levels of Evidence. [online] Available from http://www.cebm.net/index.aspx?o=5653. [Last accessed April, 2020].
6. Parab S, Bhalerao S. Study designs. Int J Ayurveda Res. 2010;1(2):128-31.
7. Schulz KF, Grimes DA. The Lancet Handbook of Essential Concepts in Clinical Research. London: Elsevier Publishers; 2006.

CHAPTER 7

Framing a Suitable Title

Piyush Gupta

■ INTRODUCTION

An author writing a thesis or paper is akin to an artist composing a painting. The key factor to bear in mind is that curiosity, and more specially, the urge to learn is what drives the human mind. The quest to engage the readers in the subject matter begins from the get-go and that starts with the *title* of your thesis. The first 30 seconds a reader (or the examiner) spends on your thesis are crucial to how he/she handles the rest of it. A good title can impress and compel the reader to read the rest of your work. Alternatively, a poorly written title may prevent people from going any further.

■ THE IMPORTANCE OF TITLE

Most people go only as far as the title. Few bother to read the summary. And even fewer proceed to read the complete thesis. The first step, therefore, is to write a concise, informative title. It not only represents the quality of thesis material but also gives an idea about the writer's character.

The title is the first thing a reader will encounter upon picking up the thesis. It should provide a concise view of the topic the thesis addresses, as well as give a sense of as to from what angle the writer is approaching the issue. Title will need to be crafted very carefully and might change many times over the course of writing the thesis protocol, as the focus of the writing shifts and the writer teases out different nuances of the subject. Authors should give themselves a chance to make a positive first impression with the title by making it descriptive and representative of the overall work.

The first thing one responds to with any work of art is the title—and it is no different with a thesis paper. A strong thesis title pulls the readers into it, making it memorable, and encouraging people to read it. A weak title dulls the reader's expectations and could negatively affect the views on your thesis, no matter how strong the contents are.

■ HOW TO FRAME A TITLE

1. Keep it Concise

Consider the following title:
"A novel study on the usefulness of typhidot M test in the diagnosis of typhoid fever in children: Analysis of clinical features and comparison with blood counts, Widal test, blood culture, with clinical follow-up in 50 patients of typhoid

fever at University College of Medical Sciences, Bharatpur." This would take ages to read! Not many people will have the patience to go through this with a clear head!

Now consider this:
"*Typhidot M for the Diagnosis of Typhoid fever in Children*"

Obviously, this title is better because it is clear and concise. It permits the reader to proceed onto the next section within his/her attention span.

2. Keep it Specific

Consider a tentative title: "*Obesity and Hypertension.*"
Despite being extremely concise, this title still lacks the power to engage the reader, the reason primarily being its vagueness. The title is too general and does not lead the reader in a particular direction. Instead, it leaves the informative work to the abstract and the paper itself, which, as we know, not many people go over.

Now consider this..."*Prevalence of Hypertension in Obese Adults.*"

Although less concise, the title is nevertheless much more specific.

3. Avoid Unnecessary Phrases

This is an extension of the "*keep it concise*" rule. Consider the following titles....
- "Role of Steroids in Nephrotic Syndrome"
- "Effects of Smoking on Lung Cancer Risk"
- "Treatment of Cholera with Azithromycin"
- "A Study on Efficacy of Beta-blockers in Heart Failure"

The underlined words in the various titles above do not add to the information provided, but instead make the title exude a certain amount of shoddiness. Avoid such unnecessary phrases (the underlined ones) in the title. Moreover, always keep important words toward the beginning of the title.

For example, *Azithromycin for Treatment of Cholera* is a better title than *Treatment of Cholera With Azithromycin*. Why? Think...

4. Whether to Include Place of Study

The same study, if conducted under the same settings, universe, and researchers, but a different location, can, at times, yield completely different results.
- "Prevalence of Obesity in Chandigarh"
- "Home-based or Facility-based Neonatal Care in Rural Bangladesh"

In the above examples, the location of the study is vital to the study itself. The prevalence of obesity at a certain geographical location is dependent on its prevalent lifestyle habits and economical/social scenario. This factor, in turn, distinguishes the study and its results as unique to Chandigarh. Similarly, a study assessing neonatal care in rural Bangladesh will be affected by socioeconomic factors particular to rural Bangladesh, which will be reflected in the results.

Now consider the following titles:
- "Daily versus Weekly Iron Supplementation in Adolescent Girls in Delhi"
- "300,000 versus 600,000 IU of Vitamin D for Treating Rickets in Mumbai"

The study of iron supplementation in adolescent girls in Delhi will not be very different from the study of iron supplementation in adolescent girls elsewhere. The affecting factor here is not the socioeconomic or political environment, but evolutionary build-up of a species, which will not differ even if we change the geographical location of the study. Same applies to the second study; the results obtained in the Mumbai study are also applicable to other geographical locations. In such studies, the name of place becomes redundant in the title.

So, when to use the place of the study in the title itself? *When it matters*. Include city, state, and country names only when essential, especially when results cannot be generalized to other locations.

5. Placing the Keywords Toward the Beginning

Let us take an example of a study being conducted to ascertain the differences in the prevalent trends of obesity between rural and urban areas. The title for this study can be composed in two ways:
- "Prevalence of Obesity: A Rural-Urban Comparison"

   OR
- "Rural-Urban Differences in the Prevalence of Obesity"

Both titles are concise, both are specific, and both are bereft of unnecessary phrases. Yet these are inherently different in their approach. The main subject of interest should always have priority over other matter in the title. In the above example, the focus of the study is not prevalence of obesity *per se*, but the rural-urban comparison of prevalence of obesity. Therefore, the second title, which emphasizes the focus of the study by placing it in the beginning, is more appropriate.

Note that by preferring the second title, you are also avoiding the use of colon, which can now be utilized for some other purpose. It is important to note that the study design usually follows a colon in the title. For example, "Azithromycin for Treatment of Cholera: A Randomized Control Trial."

6. Avoid Declarative Titles

"*Ventricular Septal Defect is the Most Common Acyanotic Heart Lesion in Children.*"

Titles like these, which reflect the hypothesis, must be avoided. While submitting the protocol before the actual study, the researcher has no way of knowing whether the conclusion will support the hypothesis or not. If it does not, the title can now not be changed in any way. A declarative title also shows an amount of bias on the part of the researcher regarding the interpretation of the data.

"*Prevalence of Ventricular Septal Defect in Children with Acyanotic Heart Disease*" is a more balanced and suitable title. It lets the reader approach the thesis with an open and unbiased mind.

7. Avoid Query Titles

Pretty basic: No title should be in the form of a query. We have a research question for the same. Consider the following two versions of a title:
"Is Endotracheal Suction Needed for Neonatal Resuscitation?"

   OR

"Endotracheal Suction for Neonatal Resuscitation: A Randomized Controlled Study"
(Which one sounds better? And why?)

> *Remember:*
> - *Research question* is a query.
> - *Hypothesis* is a declaration.
> - *Title* is a precise statement of your work; it should neither be a query nor a declaration.

8. Avoid Abbreviations and Acronyms in the Title

- MRI Findings in Autism
- Prevalence of HIV in Community
- Diagnosis of RHD
- *Khichri* or RUTF for Malnourished Children

Refrain from using abbreviations or acronyms in titles, regardless of their general awareness. For instance, "MRI" and "HIV" are terms that are better known than their counterparts, but even so, for the sake of consistency and comprehensiveness, full forms should be used.

■ ELEMENTS OF A GOOD TITLE

A Title should be SPICED

Following are the ingredients of a complete, balanced title:

- *Setting*: This is the situation in which the study takes place. The setting can be in a laboratory, in a field, or in a hospital. It can be in an uncontrolled setting with outpatient patients, unsupervised setting such as a school/community, or a detailed one (such as emergency room and inpatient facility). It is important to mention the setting in the title if results are not generalizable to other settings, or if the setting reflects the magnitude of your research. For example: "Prevalence of Anemia: A *School-based Study*." Here it is important to mention the setting because prevalence of anemia will be different in children attending school, children attending hospitals, and children who have not yet started going to school (preschool children).
- *Population*: A vital factor, population is invariably included in the title. It often forms the basis of the study, and is selected expressly in accordance with the research question. The population usually needs to be specified in terms of age and sex, if the study results are supposed to be specific to a particular segment only. For example: "Prevalence of Falls in the Elderly" OR "Hormone Therapy in Postmenopausal Women". In the first title, only age is specified because sex may not be important. The later title includes both age and sex, because of the relevance.
- *Intervention*: This may consist of a treatment, prevention, animal sacrifice, health education, etc. Intervention is an integral component of clinical trials, where the researcher introduces a *change* in the routine of the population in order to observe the outcome and effectiveness of the *change*. There might be purely observational studies with no intervention whatsoever. The title should be able to clarify the type of study (see *Design*) and the type of intervention, if it was planned.

    For example: "Local Anesthetic for Dental Procedures: An Observational Study" clarifies that this is purely an observational study; local anesthetics are given as a routine in dental procedures and this study intends to probably observe its efficacy and safety profile.
- *Condition*: This is the topic of the study, the condition on which the research is based. It is a must to include it in the title. Mostly, it refers to the clinical condition of the subjects. It also is the state which the researcher seeks to alter through intervention. It is almost always included in the title.
- *End-point*: Outcome is sparingly used in the title, and in such a way so as to avoid a declarative title. It refers to the change or type of change the condition undergoes after being subjected to intervention.

SPICED: Six Elements of the Title
S— setting
P— population
I— intervention
C— condition
E— end-point (outcome)
D— design of the study

- *Design:* It is always advisable to include the study design in the title. The study design is often preceded by a colon or an M dash, and indicates the method the researcher carries out the study in.

What All to Include in a Title?

Remember, just as when you cook a dish, it is not essential to put in all the spices you have at hand, similarly, it is not a must to have all the SPICED elements in a title. Writing the title is more of an art than a science, and you must decide, depending upon your research question and methodology, which of these elements need a definite mention in the title of your thesis.

Title should be Informative

- *The title must include*:
    o Hypothesis/problem studied (includes both condition and intervention).

"Tepid Sponging or Antipyretic for Fever".
- *The title may include, if specific*:
  - Study population or setting or both
  "Tepid Sponging or Antipyretic for Fever in Children".
- *Good to include*:
  - Research design
  "Tepid Sponging or Antipyretic for Fever in Children: A Randomized Controlled Trial".

As mentioned earlier, the outcome is sparingly used in the title, and it is also missing from the above example.

If you find it difficult to decide on your own whether your thesis title fits all the above-mentioned characteristics, take the help of your friends, peers, and teachers. Frame at least five versions of your proposed title and circulate to identify the best.

WHEN TO WRITE THE TITLE

The title should be written after everything has been finalized. At this point of time, you have all the knowledge on each SPICED element. You should have the following answers before embarking upon writing the title:
- Where is the study being done?
- Who are being studied?
- What are you doing?
- What is your main topic of interest?
- What is the important outcome being studied?
- And finally, how do you plan to do it all?

Only then will you be able to decide on the highlight of your study; which are the most important features to be included in the title, and which ones can be conveniently left out? You can, however, have a working title from the beginning, but do not finalize it until the methodology to answer your research question has been finalized. And, finally, write a title that is no more than 15–20 words.

CONCLUSION

The title reflects the soul of your study. In fact, it can make or break you. An interesting and crisp title coaxes the reader or examiner to read your thesis in detail. It forms the first impression that can be very vital for acceptance of your work. The title should be written after everything has been finalized. You should be knowing the following before writing the title: Where is the study being done? Who are being studied? What is your main topic of interest? What is the important outcome being studied? and, finally, how do you plan to do it all? As stated above, there are six important constituents of a title: Setting, Population, Intervention, Condition, End-point, and Design of the study (SPICED). Depending on the study, choose judiciously which all components are to be included in the title, keeping in mind the principles of being specific and concise.

KEY MESSAGES

- A good title must be concise and specific. It should include the main problem being studied, the population on which the study is being done, intervention, if any, and the outcome being studies.
- The title should not be in the form of a query or a declaration.
- Avoid acronyms and abbreviations in the title.
- The title for a thesis is decided at the time of submission of protocol only and is non-negotiable after the research protocol is submitted. Thus, it is important to craft it very carefully including all the elements. Revise it thoroughly before submitting the protocol.
- Title should not be of more than 15–20 words.

■ FURTHER READING

1. Bahadoran Z, Mirmiran P, Kashfi K, Ghasemi A. The Principles of Biomedical Scientific Writing: Title. Int J Endocrinol Metab. 2019;17(4):e98326.
2. Dewan P, Gupta P. Writing the Title, Abstract and Introduction: Looks Matter! Indian Pediatr. 2016;53(3):235-41.
3. Grant MJ. What makes a good title? Health Info Libr J. 2013;30(4):259-60.
4. JAMA and Archives Journals. American Medical Association. AMA Manual of Style. A Guide for Authors and Editors, 10th edition. USA: Oxford University Press; 2007.
5. Peh WC, Ng KH. Title and title page. Singapore Med J. 2008;49(8):607-8; quiz 609.
6. Tullu MS. Writing the title and abstract for a research paper: Being concise, precise, and meticulous is the key. Saudi J Anaesth. 2019;13:S12-S17.
7. Whissell C. The trend toward more attractive and informative titles: American Psychologist 1946-2010. Psychol Rep. 2012;110(2):427-44.

CHAPTER 8

Electronic Search of the Literature

Romit Saxena, Jaya Shankar Kaushik

INTRODUCTION

An effective literature search is an organized search for all the relevant literature published on the topic. An organized and systematic approach to searching literature will save time and increase the output. The three critical steps in searching the literature include identifying the problem, determining the source(s) of literature search, and search and explore the literature.

SOURCES OF LITERATURE

The available resources of medical literature can be categorized in various ways (**Flowchart 8.1**):
- *Scholarly versus nonscholarly*: Scholarly literature is usually a peer-reviewed, expert-driven information, based on verifiable sources, and focuses on research and academic discussion amongst professionals, e.g., research articles, systematic reviews, and meta-analysis, whereas nonscholarly literature is usually targeted to a wider public base, often with an intent to entertain or sensationalize, e.g., blogs, podcasts, newspapers, and magazine articles.
- *As per originality and further processing of data*: Primary literature refers to an original research material, with original research data, often published in a peer-reviewed journal such as Indian Pediatrics or New England Journal of Medicine (NEJM). It is important to understand that all journal articles may not be primary literature sources. *Secondary literature* is often an interpretation of primary literature, e.g., systematic review, meta-analysis, and practice guidelines. They can be searched from database websites such as PubMed. *Tertiary literature* is obtained from distillation and conglomeration of primary and secondary sources, e.g., textbooks and encyclopedias.

Internet as a Source of Literature

When confronted with a question, most of you tend to start your search with the most popular search engine, Google (*www.google.com*). Google references articles as per page rank, frequency, and location of keywords within the webpage. There is a vast quantity of results, but quality is often lacking. Google thereby shows the haystack rather than pointing to the

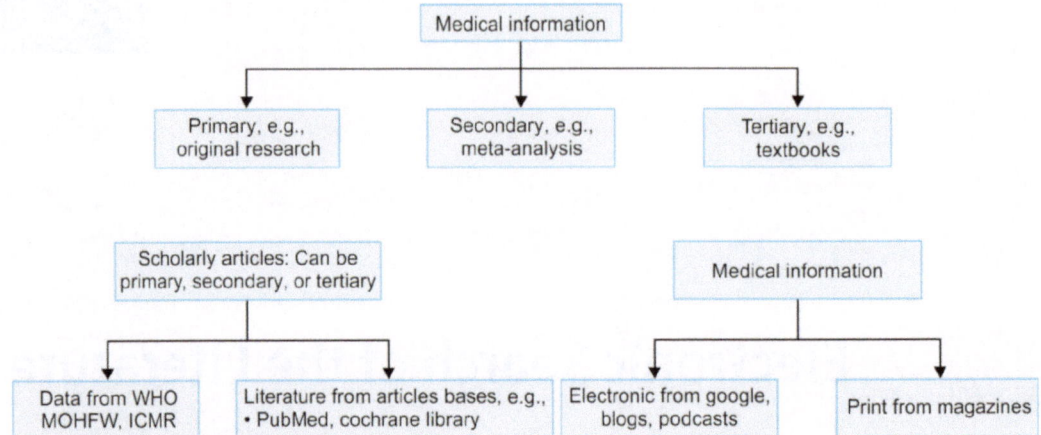

Flowchart 8.1: Sources of medical information.
(ICMR: Indian Council of Medical Research; MOHFW: Ministry of Health and Family Welfare; WHO: World Health Organization)

TABLE 8.1: Sources of medical information.

Information	Sources
Data	WHO, ICMR, Census of India, Data available on MOHFW website (as time series data on CBR, CDR, IMR, TFR)
Databases with journal references	PubMed, MEDLINE, IndMED, and Google Scholar
Full text articles	PubMed Central and Google Scholar
Evidence-based medicine database	Cochrane library
Peer-reviewed evidence based medicine	Up-to-date (available on subscription) and Clinical Key (Elsevier, available on subscription)

(CBR: crude birth rate; CDR: crude death rate; ICMR: Indian Council of Medical Research; IMR: infant mortality rate; MOHFW: Ministry of Health and Family Welfare; TFR: total fertility rate; WHO: World Health Organization)

needle in it (needle here being the Holy Grail set of articles, which might help redefine one's research).

Google Scholar, developed in 2004, goes a step further, and simplifies searches by listing articles as per ranking algorithm, based on multiple factors as citation counts (risk of Mathew effect) and words in the documents title. It accesses more multidisciplinary, scholarly, peer-reviewed work. Though it lacks Google's simplicity, it can still steer a person closer to the needle. Other search engines for medical literature include PubMed, EMBASE, Ovid, Web of Science, Scopus, Cochrane library, Science Direct, Directory of Open Access Journals (DOAJ) among others. Various sources of medical information are depicted in **Table 8.1**. The important databases as EMBASE, Google Scholar, and PubMed are further compared in **Table 8.2**.

■ HOW AND WHERE TO BEGIN

The present chapter deals with developing a plan for an effective literature search. Let us understand this method using an example of the treatment of typhoid fever.

Identifying the Problem

Typhoid fever is treated conventionally with third-generation cephalosporins and fluoroquinolones. However, there is an emergence of multidrug-resistant strains that

TABLE 8.2: Comparison between various databases.

Database	Google Scholar (https://scholar.google.com/)	PubMed Old: https://www.ncbi.nlm.nih.gov/pubmed/ New: https://pubmed.ncbi.nlm.nih.gov/	Private vendors as Embase (The excerpta medica database) (https://www.embase.com/login)
What is it?	Bibliographic database of scholarly literature on the web	Contains articles from MEDLINE® database	Embase is currently managed by Elsevier
Coverage	Started in 2004, Consists of 160 million indexed documents	Literature back to 1966 Contains over 30 million records	Literature back to 1947 Contains over 32 million records
Subscription required	No	No	Yes

Note: All database provide Abstracts, Alerts, Related searches, links to full text, and advanced search options.

do not respond to either of them. Now while we look for alternative drugs for the treatment of typhoid fever, options that we came across were azithromycin, aztreonam, carbapenems, and tigecycline. Among them, azithromycin appears to be an effective alternative to third-generation cephalosporins. So you are thinking of a research topic on "Azithromycin in typhoid fever in children." Hence you need to search the literature on how effective is azithromycin in typhoid fever? You are interested to know what all research exists on azithromycin in typhoid fever. Are there some studies in children? Hence, *the first step in searching the literature is the identification of the problem.* Once the problem is identified, you need to frame a research question. "What is the effect of oral azithromycin on the resolution of fever in the treatment of typhoid fever in children?"

Starting the Search

The moment a student is asked to search on a topic, the first page in the browser that opens is Google! Imagine when you seek the search result for "What is the effect of oral azithromycin on the resolution of fever in treatment of typhoid fever in children?" From Google, you end up getting at least 200,000 search items.

Even if you prune the sentence and search for only keywords such as "Azithromycin in Typhoid fever," you end up getting voluminous search results. It is practically not possible to go through all the relevant articles. You tend to look into the first three or four pages of Google search and end up saying that you found no research articles. Google provides everything under the sun about "Azithromycin in typhoid fever." It gives extensive coverage but is not specific. The search may also provide blogs, personal opinions, and publications in lay press on azithromycin in typhoid fever. This often obscures the authentic scientific literature that we intend to search. This can be partly overcome by the use of *Google Scholar*, but what is "scholarly" to Google Scholar might not be "scholarly" in the real sense. The actual scientific literature can be best accessed from PubMed (https://www.ncbi.nlm.nih.gov/pubmed) OR you can use Google to search for "PubMed" and open the link.

Basic PubMed Search

PubMed is an interface to help search articles from the MEDLINE database. MEDLINE (Medical Literature Analysis and Retrieval System Online, or MEDLARS Online) is a bibliographic database of life science. National

Center for Biotechnology Information (NCBI) is a part of the United States National Library of Medicine (NLM), a branch of the National Institutes of Health (NIH), which houses a series of databases pertinent to biotechnology and biomedicine.

Once you reach the PubMed webpage (**Fig. 8.1**), you are often tempted to write your research question in the search bar of PubMed. This type of searching is called "text-based search" where you are using the words directly in the search bar to arrive at the desired articles. When you type the entire research question in the search bar, this yields a very limited number of results. So, you need to identify the keywords in your research question. The keywords in the example that you are following are "Azithromycin," "typhoid fever," and "children." Once keywords are identified, the search results are broader as compared to narrow search when you use the entire stem of the research question.

Use of Filters in PubMed

You can refine the search using filters such as text availability (only abstract available or full text is available), type of article (randomized controlled trial, review article, meta-analysis, and so on), publication date (publication in the last 1 year, 5 years, and 10 years), language (English language alone or other language articles), and age and gender of the patients. These filters can be selected from the left-side panel on the webpage of PubMed. Hence, if you are keen on "clinical trials of azithromycin in typhoid fever," you can choose "clinical trials" and "randomized controlled trial" in the type of article. If you can read only the English language and keen on publications in the last 5 years, these filters can be applied accordingly.

You need to remember that once you select the filters, they remain "on" till you unselect them for your next search (**Fig. 8.2**).

PubMed Central (PMC) is the free full-text or open access branch of PubMed. Not all

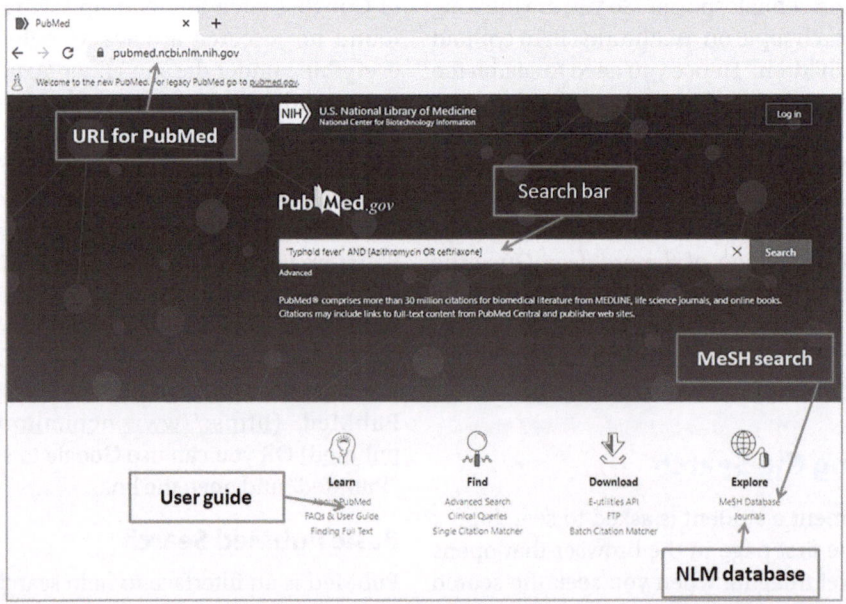

Fig. 8.1: Opening page of NCBI–PubMed revealing the search bar for text-based search, MeSH database for MeSH-based search, NLM database for searching journal, and user guide for troubleshoot. *(For color version, see Plate 1)*

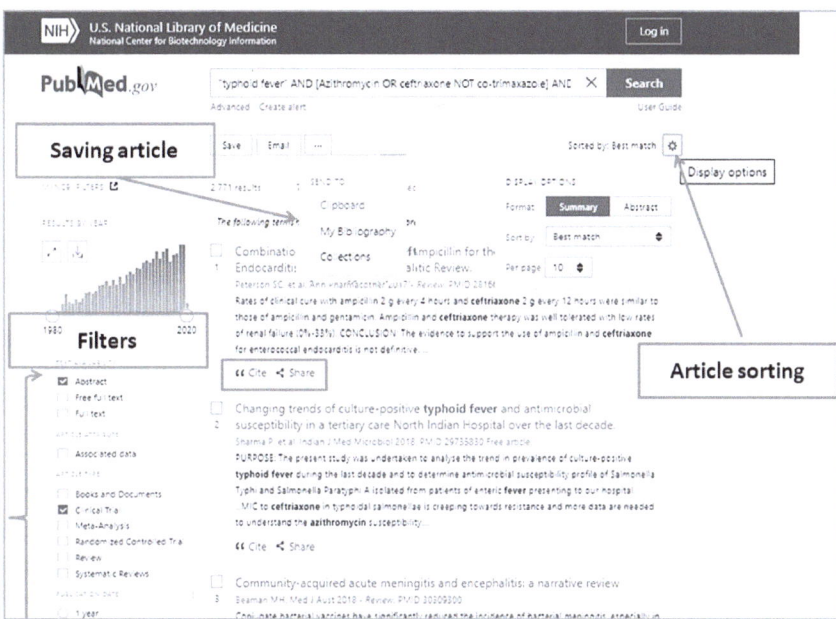

Fig. 8.2: PubMed search on typhoid fever depicting method to sort the articles, save the articles, cite and share them using appropriate filters. *(For color version, see Plate 1)*

papers indexed in PubMed are readily available at PMC to read and download. Links for full text are available either through publishers or vendors as Ovid and ProQuest.

Save the Articles

While you are searching for articles, you may encounter a few interesting and relevant articles that you would wish to retain for a full reading. To enable this, you can select these interesting articles and send them to the Clipboard. The Clipboard will be active for the next 8 hours. Once your search is finished, you can open the Clipboard and read all the relevant articles. You can save all related items in a folder of the computer as a text file. There are options for sending the selected articles to an email account. You can also save them in "My bibliography." To keep it in "My bibliography," you need to log in to PubMed. It is a good idea to create an account before you start the search. It is free! You can create folders in My bibliography and save relevant articles in relevant folders. You can also keep your search temporarily in the Clipboard and permanently in "My bibliography" or the computer hard drive.

How to Improve Text-based Search

The use of truncation, quotation, parenthesis, and the Boolean operator will refine the text-based search in PubMed.
- The use of truncation will search for all variations in the word stem. For example: when you use "child*," it will search for all articles that start with child: "child," "children," and "childhood."
- Use of quotation marks like "typhoid fever" will ensure that words are kept together instead of searching for all articles that have "typhoid" and all articles on "fever".
- The use of parenthesis will combine concepts. For example, while searching for a "comparison of azithromycin and ceftriaxone in typhoid fever in children,"

bracket can be used: child* AND "typhoid fever" and (azithromycin OR ceftriaxone). The use of this parenthesis will ensure that our search strategy will reveal articles on both azithromycin or ceftriaxone in typhoid fever in children. If you do not use the bracket, it will search for all items on azithromycin and all articles on ceftriaxone even if it is used in urinary tract infection or any other review articles on these drugs. PubMed reads your search query from left to right, and each word will stand alone without the use of parenthesis, quotation mark, and truncation mark.

- Avoid the use of stop words in the search statement. Stop words are uninformative English words that are ignored by PubMed in the mapping process. These words are not identified by PubMed. Few examples are—a, an, about, what, again, almost, although, and so on. The full list is available at *https://www.ncbi.nlm.nih.gov/books/NBK3827/table/pubmedhelp*.
- *Boolean operators:* These are the building blocks of the search strategy. There are three main Boolean operators that we need to identify: AND, OR, and NOT. These operators are always used in UPPERCASE and not be written as "and, or, not." When you search for Typhoid AND Azithromycin, it will search for all articles that have both typhoid and azithromycin. If we search for "Ceftriaxone OR Azithromycin," it will search for all articles on ceftriaxone as well as all articles on azithromycin including those which have mentioned both the drugs. Hence, use of OR will broaden the search and use of AND will narrow the search. Suppose you are interested in articles on "pregnancy" and "immunization" but you do not want articles on measles vaccine. In this case, you can use the Boolean operator NOT. The search strategy will be typed as "pregnancy AND (immunization NOT measles)".
- Avoid the use of abbreviations and acronyms in the search bar. Similarly, avoid trade names of drugs while searching.

MeSH-based Search

MeSH is a controlled vocabulary term. MeSH descriptors are organized in 16 categories: Category A for anatomic terms, Category B for organisms, C for diseases, D for drugs and chemicals, and so on. Each Category is further divided into subcategories. Within each subcategory, descriptors are arrayed hierarchically from most general to most specific in up to eleven hierarchical levels. In simple terms, MeSH is a language that PubMed understands irrespective of what we type. For example, if we type "typhoid fever" or "enteric fever", it will understand only "typhoid fever" as MeSH terms for enteric fever is also typhoid fever. So why do not we search using the language which PubMed understands, this search strategy is called MeSH-based search.

The first step in MeSH-based search is to identify the MeSH terms for the keywords that you have identified. When you scroll down the home page of PubMed, you can see the link "MeSH database" (**Fig. 8.1**). You use that link and start identifying the MeSH terms for all the keywords. When you type "typhoid fever," it will show a MeSH term "typhoid fever" with a lot of subheadings such as analysis, anatomy, and so on. Below that subheading, you can select the button on "restrict to MeSH-major topic." Click on "add to search builder." This will automatically add the MeSH term "typhoid fever" in the "PubMed search builder" that is evident on the right corner of the same page. Now in the top search bar, type Azithromycin, identify its desired MeSH term, and then add to search builder. Once all the keywords have been added as MeSH terms, you can press "search the PubMed." This icon is visible just below "add to search builder" on the right corner of the webpage. This strategy ensures that search results are specific.

Text-based or MeSH-based Search

There is no fixed rule which of the two search strategies is better. Text-based search is more useful when you are looking for some uncommon topics on which you might not expect too many articles, for example, "Gatifloxacin in typhoid fever." But when you are searching for a broad topic such as "treatment of typhoid fever," it would be better to use MeSH-based search that will narrow and provide only relevant articles. At times, you might have to hit and try both the methods to reach the desired articles.

Other Features of PubMed

You can sort your search results by "best match" or "most recent" (**Fig. 8.2**). Best match will arrange articles from most relevant articles to the least pertinent articles. Most recent searches will arrange the articles according to the time of publication starting from the latest article. You can sort the search results using a button wheel on the right corner of the webpage. Using this, you can also see the abstract instead of just the summary; you can also adjust the number of articles being displayed in a single page. You can get the citation of an article by clicking on the icon "*Cite*" below every article. You can also share an interesting article by clicking on the next button *Share* and copy its permalink and send it by WhatsApp or email (**Fig. 8.2**).

Suppose you have written an article on typhoid fever and are interested in submitting it to a relevant indexed journal. PubMed provides an *NLM catalog* where you can search for infectious disease journals or pediatric journals that are currently indexed in Medline (**Fig. 8.1**). This will help you to find a suitable journal for submitting your research. There are many other exciting features in PubMed, including clinical queries and topic-specific queries. The user guide for PubMed is available, and PubMed tutorials are available on YouTube as well.

PubMed Mobile

In this era of smartphones and secure internet access, it is a good idea to download the PubMed Mobile app from play store or apple store. You can search for articles after logging in and save them in "My bibliography." These can be later retrieved and read leisurely when you log in PubMed from your desktop.

■ OTHER SEARCH ENGINES

Other search engines for medical literature include EMBASE, Ovid, Web of Science, Scopus, Cochrane library, Science Direct, DOAJ etc. (**Tables 8.1** and **8.2**).

Google Scholar

Google Scholar is a subset of Google that allows search for indexed scholarly information. It can be incorporated as a chrome extension as well (scholar button).

- It enlists the results as title, journal name with the year of publication. It often mentions links for full text if available on the net
- Below each result, there is usually a quotation mark ("). This option enumerates the various citation formats for the study (such as Vancouver).
- There is also a link for other articles, which have cited the selected study, and the *versions* link identifies other versions of the article on other databases.
- Like PubMed, a good search can be undertaken on it using combination of keywords and Boolean characters.
- There are easy to use, advanced search options, including author name, year of publication, etc., which can help narrow the search results.

Cochrane Library

The Cochrane Library (https://www.cochranelibrary.com/) is another good place to start. It is a collection of *Cochrane Database of Systematic Reviews* (CDSR), which are prepared by Cochrane review groups. It has high quality systematic reviews on healthcare and offers good evidence for clinical decision-making.

Indian Literature

IndMED indexes Indian biomedical journals. It has been produced under the Indian Council of Medical Research (ICMR) funded project, National Database of Indian Medical journals. It is freely accessible from *http://indmed.nic.in*. It covers peer-reviewed journals from 1985 onward. Available journals are enumerated alphabetically on the website (*http://medind.nic.in/index.shtml*). Articles can be searched by author, affiliation, journal name, title, and abstract. In India, University Grants Commission (UGC) has set up a Consortium for Academic and Research Ethics (CARE) to continuously monitor and identify quality journals across disciplines. A UGC CARE list is available, which is periodically revised (*https://ugccare.unipune.ac.in*). These journals are indexed and meet a reference standard.

■ MEDICAL INFORMATICS

Medical informatics is the study of data management of patient data, clinical knowledge, population data, and other information pertinent to patient care and community health. Clinical informatics is the use of medical informatics in an interdisciplinary method to aid management of patients using clinical and information sciences. This is a relatively new field that helps one analyze the vast quantities of data generated and gets a useable distillate from the same. The components of health informatics include biomedical sciences, information technology organizational theory, among others. These suggested methods are a guide for the student to undertake a literature search, prior to embarking on a thesis, and thereafter for the review and paper writing. You are encouraged to use referencing software such as Zotero, Endnote, and Mendeley to record your search and for writing review of literature of your thesis as well.

■ CONCLUSION

Literature search becomes meaningful when you perform an organized search in a systematic manner. An effective search must begin with identifying the problem and deciding what exactly do you want to search. Your search can begin at one of the most authentic Medline database which can be retrieved using PubMed. The articles can be searched in the PubMed using text-based search for narrow and uncommon topics and MeSH-based search for broad research area. Text-based search can be improved using truncation, quotation marks, parenthesis, and Boolean operators. Effective strategy to search the article will ensure that output is increased in the limited available time window.

KEY MESSAGES

- PubMed is a powerful search engine for searching and retrieving scholarly medical literature.
- Use truncation, quotation, parenthesis, and Boolean operators while using text-based search. Avoid the use of stop words and abbreviations while searching.
- Select filters of article type, language, and free full-text availability judiciously.
- MeSH-based search is an useful alternative to text-based search to narrow the search and arrive at the most relevant articles.
- No method suits all search needs. Hit and try and keep trying as it is the practice that makes a person perfect.

FURTHER READING

1. Anders ME, Evans DP. Comparison of PubMed and Google Scholar literature searches. Respir Care. 2010;55(5):578-83.
2. Bethesda MD. PubMed Help. [online] Available from: https://www.ncbi.nlm.nih.gov/books/NBK3827/. [Last accessed April, 2020].
3. Canese K, Weis S. (2013). PubMed: The Bibliographic Database. In: The NCBI Handbook. [online] Available from: https://www.ncbi.nlm.nih.gov/books/NBK153385/. [Last accessed April, 2020].
4. Cochrane Library. (2020). About the Cochrane Library. [online]. Available from: https://www.cochranelibrary.com/about/about-cochrane-library. [Last accessed April, 2020].
5. Elsevier. (2020). Biomedical research – Embase. I Elsevier [online]. Available from: https://www.elsevier.com/en-in/solutions/embase-biomedical-research. [Last accessed April, 2020].
6. Fatehi F, Gray LC, Wootton R. How to improve your PubMed/MEDLINE searches: 2. display settings, complex search queries and topic searching. J Telemed Telecare. 2014;20(1):44-55.
7. Fatehi F, Gray LC, Wootton R. How to improve your PubMed/MEDLINE searches: 3. advanced searching, MeSH and My NCBI. J Telemed Telecare. 2014;20(2):102-12.
8. Google Scholar Search Tips. (2020). [online]. Available from: https://scholar.google.com/scholar/help.html. [Last accessed April, 2020].
9. Gray K, Sockolow P. Conceptual models in health informatics research: A literature review and suggestions for development. JMIR Medical Informatics. 2016;4(1):e7.
10. Medical Journals of India [online]. Available from: http://medind.nic.in/medind-project.html. [Lat accessed April, 2020].
11. Nourbakhsh E, Nugent R, Wang H, Cevik C, Nugent K. Medical literature searches: a comparison of PubMed and Google Scholar. Health Info Libr J. 2012;29(3):214-22.
12. Thawani R, Gupta P. Electronic search of literature: The Bare basics. In: How to Write the Thesis and Thesis Protocol, 1st edition. New Delhi: Jaypee Brothers Medical Publisher; 2014. pp. 50-61.
13. University Grants Commission. (2020). Consortium for Academic and Research Ethics. [online]. Available from: https://ugccare.unipune.ac.in/Apps1/Home/Index. [Last accessed April, 2020].
14. Wyatt J, Liu J. Basic concepts in medical informatics. J Epidemiol Community Health. 2002;56(11):808-12.

SUGGESTED WATCH

1. https://www.youtube.com/watch?v= ks46w3mNAQE
2. https://www.youtube.com/watch?v= HYW2_eUsK9E
3. https://nnlm.gov/classes/how-pubmed-works

SUGGESTED READING

1. National Center for Biotechnology Information. (2005). PubMed Help. [online] Available from https://www.ncbi.nlm.nih.gov/books/NBK3830/. [Last accessed April, 2020].

CHAPTER 9

Writing Aim and Objectives: Getting Clarity

Upreet Dhaliwal

■ INTRODUCTION

After choosing your area of research, it is time to focus on what you want to achieve through your study. It is important to give considerable thought to the question of what you want to achieve and how you plan to do it; this should be done well before research begins and all components of the research (such as research question, title, and methods) should remain faithful to it so that you do not lose focus and diverge from the questions you wish to answer. The primary focus of your research is expressed as an *Aim* (general intention) and one or more *Objectives* (specific measurable outcomes).

■ DEFINING AIM AND OBJECTIVES

Formulated in broad terms, the statement that informs the reader of your general intentions with respect to the long-term expectations from the research becomes the *"Aim"* of your study.

Aim of the study indicates broad area of interest of the research in a particular field. It gives an idea of the long-term goal and sets the stage for what you will do in the study: In other words, the *Aim* should answer the question: "What are you doing in this study?"

Example 1

> Say you want to work in the field of human immunodeficiency virus (HIV) infections and decide to focus on a specific area within these infections, such as public perception.
> Accordingly, the *Aim* of your study could be: *To evaluate public perception about HIV infections.*

"Objectives," on the other hand, are the steps taken to achieve the *Aim*; they are specific and measurable tasks that you will perform/observe in order to ensure that the *Aim* is achieved.

Objectives define specific outcome criteria of the study which the researcher intends to find out to realize the *Aim*. These impart specificity and measurability to the broad research topic, in terms of time-bound achievable targets. These answer how you are going to achieve your research goal. Objectives convert the generalizable *Aim* into practical achievable targets. They should answer the question: "What are you going to do to achieve the *Aim*?" Once objectives are set, you may define how to measure the outcome of one's objectives (outcome measures).

Table 9.1 summarizes the difference between *Aim* and *Objectives*.

Let us look at some examples showing the relationship between an *Aim* and its *Objectives*.

TABLE 9.1: Aim versus Objectives.

Aim	Objectives
What the study seeks to achieve	How the Aim is going to be achieved; the steps that are going to be taken to answer the research question or prove the hypothesis
Broad statement of long-term study outcome	Specific, focused, achievable, and immediate study outcomes
There is only one Aim of the study	The Objectives may be more than one

Notes:
The aim and objectives are interrelated.
Objectives have to fulfill the requirements of the aim.

Example 2

Aim: To investigate the relationship between lecture absenteeism and medical student performance.
Objective: To correlate the marks scored in formative assessments with the number of lectures attended.

Example 3

Aim: To evaluate public perception about HIV infections.
Objective: To estimate proportion of East Delhi population who are aware of the risk factors and prevention of HIV infections using a questionnaire.

How do you decide what Objectives to formulate for a particular Aim?

This question is answered in the following section.

■ TRANSLATING RESEARCH QUESTION INTO AN AIM AND OBJECTIVES

Aim of a study indicates broad intentions about the research topic. It may include population, intervention, comparator, and outcome (PICO) elements in it. The specific objectives of your study will depend upon what your research question/hypothesis is. The objectives must be aligned to the research question/hypothesis, otherwise you will not be able to find the right answers.

The Objectives of the study may vary as per research interest even if the aim (broad intention) is same. Objectives should define the outcome variables which contribute to realization of the broader Aim. Say, when the Aim is to find out the burden of typhoid in a hospital; the Objectives can be written as follows:

a. To calculate the proportion of patients of typhoid fever contributing to overall outpatient attendance in the hospital.
b. To find out the proportion of patients hospitalized with typhoid fever contributing to overall hospital admissions.
c. To calculate the proportion of *Salmonella* positive cultures contributing to overall blood cultures being received in the microbiology laboratory of the hospital.
d. To calculate the cost (in Rupees) per patient of typhoid fever to the hospital.

In the above mentioned example, the Aim of evaluating the burden of typhoid can be achieved in multiple ways. The key is to know how to answer the research question. The difference in research question translates into different study objectives.

■ PRIMARY AND SECONDARY OBJECTIVES

Both Examples 2 and 3 have a single objective each; this objective is directly linked to the research question/aim and will be able to answer it. Such an objective is called the *primary objective*; it must be achievable, and it must answer the research question. The choice of primary objective depends on its ability to answer the researcher's question as sometimes there may be more than one objective for a single question. For example, in the typhoid study quoted above, for a clinician the objective (*a*) is most important; for the hospital administrators, objectives (*b*) and (*d*) are most important; and for a microbiologist, objective (*c*) is the most important. Thus, the primary objective will vary as per the needs/priority of the researcher. Also have a look at the following example:

Example 4

> *Hypothesis*: Vitamin D supplementation contributes to early resolution of severe pneumonia in children <5 years of age.
>
> *Aim*: To determine the efficacy of vitamin D supplementation in severe pneumonia in children under 5 years of age.
>
> *Objectives*: To compare (*a*) the time of resolution of illness (tachypnea, chest indrawing, hypoxia, and inability to feed) in children with severe pneumonia receiving vitamin D supplementation or placebo, in addition to antibiotics and supportive therapy, and (*b*) to compare duration of hospitalization in these children.

- The study in Example 4 has two objectives; since both directly address the hypothesis, both may be considered as primary objectives. The study could have a third objective: To evaluate complications of vitamin D supplementation in these children. This objective, which does not contribute to proving the hypothesis, is a secondary objective. Secondary objectives pertain to incidental by-products of the study; the hypothesis or the answer to the research question does not depend on secondary objectives being achieved.
- *For most studies, there should be only one primary objective; however, there can be many secondary objectives (usually 2–3).*

■ ALIGNING THE AIM, OBJECTIVES, AND THE TITLE OF THE THESIS

Take a look at Example 5. Do you think the components are in agreement with each other?

Example 5

> *Title*: Comparison of fistulectomy and fistulotomy for anal fistula in adults: A randomized controlled trial.
>
> *Aim*: To establish the ideal surgery for anal fistula.
>
> *Objective*: To compare the recurrence rate of fistulectomy and fistulotomy in adults with anal fistula.

Example 5 demonstrates that the Title and the Aim are not in concordance. From the Title, it is clear that the study seeks only to compare two procedures and not to find the ideal procedure to correct anal fistula. Likewise, the Objective is too simplistic for a title that claims a randomized controlled study design. On the other hand, in Example 6, the Title, Aim, and Objective are in agreement with each other.

Example 6

> *Title*: Comparison of fistulectomy and fistulotomy in anal fistula: A randomized controlled trial.
>
> *Aim*: To compare the efficacy of two well-established operative techniques in the management of anal fistula.
>
> *Objective*: To compare fistulectomy and fistulotomy in adults with anal fistula with respect to the following parameters:
> - Duration of surgery
> - Postoperative pain at 24 hours (visual analog scale)
> - Size of wound after surgery
> - Time required for complete healing
> - Recurrence of fistula
> - Patient satisfaction

After formulating the individual components, you must revisit the Title, the research question/hypothesis, the Aim, and each Objective, to ensure that they are in concordance with each other; if they are not, you will end up confusing the reader and yourself.

■ ESSENTIAL ELEMENTS OF "GOOD" AIM AND OBJECTIVES

Once the Aim and Objectives are formulated (and aligned to the title and the research question), they must be checked to see if they are "Good Objectives." The Aim should be broad and, thus, mention the population and the outcome in general terms. The Objectives on the other hand are specific. Good objectives are "SMART." The next example demonstrates these elements.

Example 4 Revisited

Aim: To determine the efficacy of vitamin D supplementation in severe pneumonia in children under 5 years of age.

In the above Aim, the population is "children with severe pneumonia" and the outcome is "efficacy." In addition, we can identify another element, i.e., "vitamin D supplementation," which is the intervention being planned.

Objectives: To compare the time of resolution of illness (tachypnea, chest indrawing, hypoxia, and inability to feed) in under-5 years children with severe pneumonia receiving vitamin D supplementation (intervention) or placebo (control or comparator), in addition to antibiotics and supportive therapy, and to compare duration of hospitalization in these children.

Let's first identify the **PICO** elements for Objectives:
Population = children with severe pneumonia
Intervention = vitamin D supplementation
Comparator = placebo
Outcomes = time of resolution of illness and duration of hospitalization.

And then see whether they fulfill the attributes of SMART objectives:
S = *Specific* (clear, well-defined; all PICO elements specified).
M = *Measurable* (outcomes are measurable) (time; duration).
A = *Achievable* in terms of resources, knowledge, and expertise.
R = *Relevant* to departmental and national goals (to reduce pediatric mortality).
T = *Time bound*; can be achieved in the usual time frame available to postgraduate students.

Table 9.2 summarizes the steps that you should take to ensure you have formulated Aim and Objectives that are relevant and appropriate for your study.

Some more examples of Aim and Objectives for different study designs are given below.

Example 7

Research question: What is the role of safe and clean drinking water supply in causation of typhoid fever?

Design: Analytical cohort OR case–control
Aim: To identify the protective role of safe water supply in causation of typhoid fever in a slum.
Primary objective: To compare the incidence of typhoid fever in population with and without access to safe water supply.
Secondary objective: To compare stool positivity for *Salmonella* in both populations.

Example 8

Research question: What is the efficacy of oral azithromycin in treatment of typhoid fever?

Design: Experimental, randomized clinical trial.
Aim: To compare the *efficacy* of azithromycin vs. ciprofloxacin for treatment of uncomplicated typhoid fever.
Primary objective: To compare the proportion of nonresponse in patients receiving azithromycin or ciprofloxacin for treating uncomplicated typhoid fever.
Secondary objectives:
1. To compare the mean duration of resolution of fever in both groups.
2. To compare the rate of hospitalization in both groups.

TABLE 9.2: Steps to formulate Aim and Objectives.

Steps	Example A	Example B
Step 1: Choose a broad area	Cataract	Cataract
Step 2: Focus on a specific area within that	Barriers to surgery	Vision-related quality of life
Step 3: Formulate a research question (RQ) or hypothesis (H) as appropriate	RQ: Why do some patients delay cataract surgery even when they have visually disabling cataract?	H: Vision-related quality of life in patients with marked visual deprivation due to cataract is poorer than in those with moderate deprivation
Step 4: Specify what you plan to do (Aim)	To contribute to the understanding of barriers to surgery for cataract	To determine vision-related quality of life in patients with cataract
Step 5: Specify how you plan to achieve the Aim (Objectives)	Primary objective: To identify nature of barriers for the acceptance of surgery among hospital-based patients with visually-disabling cataract, using an open-ended questionnaire	Primary objective: To measure quality of life in patients with visually-disabling cataract using the Indian Visual Function Questionnaire Secondary objectives: 1. To compare quality of life scores between patients with low vision and those with blindness due to cataract 2. To compare quality of life scores between patients with low vision due to cataract and those with low vision due to other causes
Step 6: Revisit the Aim and Objectives to check whether they are "good"	Are they *aligned* to the title? Will they *answer* the research question? Are they SMART and do they have PICO elements?	

Example 11

Research question: What is the role of Typhidot M test for the diagnosis of typhoid fever?

Design: Study for diagnostic accuracy, cross-sectional.

Aim: To ascertain the *diagnostic accuracy* of typhidot M vs. blood culture for early diagnosis of typhoid fever.

Primary objective: To calculate the sensitivity and specificity of typhidot M vs. blood culture for diagnosis of typhoid fever.

Secondary objective: To calculate the positive and negative predicative value of typhidot M vs. blood culture for diagnosis of typhoid fever.

◼ CONCLUSION

The Aim and its Objectives are formulated early in the study right after you have chosen the area of research. This enables you to focus your attention on what you are planning to do/find out (the Aim) and what actions you will take to achieve it [the Objective(s)].

Stating the Aim and Objectives upfront helps give direction to the methods and the outcome measures: they should all be aligned to each other.

> **KEY MESSAGES**
> - Formulate Aim and Objectives early in the research to avoid a mismatch with the methods and, later, with the results.
> - The primary objective should be carefully framed; it reflects directly on the research question/hypothesis; therefore, it must be achieved otherwise you will fail to answer the research question or prove the hypothesis.
> - While framing Aim and Objectives, keep your focus on the PICO elements relevant to your research and to the SMART attributes.

FURTHER READING

1. Bjerke MB, Renger R. Being smart about writing SMART objectives. Eval Program Plann. 2017;61:125-7.
2. Solent University. Dissertations and major projects: Proposal. [online] Available from ahttps://learn.solent.ac.uk/course/view.php?id=31634&section=2. [Last accessed April, 2020].
3. Lempriere M. What are you doing and how are you doing it? Articulating your aims and objectives. [online] Available from https://www.thephdproofreaders.com/structuring-a-thesis/writing-your-research-aims-and-objectives/. [Last accessed April, 2020].
4. University of Southampton. Research methods: Process and design. [online] Available from https://generic.wordpress.soton.ac.uk/researchmethods/research-toic/process-and-design/. [Last accessed April, 2020].

CHAPTER 10

Writing the Introduction: Justifying Your Research

Naveen Sharma

■ INTRODUCTION

Have you ever finished reading a book that did not grip you right at the beginning? If that book was not a compulsory read as a part of a syllabus, it would have been immediately discarded as being unworthy of the time required to read it. In order to ensure that the fruit of your labor over the better part of the last 2 years—your thesis—does not suffer the ignominy of being junked by the reader (and above all, the examiner!), you must ensure that the Introduction is written well.

■ WHEN TO WRITE INTRODUCTION?

Even though the Introduction is placed at the beginning of the protocol or thesis, it does not have to be the first portion of the text that you write. In fact, it may be a better idea to write the Introduction after writing the "Review of Literature." You are better placed to justify the rationale of the thesis after having reviewed the literature completely and organized your thoughts during the actual writing of the "Review of Literature."

Length

The length of the Introduction can vary from one page to two pages. Very few people would be interested in reading a long drawn, shoddily meandering Introduction. You must be able to grasp the reader's attention through the Introduction while remembering that the real meat of the thesis lies beyond the Introduction.

■ PURPOSE OF INTRODUCTION

The Introduction answers "*Why*" this research deserves to be performed. It serves the purpose of acquainting the topic to the reader. It must inform the reader about the background and importance of the topic that you have chosen to study. It must be crisp and should arouse the reader's interest in the topic. In a few sentences, the area of study must be made absolutely clear. A brief summary of the reviewed literature serves to establish that the topic under study will indeed fill a lacuna in the existing knowledge. The Introduction should convince the reader that the research question is important and worth the effort of conducting a study to answer it.

Funnel Approach

A "funnel approach" can be a good way to write the Introduction. A general statement pertaining to the area of research is followed by sentences which elaborate on the topic but progressively narrow down the area of interest and finally take the reader closer to the topic of research. Needless to say, the language has to be free of grammatical errors. One sentence should lead on to the next smoothly and ideas should flow logically. Lets see an example:

Acute abdominal pain is one of the most common reasons for emergent surgical consultation. A common cause of acute abdominal pain is acute appendicitis. The usual management of acute appendicitis is appendectomy; however, recent reports have suggested that a nonoperative approach may be as safe and effective as appendectomy. Whether nonoperative management is safe in patients above 60 years of age has not been studied till date. We examined whether the nonoperative management is safe in the geriatric population.

In four sentences, we have been able to focus the attention of the reader to why our area of study serves to fill an important gap in literature. See **Figure 10.1** and try to correlate it with the example given above.

■ STRUCTURE OF INTRODUCTION

Now that you have understood the importance of writing a concise Introduction and what an Introduction is supposed to do, let us discuss about the structure of the "Introduction."

- Essentially, the first one or two paragraphs of the introduction should provide a brief summary of the review of literature (that is why it is a good idea to write it after the review of literature). This constitutes "What is known." Use appropriate and relevant references here.

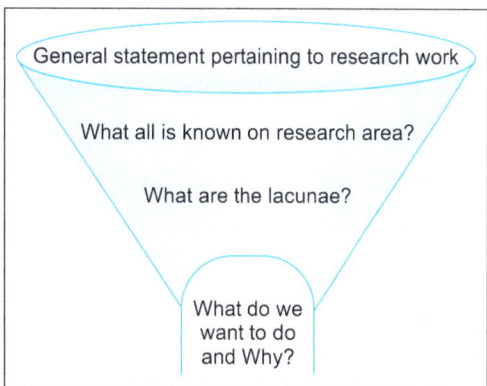

Fig. 10.1: The funnel approach for Introduction.

- The next paragraph should point out the lacunae in the current knowledge/understanding of the subject and how your research will contribute to the filling of the gap in current knowledge.
- And finally, the Introduction should end with a paragraph which informs the reader what you propose to find, (i.e., your research question) to fill up the lacunae stated in the previous paragraph.

What Not to Include in the Introduction?

It is equally important to know what *not* to include in the Introduction. The Introduction is not a summary of the thesis. Introduction should not front load your thesis: You should not be certain of your conclusion while introducing the chapter, for example, avoid *"This study will prove that duration of antibiotics for acute cholangitis is 14 days and NOT 21 days."* This is not the place to report or discuss results, or to state the conclusion. Doing so would be tantamount to revealing the climax of a movie in the trailer.

Most importantly, the aim highlighted/stated in the Introduction should be the same as stated under section "Aim and Objectives." Please double-check.

Do not write Introduction in a hurry. This may be the reason why the Introduction does not come across as the well-written, eyeball-grabbing, crisp piece that it ought to be. Please ensure that you have adequate time left for writing this vital piece. Start early, and finish well! Happy writing and good luck!

■ CONCLUSION

The basic purpose of the Introduction section in thesis is to capture attention of readers toward a particular topic, and to explain why the present research needs to be performed. A good Introduction is short, focused, and takes readers from known (broad) to unknown (narrow) aspects of a topic, maintaining a continuity between sentences. You must avoid a detailed review of literature in this section and cite only few references that are important to highlight the problem and the lacunae in existing literature.

SAMPLE INTRODUCTION

Inguinal hernia repair in adults is one of the commonest surgical procedures performed worldwide. Open mesh repair is the most commonly performed procedure for inguinal hernia. Laparoscopic repair of inguinal hernias is also commonly performed nowadays.

The best hernia repair procedure should be simple, rapid and safe; it should result in less surgical trauma, postoperative pain, and low recurrence rate. Compared with open hernia repair, laparoscopic hernia repair may result in less pain and shorter convalescence.[1] Laparoscopic repair is technically more difficult than open repair and there is evidence of a "learning curve" in its performance.[2]

Total extraperitoneal (TEP) laparoscopic inguinal hernia repair is preferred to transabdominal preperitoneal (TAPP) repair since it preserves peritoneal integrity. However, it is considered to be more difficult than TAPP because of the peculiarity of anatomy and limitation of working space.

In extraperitoneal repair, the initial extraperitoneal space can be created either by telescopic dissection or by balloon dissection. In telescopic blunt dissection, the space is created under vision; whereas, in case of indigenous balloon dissection, it is a blind technique. It is not known which of the two modalities provide a better working space to the surgeon.

The present study attempts to fill up this void in literature. The aim is to compare the initial space creation between the two groups undergoing telescopic dissection and balloon dissection in TEP inguinal hernia repair.

KEY MESSAGES

- Introduction should take a reader from "What is known" to "What is less known" and then should justify the need of study by pointing out lacunae in existing literature.
- Provide a brief summary of the problem in the beginning (first paragraph) of the Introduction. This should be focused toward a specific aspect of the exact problem being studied, for example, diagnosis or therapy rather than epidemiology every time.
- The next paragraph should point out the lacunae in the current knowledge of the subject and how you plan to contribute to fill this gap.
- The final part of the Introduction should be a paragraph that informs the reader what you propose to study, (i.e., your research question and hypothesis) to fill up the lacunae stated above.

■ FURTHER READING

1. Freedman L, Plotnick J. Writing Introduction and conclusions. [online] Available from: http://www.writing.utoronto.ca/advice/planning-and-organizing/intros-andconclusions. [Last accessed April, 2020].
2. USC Libraries. Organizing Your Social Sciences Research Paper. [online] Available from: https://libguides.usc.edu/writingguide/introduction. [Last accessed April, 2020].
3. Seven Ways to Write an Introduction. [online] Available from https://web2.uvcs.uvic.ca/encomium/writingdemo/wa/unit1/u1_l1b_a.htm. [Last accessed April, 2020].

CHAPTER 11

Review of Literature: Recalling the Past

Sanjay Gupta

■ INTRODUCTION

Review of literature, in the context of medical research, may be defined as the process of reading, analyzing, evaluating, and summarizing scholarly material about a given topic. It aims to review the critical points of current knowledge in the area of study. Additionally, it also (1) lays groundwork for the present research; (2) brings clarity and focus to the research problem; (3) improves the methodology; and (4) shows to the reader that relevant literature has been critically analyzed and the intended research is justified.

In a thesis, the review of literature follows the introduction; and precedes the objectives, methodology, results, and discussion, though this is strictly not the chronological order in which one does scientific research. Instead, after the broad area of research is decided upon, review of literature is the first step undertaken to understand the currently accepted level of knowledge and identify the areas of deficiency, conflict, or lack of clarity of information. Introduction to protocol or thesis is written only after reviewing the literature.

■ WHAT CONSTITUTES THE LITERATURE?

All the scholarly articles (research papers, reviews, case reports, etc.), chapters in books, scientific conferences and their published proceedings, earlier theses and dissertations, scientific work available on the internet as well as unpublished information obtained by personal correspondence constitute "Literature."

Primary, Secondary, and Tertiary Literatures: Their Strengths and Weaknesses

Depending upon the originality of the information presented and closeness to the source of information, medical literature may be considered as primary, secondary, or tertiary.

Primary Literature

This is the published work of original researcher. Research papers, dissertations, case reports, and conference proceedings represent primary literature.

The quality of the primary literature is variable. Research articles published in good scientific journals are rigorously peer reviewed and constitute strong evidence, suitable for inclusion in literature review. On the other hand, published conference proceedings often include preliminary data and are usually not peer reviewed. Thus, while being a good source of research ideas, these do not constitute strong evidence. Case studies are usually peer reviewed, and, though not as good quality as a research article, may be the only source of literature for uncommon problems.

Secondary Literature

It analyses, interprets, summarizes, or reorganizes the information reported by the primary sources. Review articles and meta-analysis published in scientific journals and literature reviews from theses and dissertations constitute secondary literature.

While not being original research work, these are often peer reviewed and bring together important articles pertaining to the topic under consideration. Often written by experts in a given field, these reviews highlight the strengths and shortcomings of various studies. The areas of consensus as well as disagreement are commented upon. It must be kept in mind that, occasionally, the review may be influenced by the reviewer's bias.

Review articles are a good point to start studying literature pertinent to a given field. This way, with much less effort, one can identify important primary literature which the researcher needs to study in detail, and the possible direction in which fresh research is worthwhile.

Tertiary Literature

Textbooks, encyclopedias, and guidelines issued by competent bodies constitute the tertiary literature. These present the currently accepted knowledge rather than contribute to it.

In a literature review, tertiary sources do not need critical analysis and are good for referencing well-established facts. However, care must be taken that these tertiary sources are not extensively reproduced in the literature review. As an example, while reviewing the anatomy of inguinal region in a thesis pertaining to a new method of inguinal hernia repair, rather than repeating the description of inguinal region from a standard textbook of anatomy, one may write only those facts which are relevant to the current research, and refer the reader to the textbook for full description.

■ COMPONENTS OF LITERATURE REVIEW

Literature reviews could be categorized into various types, based on the following characteristics of the review:
1. *Focus:* Where is the exact emphasis?
2. *Goal:* What the author wants to achieve?
3. *Perspective:* Whether author is neutral or taking sides?
4. *Coverage:* How exhaustive is the literature search?
5. *Organization:* What is the flow of thoughts?
6. *Audience:* For whom it is meant?

1. Focus

The focus of a literature review could be on the outcome, methodology, theories, or practice in a given area.
- *Outcome-oriented literature review:* The focus is on the results of different studies. It may identify discordance or ambiguity in a particular research outcome amongst these studies, justifying the need for additional research.
- *Methodology-oriented literature review:* If the focus is on the methodology, the review would critically analyze various methods to research a given problem, compare them and justify a different methodology.
- In theoretical or social research, the focus is usually on different theories or prevalent practices.

- In the field of medicine, most of the research is experimental, and focus is on methods as well as outcome.

2. Goal

The goal of literature review is what the author expects the review to accomplish. This may be to integrate the results of the past studies and bring out the essence of knowledge. Such reviews resolve the conflicts of earlier studies and bring out general statements. A meta-analysis is one such review which synthesizes results of many studies using statistical methods.

As against this, a review may critically analyze the previous studies, focusing on their limitations. The author of such reviews often supports a particular opinion and highlights the shortcomings of contrary views.

A third goal may be to identify central issues addressed in the earlier works, focusing on the questions that need answering in the future. It thus suggests the way for future research. Reviews in majority of medical research are of this type.

3. Perspective

The researcher could take a neutral position in the review, not favoring one view or the other. This is often the case in medical research. Conversely, as happens in theoretical research, the researcher could favor a particular theory, bring out literature in its support and highlight the shortcomings of contrary views. For the medical thesis, it may be more appropriate to remain neutral and just present the facts as they are.

4. Coverage

Coverage of the literature could be exhaustive, extensively reviewing the literature under consideration. Alternatively, the review could be focused, critically analyzing only the important literature in the field. It may be advisable to take the latter approach in medical research. Meta-analyses and well-designed research articles, which constitute strong evidence, should be preferred in the review.

5. Organization

- There are three broad ways in which the literature could be organized in a review.
  i. Chronological arrangement of information
  ii. Conceptual organization
  iii. Methodological organization

In the *chronological organization*, the reviewed literature is arranged in the sequence of publication date. This type of review is more suited for theoretical or social research topics, where various theories and concepts are reviewed in the order in which they were developed.

In the *conceptual method* of arranging literature review, all the literature pertaining to each concept is presented together, usually under a separate heading. In a medical thesis, while the entire literature review may be written in the concept-based format, quite often this format is used along with the chronological arrangement.

In the *methodological organization*, work employing similar methods are grouped together. Thus, the review may begin with introducing the research topic, and then discuss various methods employed in the earlier research, followed by results and conclusions of these studies. Within these broad headings, the reviewed articles could be arranged chronologically or conceptually.

For example, when writing the literature review on the role of pesticides and genetic factors in patients suffering from urinary bladder cancer, one could have the broad categories of introduction (theories of carcinogenesis), specific literature pertaining to role of pesticides, and genetic make-up of the individual and methods available for studying these factors. Within these broad categories, the reviewed literature could either be arranged in a chronological order of publication or these broad categories could be further subdivided. Thus, in the section dealing with genetic factors in urinary bladder cancer, the reviewed literature could be further subdivided into gene studies and proteomics.

6. Audience

The style of writing the review would depend upon the intended readers. Thus, a review written for the experts in the given subject may contain more technical terms and less explanatory notes, when compared to a review intended for general reader.

■ PROCESS OF "REVIEWING" THE LITERATURE

After the relevant literature has been collected, the next step is to review it. The aim should be to identify major themes and concepts in the selected literature and discover relationships as well as disagreements and critical gaps among various studies. The steps involved in this review process are summarized in **Flowchart 11.1**.

Sorting and Prioritizing the Retrieved Literature

With the online availability of scientific literature, it is not difficult to quickly collect the relevant articles. We have already discussed in Chapter 8 how to search the literature online. However, the major problem in internet search may be that of plenty. It is important that these articles are scrutinized to identify those which are most likely to be relevant to the present research and need to be studied in depth. Reading of abstract, introduction, and conclusion gives enough idea about the usefulness of the article for the researcher.

It is helpful to identify and study review articles in the first instance. Those published in good scientific journals and written by experts in the field should be preferred. Going through these, one can identify important primary articles which have contributed significantly to a given field and are cited frequently. These primary articles should next be studied in detail, identifying their methodology, results, and conclusions.

The researcher should then identify those studies which are based on these primary seminal works. The aim of these secondary studies could be to see if the results are reproducible in different settings or they may address an area of interest based on, but not addressed in, the primary studies. The researcher is thus able to identify the areas already covered and that where further research is required. In addition, identifying studies in this way helps in building up the argument justifying the need for the present research. See **Flowchart 11.2** for a diagrammatic depiction.

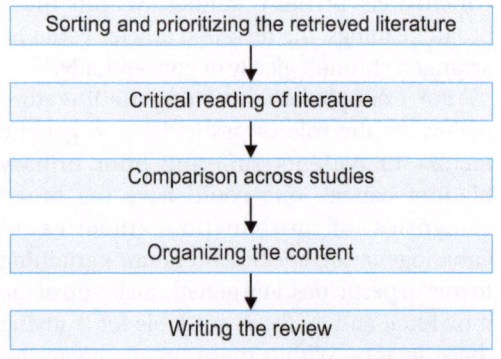

Flowchart 11.1: Process of reviewing the literature.

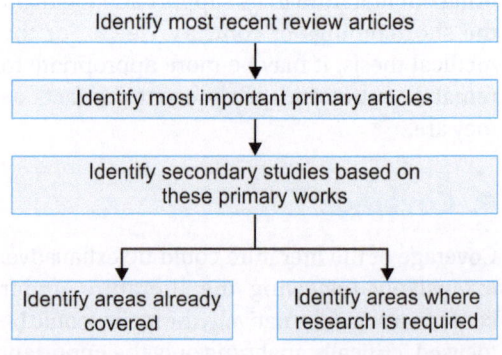

Flowchart 11.2: Steps in sorting the relevant literature.

Critical Analysis of Literature

Critical reading implies that the selected literature is not accepted on its face value. The researcher determines the accuracy, reliability, and significance of the information presented. The suitability of methodology, internal consistency of results, and accuracy of data analysis must be kept in mind while accepting the conclusions. These should be based on the facts presented rather than unsubstantiated opinion. It is essential, therefore, for you to have a reasonable grasp of research methodology to avoid including unsuitable literature in the review.

Comparison across Studies

The next step in reviewing is comparing different studies pertaining to a given aspect of research. Emphasis is given to similarities and differences among their aims and hypotheses, design and sampling, methodology, results, data analyses, and conclusions.

Unlike an annotated bibliography, in which only the summaries of these articles are listed, a literature review must include comments of the researcher. Take care not to reproduce the textbook material extensively. Only the relevant concepts should be mentioned and referenced. Based on this comparison, the researcher justifies the need, aim, and methodology for the present research.

Organizing the Contents of Review of Literature

As discussed earlier in this chapter, the collected literature could be organized chronologically, conceptually, or methodologically. A conceptual arrangement of the review is often preferred in writing medical thesis. This is depicted in **Flowchart 11.3**.

WRITING THE LITERATURE REVIEW

After you have collected the relevant literature, critically analyzed it, and decided on the style of organizing it, the last and the most important step is to actually write it down. The reason for choosing the research topic, writing the background information, presenting the important work done in the chosen area, and justifying aim and methodology of the proposed research should all come out clearly and concisely. It is useful to divide the literature review into the following broad sections: introduction, main body, and conclusion.

Introduction

Outline the research question and state your point of view, so that the reader can understand the line of argument being followed in the subsequent paragraphs. Define all the key terms so as to avoid any ambiguity. Provide adequate and appropriate references.

Main Body

In this section, the researcher summarizes relevant literature. In a medical thesis, research articles pertaining to one aspect or concept are grouped under one heading. For this concept, the articles may be either presented in chronological order or grouped according to their conclusions. For example, all studies in favor are discussed together, followed by all studies against. Such information can also be organized in a tabular form by mentioning important elements such as place of study, sample size, type of participants, key outcomes, and comments. Summarize each article. Provide your comments and analysis in brief. Do not offer detailed comments here. Reserve them for the Discussion section.

In an experimental research, the available methods and tools should also be reviewed. The justification for using these methods should be given in the Discussion section.

Conclusion

This section summarizes the researcher's reason for doing research on the given topic, briefly reviews the proposed methodology,

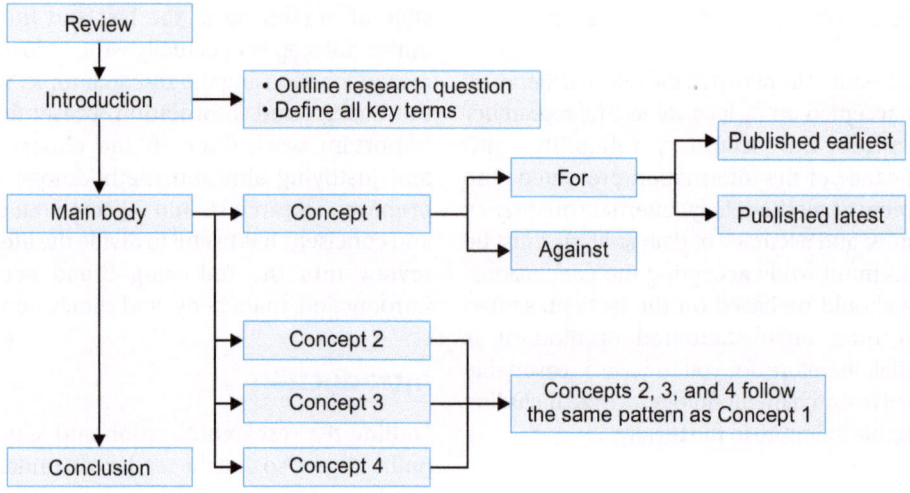

Flowchart 11.3: Writing the literature review.

and leads to the following sections on aim/objectives and methodology.

MISTAKES IN WRITING REVIEW OF LITERATURE

While writing literature review, the following should be avoided:
- The method of conducting literature search is not stated.
- A primary article is not reviewed. Instead, secondary sources are relied upon to collect information about the primary article. For example, if a primary article "A" is quoted by a review article "B," the researcher does not read "A," instead quotes the information about "A" based on reading of "B" and then cites "A" in the reference. In case the full text of the primary article is not accessible, it may be better to clearly state that the information of "A" is based on "B" and give reference of "B."
- Only a summary of the cited article is given in the literature review, quite often copied verbatim from the original article. Since different primary articles are written in different styles, there is no uniformity in the language style of the final review. A critical reader can very easily identify this "copy and paste" job.
- All aspects of research design and analysis of the reviewed article are not critically examined. There are no comments from the reviewer.
- Only those articles which support the researcher's point of view are reviewed.
- The review is not written in a consistent style with logical headings and subheadings.

CONCLUSION

Clearly, rather than just being an unavoidable part of writing a thesis, review of literature is a vital part of any research. In the absence of a good review, the research may end up being aimless, repeat of an earlier work, or done using an unsuitable method.

> **KEY MESSAGES**
>
> - Review of literature forms the main bulk of thesis, and thus should be exhaustive, simultaneously focused to the topic.
> - The first step in the process is to collect all the relevant literature, go through their titles and abstracts, identify the literature to be reviewed and cited, and read their full text.
> - Primary literature (research articles) and secondary literature (systematic reviews and review articles published in peer-reviewed journals) should be preferred over tertiary literature (e.g., textbooks and online medical resources) while writing this section.
> - The next step is to organize and write the content in a proper chronology, often based on the concepts being presented. Use headings, subheadings liberally, maintaining uniformity of the style. Use tables and figures liberally to organize and explain the concepts.
> - It is important to include all relevant literature on the topic rather than choosing what suits your hypothesis. Write in your own words, using information and data from published research articles and reviews; copy and paste is a strict NO.

■ FURTHER READING

1. Baker JD. The purpose, process, and methods of writing a literature review. AORN J. 2016;103(3):265-9.
2. Boote DN, Beile P. Scholars before researchers: On the centrality of the dissertation literature review in research preparation. Educational Researcher. 2005;34(6):3-15.
3. Carnwell R, Daly W. Strategies for the construction of a critical review of the literature. Nurse Edu Pract. 2001;1(2):57-63.
4. Connelly LM. Reviewing the literature. Med Surg Nurs. 2010;19(4):245-6.
5. Kearney MH. Moving from facts to wisdom: facilitating synthesis in literature reviews. Res Nurs Health. 2016;39(1):3-6.
6. Kowalczyk N, Truluck C. Literature reviews and systematic reviews: what is the difference? Radiol Technol. 2013;85(2):219-22.
7. Pautasso M. Ten simple rules for writing a literature review. PLoS Comput Biol. 2013;9(7):e1003149.
8. Randolph J. A guide to writing the dissertation literature review. Pract Assess Res Eval. 2007;14(13):1-13.

CHAPTER 12

Material and Methods: How will I do it?

Dheeraj Shah

■ INTRODUCTION

The "Material and Methods" section provides information on how you will approach (for thesis protocol) or how you approached (for full thesis report) your research work, including the source of the materials you used in this work. This section is often rated as the most important section of the thesis or thesis protocol as it is usually evaluated most carefully by experts who review your protocol or thesis. The methodology mentioned in the protocol has to be strictly followed while carrying out the research and any deviations, unless with written permission, can have serious repercussions on the acceptability of the work. You should take extreme care in planning and writing this part of your study, giving importance to all the necessary details.

> Methodology remains the same for both thesis protocol and the final thesis.

■ COMPONENTS OF MATERIAL AND METHODS

It is a common practice to describe "Methods" and "Material" in the same section. "Material" implies all items such as equipment, reagents, proformas/questionnaires, computer software, and, above all, human/animal participants and/or their body tissues/fluids. "Methods" refer to how, when, and where are you going to use this material and carry out the procedure to fulfill your objectives. You should mention enough details to enable someone else to exactly replicate the experiment. The details under this section should be preferably organized into various subheadings. Structure of "Methods" section according to different types of study designs is presented in **Boxes 12.1** to **12.4**. The details of the subheadings are given in the following text.

Please note that the methods are written in future tense in thesis protocol, and in past tense in final thesis report for obvious reasons. The description below relates to writing "Methods" section for the thesis protocol.

Preliminary Information

Study Design

It is either descriptive or analytical. If descriptive, subclassify accordingly as survey, case series, diagnostic study, or cross-sectional study. If analytical, whether observational (cohort, case-control, or cross-sectional) or

Guidelines on Reporting different Study Designs

Box 12.1: Interventional studies [including randomized controlled trials (RCT)].

Suggested subheadings (sequential)
- Study design
- Study setting
- Study duration
- Ethical aspects
- Participants
  - Eligibility (inclusion and exclusion criteria)
  - Process for selecting participants (sampling) and assigning them to intervention or comparator treatment (equivalent to randomization in RCT) (type of randomization, sequence generation, allocation concealment, and blinding)
- Intervention(s) along with standard clinical, diagnostic, and therapeutic procedures
- Outcomes, including plan for their recording
- Sample size
- Statistical analysis

CONsolidated Standards Of Reporting Trials Statement
CONSORT
http://www.consort-statement.org/

Box12.2: Diagnostic accuracy studies.
- Study design
- Study setting
- Study duration
- Ethical aspects
- Participants:
  - Eligibility (inclusion and exclusion criteria)
  - Participant recruitment (sampling)
- Test methods:
  - Reference and Index test
  - Other diagnostic/therapeutic considerations
- Sample size
- Statistical analysis

STAndards for Reporting of Diagnostic accuracy
STARD
http://www.equator-network.org/index.aspx?o=1050

Box 12.3: Observational studies (descriptive, cohort, cross-sectional, case–control).
- Study design
- Study setting
- Study duration
- Ethical aspects
- Participants:
  - Eligibility criteria
  - Sources and methods of selection (in descriptive and cross-sectional studies), and of case ascertainment and control selection (in cohort and case–control studies)
  - Matching criteria (for matched studies)
- Variables (exposure, outcomes, and confounders), including plan of their recording
- Data sources/measurement
- Sample size
- Statistical methods

STrengthening the Reporting of OBservational studies in Epidemiology
STROBE
http://www.strobe-tatement.org/index.php?id=available-checklists

Box 12.4: Systematic reviews/meta-analyses.
- Study design
- Eligibility criteria:
  - Types of studies, participants and interventions
  - Outcome measures (primary/secondary)
- Search methods
- Data collection and analysis:
  - Selection of studies
  - Data extraction and management
  - Assessment of risk of bias
  - Measures of treatment effect
  - Assessment of heterogeneity
  - Data synthesis
  - Subgroup analysis
  - Sensitivity analysis

Preferred Reporting Items for Systematic reviews and Meta-Analyses
PRISMA
http://www.prisma-statement.org/

interventional [randomized controlled trial (RCT), nonrandomized comparison, or crossover] (See Chapter 6 for details of various study designs).

Study Setting

Where will the study be carried out? Mention the name of principal department and institution along with all other participating departments/institutions. Also mention whether the study would be hospital-based or community-based. If in hospital, mention the setting of participant enrollment (outpatient/emergency/inpatient). Similarly, mention the exact setting of a community-based study (i.e., home and school).

Study Duration

When (from........to) the study will be carried out—this period should include separately the stipulated duration for participant enrollment, their follow-up, statistical analysis, and report writing.

Ethical Aspects

Every research project must be cleared by a properly constituted ethics committee in human or animal research. Mention the name of ethics committee to which you will submit the protocol for ethical clearance. Mention how patient confidentiality is being maintained. Mention about the informed consent and attach the proposed informed consent form (in English as well as in local language) as Annexure. Also, enclose the patient information sheet that details the information about the project in simple and local language. The patient information sheet should give some details of the disease/condition to be investigated, the purpose of the research work, some details of the procedure, which are relevant for patients/parents such as amount of blood to be withdrawn and nature of intervention (if any), and benefits/harms (if any) to the participants (See Chapter 14 for details). A sample of (1) informed consent form and (2) patient information sheet are also provided in Chapter 14.

Participants (Population)

This section outlines the criteria that make a person (or his/her body part/fluid) eligible or ineligible for inclusion into the study, from where you would be choosing them, and how are you assigning one or other intervention to these participants (in controlled interventional studies). For most studies, the participants would be humans or animals but for some type of studies, participants of research could be inanimate (e.g., blood samples and culture plates). For a systematic review, the participants of research are studies such as RCTs.

Inclusion Criteria

What makes the person eligible for inclusion? Define ages, sex, (if applicable) and criteria for defining disease condition under question. Also, mention the place from where the participants will be enrolled, e.g., from outpatient department of a hospital or from a particular geographic area. For example, if you are planning to conduct a study assessing proportion of hypertensive young adults having hyperlipidemia, you need to define "hypertension" and "young adults" as planned in your study. The inclusion criteria for such a study could be:

> *All young adults (aged 20 to 40 completed years) presenting to the cardiovascular disease clinic of the ABC Hospital with hypertension will be eligible for inclusion in the study. Hypertension will be defined as systolic blood pressure of ≥ 140 mm Hg and/or diastolic blood pressure of ≥ 90 mm Hg, measured on two separate occasions with a minimum interval of at least 5 minutes between the two measurements [Ref] or a self-reported history of receiving antihypertensive medications for >1 month before enrollment.*

Note that you do NOT need to define "hyperlipidemia" here as it is the outcome and would be dealt in a different subheading later.

Exclusion Criteria

This should include persons who otherwise are eligible for inclusion but would not be included because of various reasons. Possibility of introducing bias, ethical issues, and feasibility issues could be some of the reasons for exclusion. Remember that "exclusion criteria" is not just the opposite of "inclusion criteria"; for exclusion, the person should first satisfy the inclusion criteria.

In the above example of study on proportion of hypertensive young adults having hyperlipidemia, you may want to exclude persons with secondary causes of hypertension such as chronic kidney diseases and aortoarteritis (as they may form a distinct group of patients, not related to your objectives), those who are already receiving hypolipidemic drugs (as the lipid profile will be modified by these drugs), or those who have other comorbid conditions affecting lipid profile (e.g., hypothyroidism). The statement for exclusion criteria in the above example would be:

> *Persons with known secondary causes of hypertension (e.g., chronic kidney diseases, aortoarteritis, and coarctation of aorta), comorbid conditions that affect lipid profile (e.g., hypothyroidism), those already receiving hypolipidemic drugs (any duration), or those receiving oral contraceptives, corticosteroids, or anticonvulsant medications for at least 1 week before enrollment would be excluded from the study.*

You should NOT write age <20 years or >40 years as exclusion as these persons do not fulfill inclusion criteria; a common mistake done by the students and naïve researchers.

Sampling (Different from Sample Size, which is Discussed Later)

Out of all eligible population, which all people will you include? These could be all consecutive participants till the sample size is met (sequential sampling), or selective sampling decided on the basis of some random process such as *simple random sampling* (based on random number table or some other procedure such as tossing of a coin), *systematic random sampling* (every second or every third eligible person) or *stratified sampling* (e.g., equally divided into various age groups or equal number of males and females). Many a times, the sampling could be decided on the basis of feasibility (*convenience sampling*) such as whenever the investigator is available or on some select days of the week. Random sampling is more often used in studies in community where you have large number of eligible persons, and you need to select a representative sample. In hospital-based theses, you can use feasibility sampling (for common conditions) or consecutive sampling (for uncommon conditions).

Note that this "sampling" procedure is also different from randomization that is an integral part of RCT. Sampling is used in all studies, whereas randomization is used only in RCTs.

Comparison Group

In many interventional and observational studies, there would be a comparator or control group, which may receive no intervention, a placebo, or some other intervention. You need to clearly specify the criteria for considering a participant as control (in observational studies, e.g., cohort, case–control, and cross-sectional) or the basis of deciding which participant would receive intervention under research or comparator treatment (in interventional studies). The comparator group in interventional trial could be decided on the basis of some nonrandomized procedure [such as alternate (odd–even) allotment, based on the presentation on certain days of week or just convenience]; the best method is when you ensure that it is only chance that decides the allocation to intervention or comparator group, the latter is termed *randomization*.

Randomization (Sequence Generation and Allocation Concealment) and Blinding

If you are planning to conduct an RCT, you need to clearly mention the process of randomization. If you write "randomization into two groups" without any details, it does not mean anything. If you do not plan any randomization, honestly declare that your study will be a nonrandomized comparison and mention the basis on which you plan to assign the index or comparator intervention. Masquerading nonrandomized studies as randomized trials can have serious repercussions for medical research. If you plan randomization, mention the following details:

- *How will you generate the sequence?*
  It could be by use of a random number table, some computer program, or an online randomization generator. Also, mention the type of sequence generated (e.g., simple randomization and block randomization).
- *How will you conceal the allocation?*
  It means how will you ensure that the person who allocates one intervention or the other to a particular participant is completely unaware (and has no control) of what is coming next. It is an integral part of an RCT and is different from blinding. The common methods of allocation concealment are sequentially numbered opaque sealed envelopes (SNOSE) and pharmacy-coded medicine bottles and strips.
- *Write details of any blinding of participants, treating physicians and outcome assessors*
  If there is no blinding, declare study as *open label*. The most common method of blinding is by use of placebo with a similar appearance, taste, and smell as a drug. Note that "blinding" is different from "allocation concealment" as in the former, the participants as well as treating physicians (those delivering the intervention and those assessing the outcomes) are unaware of the nature of intervention (index or comparator) throughout the study. Blinding may not be possible in many studies (e.g., medical vs. surgical management of acute appendicitis) whereas "allocation concealment" is a must in all RCTs.

Procedure

Procedures could be diagnostic (e.g., collection of blood or sputum samples to validate a diagnostic test), observational (e.g., conducting a questionnaire-based survey and observation of the participant's environment), or interventional. Interventions could be therapeutic (e.g., antihypertensive medications), preventive (e.g., breastfeeding promotion and handwashing), or in the realm of social sciences such as providing training or information to groups of individuals.

Baseline Data Recording

Write about the information you are going to collect from the enrolled participants (both cases and controls) such as:
- Clinical methods (history and examination)
- Measurements
- Laboratory investigations:
  - Details if using a new method
  - Quote reference for standard method
  - Describe any modifications
  - Mention exact quantitative aspects
  - Machine specifications

For standard methods, appropriate references are sufficient, but if standard methods are modified, these should be clearly brought out. Provide complete details of any new methods or apparatus used (manufacturer's name and address in parentheses).

Intervention (if any) and Comparison

Write precise details of the intervention such as:
- Description of drug/device/vaccine/educational program that is being tested
- Dosage, formulations, and schedules
- Duration of intervention
- Similar details for comparator agent/method

In observational studies, "exposure" will replace intervention. In diagnostic studies, investigational test (index test) and standard test should be described in detail, including criteria for considering the tests as positive or negative.

Data Collection and Monitoring

This should include plan for managing and monitoring the participants during their period of enrollment into the study such as frequency of clinical assessment, schedule of laboratory investigations, and treatment plan. What steps are being taken to ensure quality control for assessments?

Use a flow diagram (**Flowchart 12.1**) to explain the monitoring plan, including timing of assessments.

Outcome Measures

These are the parameters which will fulfill the objectives of the study. Outcome measures can be divided into primary and secondary.

Primary Outcome Measure

This is the outcome on which study hypothesis is based; the main thrust of interest in the protocol. You should also base your sample size on the basis of primary outcome. For example, if the objective of the study is to assess the impact of antenatal zinc supplementation on birth weight, the birth weight becomes the primary outcome measure. Proportion of low birth weight (<2,500 g) may be another primary outcome measure in such a study. The number of primary outcome measures should be restricted to one or two as the sample size and study hypothesis is based on this measure.

Secondary Outcome Measures

These are the other outcomes of possible interest. For example, if you are planning to do a study of antenatal zinc supplementation on birth weight, you may also be interested in knowing whether there is an impact on length or if there are any adverse effects of supplementation on mother or baby. These become the secondary outcomes.

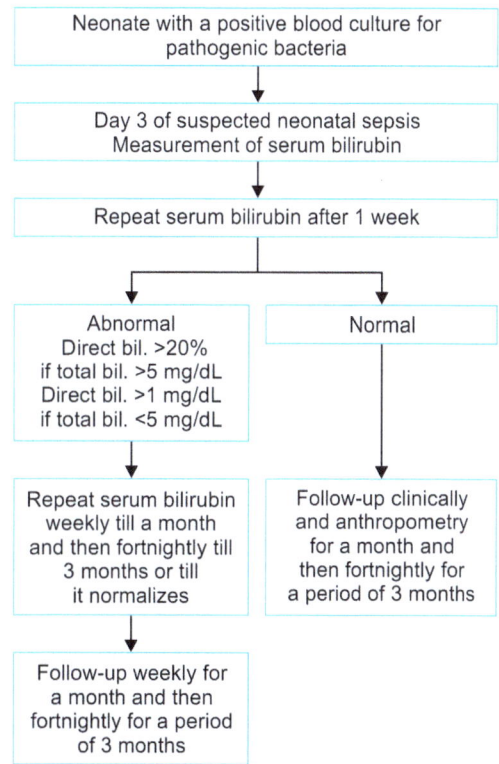

Flowchart 12.1: Evaluation and monitoring of study participants.

Clearly define the outcome measures. In an earlier example of a study of finding proportion of young hypertensive adults having hyperlipidemia, the outcome measure is hyperlipidemia (or proportion of participants with hyperlipidemia). Here, you need to clearly define hyperlipidemia, providing a reference if the same definition has been used earlier, or is based on some recommended guideline.

Mention clearly about who will make the assessment for the outcome measures and using what tools. The method for measuring the outcome variable should also be detailed here if it has not been outlined earlier in "Data collection and monitoring."

Sample Size

Whenever you start a research work, you must know (and write too) how many participants you plan to enroll in the study. While writing the final report, people are often tempted to write the final sample size achieved in "Methods" section. This section should just include "how many participants you planned to enroll" and NOT how many you finally enrolled. The latter is described with "Results." Similarly, you should not write the details of the participants (e.g., age and sex distribution) here.

The protocol should inform and justify how you decided this sample size. Sample size calculations are based on the type of study, the effect size you are looking for, and the levels of errors acceptable to you. Clearly explain the basis on which you arrive data sample size at the protocol level. As the postgraduate thesis is a time-bound research activity, the sample size may sometimes be based on feasibility depending on the expected patient load in their facility during the study duration. If this is the case, it should be stated explicitly. The principles underlying the estimation of sample size are detailed in Chapter 13.

Statistical Analysis

At the level of protocol itself, provide enough detail to enable a knowledgeable person with access to original data to verify the reported results.

- Use statements specific to the study. General statements are NOT recommended; you already know what outcomes you are going to record and compare. Present a plan for the assessment of all outcome measures outlined earlier. Mention the level of significance or the level of confidence.

General statement (NOT RECOMMENDED):

> Mean values between two groups will be compared using student's t-test and proportions will be compared using Chi-square test.

Specific statement (RECOMMENDED):

> Mean (SD) birth weight and length between the zinc supplemented and placebo group will be compared by using student's t-test. The proportion of low birth weight infants between the two groups will be compared by using Chi-square test or Fisher's exact test, as applicable. A P value of <0.05 will be considered significant for all outcomes.

- *Specify data management issues*: How are you going to tabulate the collected information? Which computer software will you be using for data analysis? For example: *Data will be tabulated in Microsoft Excel sheet. All analyses will be performed by SPSS Statistics Version 26.0 software.*

■ GENERAL TIPS FOR WRITING "MATERIAL AND METHODS" SECTION

Use Appropriate "Tense"

While writing the protocol, use "future tense" throughout this section. In the final thesis report, write all the procedures in the "past tense" as the work has already been completed. You have to be very careful about the tense; any error will reflect carelessness on your part. A well-written "Methods" section in the protocol can be taken as such in the final report after changing the tense but be careful to include any modification/deviation in methodology or any later change in statistical analysis based on the distribution of data.

Provide Enough Details

The details should be enough and elaborate enough to enable other researchers to replicate your study. Avoid details that are not relevant to the outcome of the experiment. For example, in the study on assessing the proportion of young hypertensive adults having hyperlipidemia, you should mention details of procedure for recording blood pressure and for measuring lipid profile. In this study, you might also be collecting other samples (e.g., blood sugar and hemoglobin) or taking some measurements (e.g., weight, height, and body mass index); the details related to these may be unnecessary.

Check the Formatting and Flow, Proofread

- *Formatting*: Be consistent with the font size and the line spacing. Take care to be uniform in the style of headings/subheadings. Ensure that headings and subheadings have different style.
- *Check* whether you have taken care of all relevant subsections and have not omitted any important information. **Box 12.5** presents a checklist for "Material and Methods."
- *Proofread* your protocol for any errors, ambiguity and disagreement with other sections. Ask a colleague to go through it once you are through. Your procedures

---

Box 12.5: Checklist for "Material and Methods".

Checklist for "Material and Methods"
- Type of study: Descriptive or analytical. If descriptive, classify into survey, diagnostic study, case series, or cross-sectional study, as appropriate. If analytical, whether observational (cohort, case-control, or cross-sectional) or interventional [randomized controlled trial (RCT) and cross–over]
- When (…….. to …….) and where the study will be carried out
- Ethical aspects: Name of the ethics committee providing ethical clearance, informed consent, patient information sheet, trial registry (if any), regulatory clearance (if any)
- Participants: Target population (age group and sex). Inclusion and exclusion criteria. Details about the control group (if any)
- Place where participants will be recruited from
- Inclusion criteria: Define ages, criteria for defining disease condition/normalcy
- Exclusion criteria: Persons who fulfill inclusion criteria BUT would be excluded because of other conditions that could possibly introduce bias
- Criteria for assigning a participant to index or comparator intervention (in interventional studies)
- Method of randomization (if RCT): How will you generate the sequence? How will you do allocation concealment and blinding (if any)?
- Procedure:
    - Detail if using a new method; or else quote standard reference, if anybody else has already described the method you are going to use
    - Describe modifications you have made to a standard or published method
    - Quantitative aspects: Masses, volumes, incubation times, concentrations, and machine specifications (include manufacturer's name and location)
    - Who will make the assessments and using what tools?
    - Frequency and duration of intervention
    - Procedures and schedules of examination/investigations/treatment, and observation of outcome measures
    - Dosage, formulations, schedules, duration of drug treatments (if any)
- Outcome Measures:
    - Primary outcome measures: These are the outcomes on which study hypothesis is based; the main thrust of interest in the protocol
    - Secondary outcome measures: These are other outcomes of possible interest
- Sample size with justification
- Data management and statistical analysis
- Procedure and computer program for data handling/statistical tests planned/statistical software

(especially outcome measures) should match your objectives.
- *Abbreviations*: Use only standard abbreviations and write full form on their first use. Do not abbreviate the same word differently throughout the report.

What Not to Include in the "Methods" Section

- *Results*: The number of participants actually enrolled in your study, the percentage loss to follow-up, and number followed up till the end-point are all your results. Do not include this in "Material and Methods" section; a common error. "Methods" section should include only proposed sample size, not what you actually achieved.
- *Discussion*: The reason why you chose a particular method over the other or why your methodology is free of bias should not be a part of "Material and Methods." This should be a part of the discussion. Remember "How you did it" is "Methods"; "Why you did so" is "Discussion."

■ FURTHER READING

1. Arora SK, Shah D. Writing methods: How to write what you did? Indian Pediatr. 2016;53(4):335-40.
2. Duke T. How to do a postgraduate research project and write a minor thesis. Arch Dis Child. 2018;103(9):820-27.
3. Equator Network. Reporting Guidelines for Main Study Types. [online] Available from https://www.equator-network.org/reporting-guidelines/. [Last accessed April 30, 2020].
4. Jackowski MB, Leggett T. Writing research proposals. Radiol Technol. 2015;87(2):236-8.
5. Vealé BL, Moore QT. Writing a methods section: Detailing your approach. Radiol Technol. 2016;88(1):111-2.

CHAPTER 13

Sample Size Estimation

Amir Maroof Khan

■ INTRODUCTION

A study was done in which two drugs were compared for controlling bleeding in children with hemophilia. The sample size was 20 in each group. It was found that 30% and 50% of the subjects were benefitted by the two drugs, respectively. The difference was found to be statistically nonsignificant, P = 0.80. Should we believe this result that the difference was statistically not significant? Another way to put this is: Was the sample size enough to detect a difference of this magnitude?

The power of this study was found to be 24.7%. This meant that, with the given sample size of 20 in each group, the ability to detect a difference of this magnitude as statistically significant was only 24.7%. Or in other words, the sample size was not large enough to detect the difference between the effects of two drugs.

So, how large should the sample size be for this study. On calculation, it was found to be 93 subjects in each group. This implies that at least 93 subjects were required in each group to detect the observed difference with 80% probability (power).

The point is that a study with an inadequate sample size is to be interpreted with caution because even if there is a difference between the interventions, it will not be able to detect it.

■ WHY CALCULATE THE SAMPLE SIZE?

Sample size is the number of subjects that are needed to be studied in a given research. During the research protocol presentation, this is one of the most important questions asked to the researcher. As has been discussed in another chapter, you know that it is not possible to study the whole population under consideration and, hence, a sample is selected from the population in a random manner. The sample size should be "just large enough" to be able to detect the difference, if it exists.

- Studying a sample size larger than that is required for the study will lead to wastage of resources, such as time, money, and manpower. It may also lead to very small clinically insignificant difference/s being detected as statistically significant results, which may not be useful at the practical level.
- If the sample size is smaller than that required, it may not be possible to detect a significant difference/association, even if it exists. Thus, it may not be appropriate also to attempt a study with a smaller or a larger sample size, when we know a *priori* that it may lead to results which may be erroneous or not relevant at the practical level.

- Calculating sample size also helps in planning of the study. It will help you in estimating the resources, i.e., man, money, material, and time required to accomplish the research.
- Sample size calculation helps to ensure scientific (validity and reliability) and ethical integrity of the research study.

■ HOW TO CALCULATE THE SAMPLE SIZE?

When you will ask the statistician, "how much sample size is needed for my study?," he will not give you a magic number immediately, because in order to arrive at that number, the statistician needs your responses to the five questions. These questions are listed in **Box 13.1** and discussed in the following text.

1. What is the Type of Study?

For the sake of simplicity in calculation of sample sizes, be sure which of the following you are interested in: (*a*) Finding an estimate; or (*b*) testing a hypothesis.

Studies on Determining an Estimate

You are interested in estimation when you are doing a descriptive or a prevalence study. You may be interested in estimating a mean or a proportion of the given variable in the population. Here you do not want to compare two variables and so there is no null hypothesis involved, e.g., *Prevalence of hypertension among adults in East Delhi*. It is important to note that here we do not intend to compare or find some association between the variables. We just want to estimate the prevalence of hypertension of the population of East Delhi from a randomly selected sample.

Exact prevalence can be determined only if you study each subject in the population. As studying the entire population is not possible, you will study a randomly selected sample. The prevalence that will be calculated from the sample will not be exactly similar to that of the population and there will be some difference. If you want it to be very precise (or confidence interval is smaller), then a larger sample size will have to be studied. If a smaller sample size is studied, the results will be imprecise (confidence interval is larger). Therefore, you will have to specify the level of precision (confidence interval) that you want for the estimate, in order to decide on the sample size.

> Confidence interval = Point estimate (obtained from sample studied) ± margin of error (this determines sample size and vice versa).

A 10% margin of error can be achieved with a sample size of 100, whereas for getting a lesser margin of error (that is making the point estimate more precise) of say 5%, a sample size of 400 will be required. So, we see that for reducing the error or increasing the precision by two times, there is four times increase in the required sample size.

Studies to Test a Hypothesis

In studies involving hypothesis testing, you intend to compare the effect of two or more interventions. This effect is measured in terms of proportion of success/treated, etc., or in terms of a mean value of a variable. The null hypothesis states that the two interventions have an equal effect and your aim is to be able to reject this null hypothesis if it is false. This

---

Box 13.1: Sample determination: Five requirements.

1. What is the type of study: (a) Determination of estimate; or (b) Hypothesis testing?
2. What is the primary outcome variable?
3. What is the estimated value of primary outcome variable, and acceptable precision? This is applicable for studies of type (a) above
4. What is the acceptable type I (alpha) error and type II (beta) error? These values are needed for studies on hypothesis testing, i.e., type (b) above
5. What is the desired effect size? [For studies of type (b) above]

will be discussed further when we discuss the relationship of sample size with type I and type II errors.

2. What is the Primary Outcome of your Study?

In trials where two interventions are compared, the outcome of the interventions can be assessed in different ways, e.g., death of the patient, costs involved, duration of stay in the hospital, etc. Avoid overloading the study design with too many objectives and, thus, measurement and comparison of too many outcomes. A single primary question which leads to an outcome measure—used to make the decision on the overall result of the study— is the best approach. This will then serve as the basis to determine the number of patients needed for the study. Thus, *each clinical trial should preferably have only one primary endpoint,* which should be defined before initiating the study and it will also decide the sample size needed. However, if you choose to have more than one primary outcome variable, you will have to calculate sample size for all of them, separately. The final sample size in this case will be the "larger" number.

3. What is the Estimated Value of Outcome Variable and Margin of Error Acceptable to you?

Specify (a) the estimated baseline prevalence of the variable of interest, and (b) margin of error or the level of precision acceptable to you. These data are needed for all studies for determining the estimates.

- *Estimated value of the outcome variable*: Suppose you want to find out the prevalence of hypertension in a slum of East Delhi. So, what will be the sample size required for that? For estimating the sample size, you need to know an estimate of the prevalence of hypertension in that slum area. You may say that if I have a rough estimate of the prevalence, why should I be doing this study.

But that is the irony of the situation. It is vital to have an estimate of the prevalence, if you want to estimate the sample size. Similarly, if you want to find a mean of some variable, in your study, you should have an estimate of the expected mean. For determining odds ratio, you need to provide the estimate of the expected odds ratio. These estimates can be found out from previously published studies or from your hospital records. If you do not have these, then you conduct a small pilot study to find out the estimates and then use these figures for sample size calculation.

- *Margin of error*: If you do not study the whole population and study a sample of it, you know that the mean of the population will be different from that of the sample studied. So, error will be there, which is called as *sampling error*. How much error you can tolerate in the result that you get from the sample is to be decided by you for calculating sample size. For zero sampling error, you need to study the whole population and as you go on increasing the error, the sample size decreases.

4. What are the Acceptable Type I and Type II Errors?

These data are needed for studies to test a hypothesis. We start with a null hypothesis that there is no difference between the two groups, i.e., say there is no difference between the effect of two drugs.

The truth may be one of the following two: *No difference exists* or *A difference exists.*
Errors may be of two types:
1. If no difference exists in reality and our study finds a difference, we say that an error (*type I or alpha error*) has been committed.
2. If there is a difference existing in reality and our study is not able to find it, we say that an error (*type II or beta error*) has been committed.

Type I error is usually fixed at 5%. This implies that the probability of finding a difference when there is no difference should be <5%.

Type II error is by convention taken as 20% in calculation of sample size. This implies that the probability of not finding a difference when there is a difference should be <20%. This also means that there is 80% (100–20) probability of making a correct decision of not reporting a difference, when there is no actual difference. This is also known as **Power** of the study.

5. For Studies Involving Hypothesis Testing, What is the Effect Size that you Intend to Detect?

Let us start with an example. A study is being conducted to find out the effect of a drug on the systolic blood pressure (SBP) (measured in mm Hg) when given daily for 1 week in a group of hypertensive patients. The SBP will be measured at baseline and after 1 week to see if there is any difference or not. So here it is to be seen whether the difference in SBP (from baseline to 1 week) is statistically significant or not. But what is the minimum difference that we want to capture. Is it 1 mm Hg, 50 mm Hg, or some other value? Suppose you say that a 10 mm Hg difference (mean of SBP before the drug minus mean of SBP after 1 week of drug administration) is clinically relevant and the sample size should be sufficient enough to detect this means difference statistically. This 10 mm Hg difference is the absolute effect size. However, this is not the only thing required to assess the difference in the effects of the two drugs for SBP. Let us explore further.

You also need to look at the "measure of dispersion" of the two curves. You very well know that standard deviation is what you use as a "measure of dispersion". Try understanding it by comparing the two figures above. Out of the two (**Figs. 13.1A** and **B**), in which figure do you find the curves more overlapping?

In **Figure 13.1B**, the curves seem to be overlapping more as compared to those in **Figure 13.1A**.

Even though the difference between the means of the two curves in both the figures is equal, the overlap is more in **Figure 13.1B**, because of greater area under the curves in **Figure 13.1B**. This further implies that you must take both the mean and standard deviations into consideration when you want to decide what difference you expect in the two groups that you want to compare.

- Exact mean/proportion is important. Just telling the value of mean difference or the difference in proportion that is clinically relevant for your study is not going to help in deciding the sample size.
- You also need to tell the standard deviations of the two groups. To detect the difference between the two curves of **Figure 13.1B** will require a larger sample size as compared to

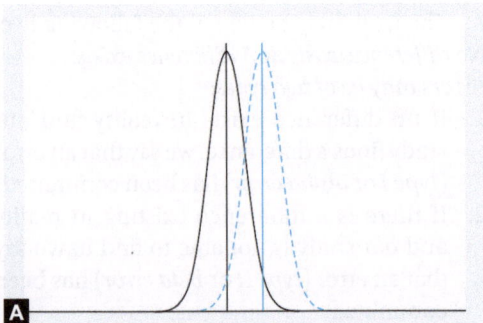
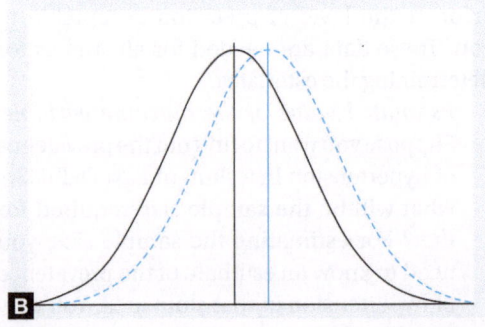

Figs. 13.1A and B: The graphs depict the mean, and dispersion around the mean. Group A is represented by complete line while the dotted curves denote Group B.

that required for **Figure 13.1A**. This is to highlight the fact that the spread of the curve (standard deviations) is also important in the effect size. Mean and standard deviation can be ascertained from earlier published literature or some pilot studies done using the variables in question.

Effect Size

A measure that has been devised, which takes both the difference in means and the standard deviations into account is called *effect size*. Effect size is not just a difference in means; it is the standardized difference in means. Effect sizes are used in calculating sample sizes.

Let us try to understand the relationship between effect size and sample size with an analogy. Sample size is like the magnification of a microscope. By increasing it you will be able to detect even smaller differences (effect sizes). In order to decide on the minimum sample size needed, decide on the maximum size of difference (effect size) that you want to detect. Thus, you can say that *sample size is inversely related to effect size*.

The formula for effect size for means between two groups A and B is as follows:

$$\text{Effect size (Cohen's d)} = \frac{[\text{mean of A} - \text{mean of B}]}{\text{pooled standard deviation}}$$

This standardized mean difference is known as the Cohen's d.

As there are two curves to compare, the question is which of the two standard deviations to use the denominator in the above equation of effect size. Here instead of any one curve's or variable's standard deviation, a pooled standard deviation which is calculated by taking both the standard deviations into consideration is used. Pooled standard deviation for two means

$$= \sqrt{[\{(n_1 - 1) \times s^2 + (n_2 - 1) \times s^2\}/\{(n_1 + n_2)/2\}]}$$

Where n_1 and n_2 are the sample sizes of the two groups and s_1 and s_2 are the standard deviations of the two groups.

For the sake of simplicity, here we have considered difference in means for explaining effect size. But effect sizes (the magnitude of the effect that the intervention has) can be measured even in terms of relative risk, odds ratio, difference in proportions, etc. So, in certain types of studies, you may like to have some other effect size and not difference in means described above.

Effect size should be specified for estimation of the required sample size for a given study. This can be found from the previous studies done on that topic or a pilot testing can be done to find out the mean and standard deviation for the two groups so that you can yourself calculate the effect size. Remember that sample size can be minimized by increasing the difference that you are interested in detecting (effect size).

ADJUSTING THE SAMPLE SIZE

Several factors affect the final sample size. These factors include feasibility, nonresponse rates, and dropouts. They should also be taken into consideration before deciding on the final sample size for the study.

Feasibility

Feasibility is what is possible, what you can do, depending upon the resources available to you. Getting a sample size as 10,000 for a research study may not be feasible for you as you have limited time for data collection, i.e., 9-12 months. So, this sample size is not feasible for a thesis. The time required to study and collect data from one subject, and the number of subjects that you will be able to cover in a single day should be known to you before committing on the sample size. These estimates should be realistic and one way to make it so is to do a pretesting of the questionnaire, wherein apart from noting down the modifications required in it, you can also know the time required for the given task. Similarly, cost factor should also be estimated when you require some kits or traveling costs, etc. for your study. The total cost will depend upon the final sample size that you have arrived at and committed to.

Nonresponse and Dropout Rates

Not everyone whom you select for including in your sample will respond. Some will be nonresponders. Nonresponders can vary a lot depending upon the type of research. Also, not all of those who are randomized and included in the study will complete the whole course of trial. There may be some who may dropout in between and the final sample size you are left with will be less than that required for that study. Nonresponse rates and dropouts lead to a reduction in the sample size studied and, thus, the power of the study will also decrease resulting in incorrect results, if these are not accounted for in the initial calculations.

Your sample size tells you how many subjects should be studied for the given objective. If your sample size is 100 and you approached the 100 subjects and found that 20% were nonresponders, then that means you have been able to study/collect data from 80 subjects only and you are short of 20 subjects. An estimate about the nonresponse rates/dropout rates can be made by either past experiences of you and/or your supervisor or published literature on the research topic. If adjustment in sample size is not made for nonresponse and dropout rates at this stage, then the final sample size may be lesser than what was required in the study.

Formula for Estimating the Sample Size Taking into Consideration Nonresponse Rate and Dropouts

First take into consideration nonresponders and calculate the sample size:

$$n_1 = n/(1 - \text{nonresponse rate})$$

Then calculate the sample size by considering the dropout rate:

$$n_2 = n_1/(1 - \text{dropout rate})$$

In randomized controlled trials (RCTs), when you commit for intent-to-treat analysis, the methods of handling missing data or dropouts are different. For further discussion, do consult your statistician regarding these aspects.

The main thing is that you should not promise the moon when it comes to committing sample size for your research. Taking decisions based on available logical evidence will be the best approach in sample size estimation.

■ SOFTWARE FOR CALCULATING SAMPLE SIZE

The software that are used for calculating sample size are given in **Box 13.2**.

Example 1

A study is being planned to find out the prevalence of hypertension among the adults of North India. What would be the sample size required for this study?

Now, there are two ways to do it. You can either use a formula to do it or use a software available on the internet. First, let us calculate the sample size using the Epi Info software. You can access this by typing and clicking "https://www.cdc.gov/epiinfo/index.html" in your browser. You will be directed to the Epi Info

---

Box 13.2: Software for calculating sample size.

- Sample size calculators that can be downloaded for free and used to find the sample sizes:
    - Epi Info 7 for Windows can be downloaded from: *http://wwwn.cdc.gov/epiinfo/7/*
    - Power and sample size (PS2) calculation can be downloaded from: *http://biostat.mc.vanderbilt.edu/wiki/Main/PowerSampleSize*
    - G Power 3 for sample size calculation can be downloaded from: *http://www.psycho.uni-duesseldorf.de/abteilungen/aap/gpower3/download-and-register*
- Online calculators for sample sizes:
    - *http://www.openepi.com/OE2.3/Menu/OpenEpiMenu.htm (based on Epi Info)*
    - *http://www.raosoft.com/samplesize.html*
    - *http://www.stat.ubc.ca/~rollin/stats/ssize/*

software of Centers for Disease Control (CDC), USA. After downloading and installing it in your computer it looks like the picture shown in **Figure 13.2**. Epi Info is compatible with Windows operating system computers.

Using Epi Info

Click on "StatCalc" → "sample size and power" → "population survey" and the next box pops up (**Fig. 13.3**). Note that there are three values to fill here before you get the sample size:
1. Population size
2. Expected frequency
3. Confidence limits

1. Population Size

The first is your *population size* from which you want to draw your sample. For a large population, or statistically we say an "infinite" population, put it as 99,999. It is advised that you see for the variation in the sample sizes by changing the population sizes and then you will appreciate that after a certain population size (9,999), the sample size does not change much. But for smaller population sizes, *e.g.*, a study on prevalence of hypertension among medical students of a particular batch of 100 medical students, we have to put the population size as 100 in the software and it will return the appropriate sample size. It is recommended to put >20,000 in the population size, and calculate sample size for "infinite" population. Sample size for a "finite" population will be less than that for "infinite" population.

2. Expected Frequency

The next value to be filled is of *expected frequency*. As has been discussed earlier, you should have an estimate of the prevalence of hypertension among the adults in North India

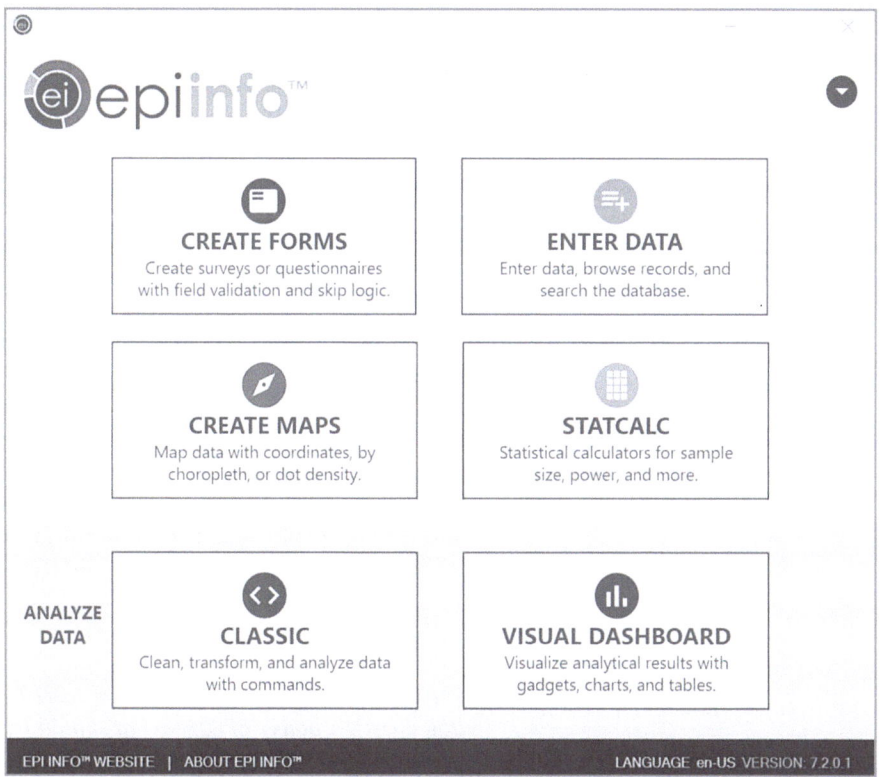

Fig. 13.2: Epi Info 7 software for Windows-based calculation of sample size.

before you can get the sample size for this study. Note that you should have an estimate only and not the actual thing. If you do not have an estimate, then you can do a small pilot study of, say, 50 adults in North India or search the review of literature. In this case, suppose it is 15% by one published study on hypertension in India. We put the expected frequency as 15%.

3. Confidence Limits

The third value to be put is "*confidence limits*". In this example, it has been mentioned as 5%. This is also known as acceptable margin of error and we notice here that Epi Info also uses this term. As you decrease the confidence limits, you increase the accuracy of your finding and so the sample size increases. You can also notice in **Figure 13.3** that as confidence level increases (the surety with which you can tell that the population prevalence lies within the confidence interval), the sample size also increases. By convention, we take the confidence level as 95%.

Here we get the sample size as 196.

Formula-based Calculation

$n = [(z_{\alpha/2})^2 \times P \times (100 - P)]/e^2$, where $z_{\alpha/2}$ is the z value for a particular confidence level determined by α value, P is the estimated prevalence and e is the acceptable absolute error.

$= [(1.96)^2 \times 15 \times (100 - 15)]/(5)^2 = 196$

Fig. 13.3: Epi Info: Values needed to calculate sample size.

Example 2

The objective of this study was to test the hypothesis that administration of a daily iron supplement from enrollment to 28 weeks of gestation to initially iron-replete, nonanemic pregnant women would reduce the prevalence of anemia at 28 weeks. What is the sample size required for this study?

This can be calculated using power and sample size (PS2) software.

Let us use PS2 Software for Calculating this (Fig. 13.4)

Figure 13.4 shows that 120 subjects are required per group. Taking the rate of loss to follow-up as 10%, 120/(1 − 0.1) = 120/0.9 = 133 per group. This means a total sample size of 266, i.e., 133 cases, which will receive iron tablets and 133 placebo group.

Formula-based Calculation

$n = [z_{\alpha/2} + z_\beta]^2 \times [p1(1 - p1) + p2(1 - p2)]/(p1 - p2)^2$ where $z_{\alpha/2}$ is the z score for a particular confidence level, z_β is the z score for a particular type 2 error, p1 is the proportion in group 1 and p2 is the proportion in group 2. Substituting the values as follows:

$z_{\alpha/2}$ for 95% confidence level = 1.96
z_β for 20% type 2 error = 0.84
p1 = 0.3 and p2 = 0.15

We get a sample size of 118 in each group. This is nearly equal to what has been achieved by using the software described above. Slight difference in sample size estimated by manual calculation and software use is expected as there are many ways to calculate sample size and different softwares use different formula for this task.

Example 3

On the basis of a 5% significance level (two-tailed test), a power of 80%, what should be the sample size to detect a difference in hemoglobin concentration of 5 g/dL and a standard deviation

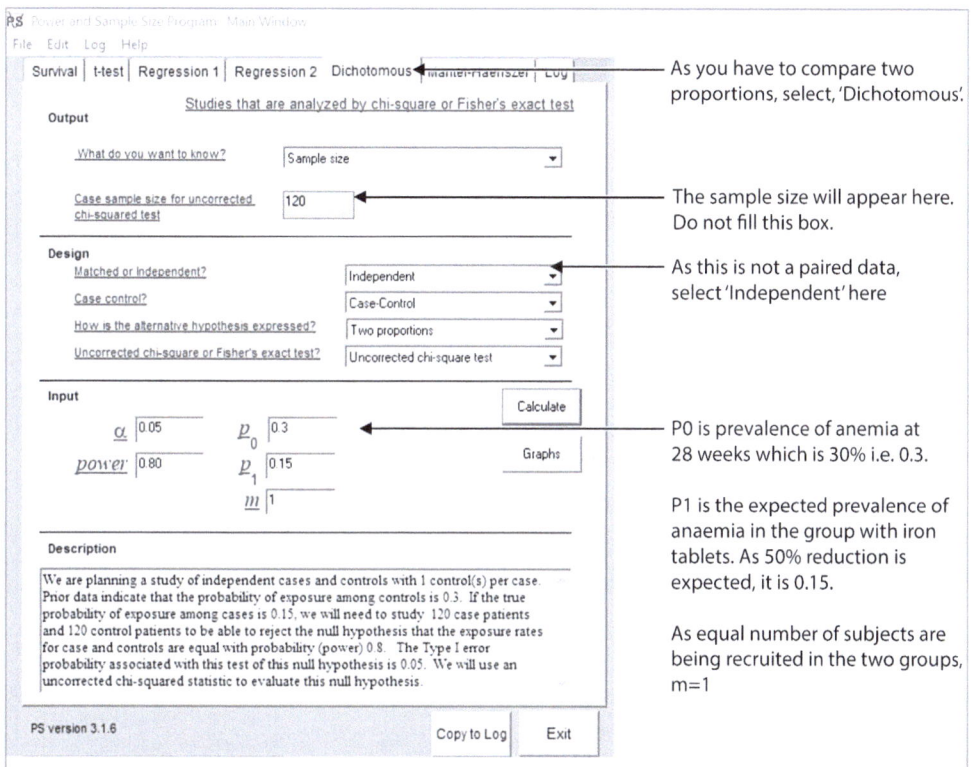

Fig. 13.4: Calculating sample size for a case–control study on hypothesis testing for comparing of proportions between two groups in PS2 software.

of 10 g/dL (standard deviation of hemoglobin concentration of the population under consideration obtained from a past study).*

PS2 Software Calculating Sample Size

As you can see in **Figure 13.5** that after putting in the values for mean difference, alpha error, power (1–beta error), mean difference, standard deviation and the ratio of the group sizes, you get a sample size of 64 in each group. See what happens as you increase the mean difference, or you change the power. This will help you develop further understanding of the relationships of power and effect size with sample size.

Formula-based Calculation

$$n = [z_{\alpha/2} + z_\beta]^2 \times 2 \times \sigma^2/\delta^2$$

where $z_{\alpha/2}$ is the z score for a particular confidence level, z_β is the z score for a particular type 2 error, σ is the standard deviation of the population and δ is the difference in mean that is clinically relevant for us to determine. Substituting the values as follows:

$z_{\alpha/2}$ for 95% confidence level = 1.96
z_β for 20% type 2 error = 0.84
$\sigma = 10$ and $\delta = 5$,

---

*(Muslimatun et al. Weekly supplementation with iron and vitamin A during pregnancy increases hemoglobin concentration but decreases serum ferritin concentration in Indonesian pregnant women. J Nutr. 2013;131(1): 85-90.)

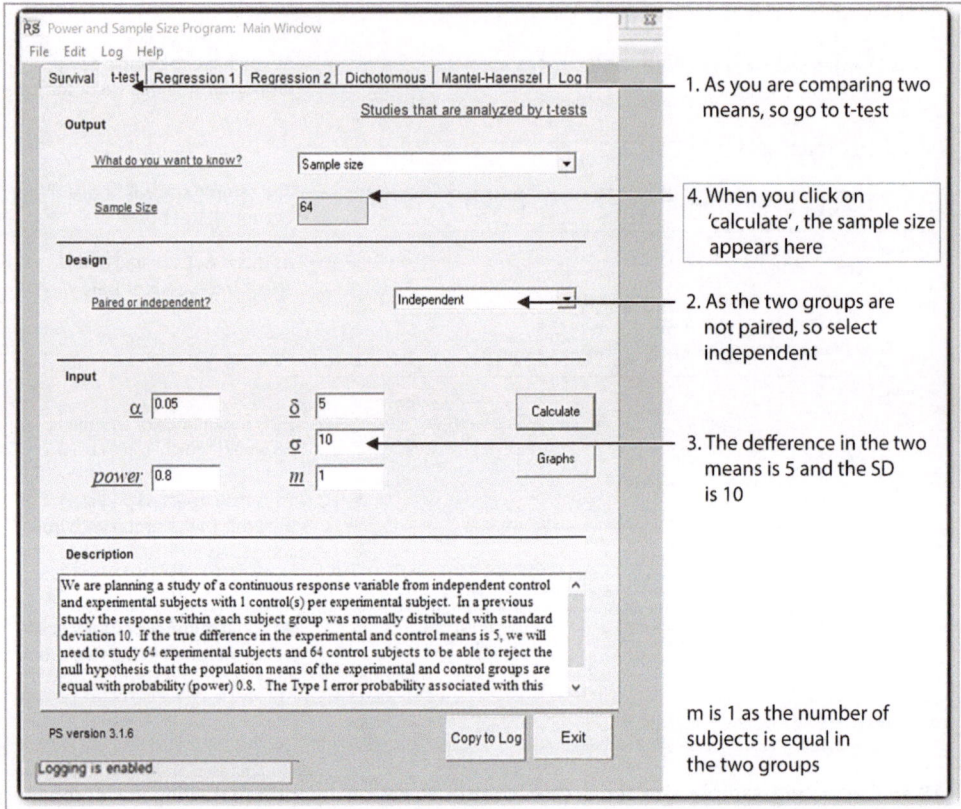

Fig. 13.5: Calculating sample size for a randomized trial, for hypothesis testing to detect difference between means of the groups in PS2 software.

We get a sample size of 63 per group, which is nearly the same as obtained by using the software mentioned above.

In case you were not having the standard deviation of the population for the variable to be studied, and from review of literature, found out the standard deviation of the two groups to be studied, then you can substitute pooled standard deviation of these two standard deviations and put in place of the standard deviation of the population in the abovementioned formula. How to calculate pooled standard deviation has been mentioned above in this chapter itself.

Example 4

What sample size is needed to detect the association of smoking and lung cancer? From previous studies, the odds ratio of the association between smoking and lung cancer is 2. It is also known from previous studies that around 20% of the non-lung cancer patients are exposed to smoking. The type I error and type II error are to be kept at the default values, i.e., 5% and 20% respectively.

Epi Info Software Calculating Sample Size

As you can see in **Figure 13.6** that after putting in the values for odds ratio, percent of controls,

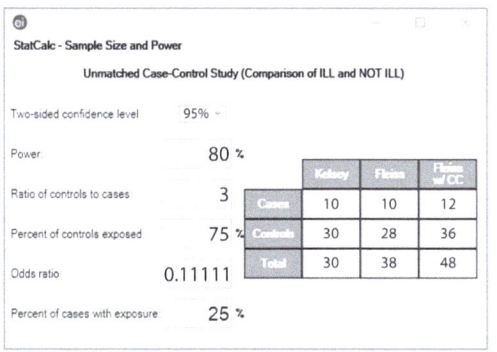

Fig. 13.6: Calculating sample size for a case–control study to detect odds ratio in Epi Info 7 software.

i.e., non lung cancer exposed to smoking, considering ratio of cases to controls as 1, and for a power of 80% and 95% confidence level, you get a sample size of 172 in each group.

Formula-based Calculation

$n = [(r + 1)/r] \times (p^*)(1 - p^*)(z_{\alpha/2} + z_\beta)^2/(p_1 - p_2)^2$ where $z_{\alpha/2}$ is the z score for a particular confidence level, z_β is the z score for a particular type 2 error, r = ratio of control to cases, p^* = average proportion exposed, i.e., proportion of exposed cases + proportion of control exposed/2; $p_1 - p_2$ = effect size of different proportion expected based on previous studies. p_1 is proportion in cases and p_2 is proportion in controls.

Substituting the values as follows:

$z_{\alpha/2}$ for 95% confidence level = 1.96
z_β for 20% type 2 error = 0.84
r = 1
p_2 = 20% = 0.2
p_1 = OR × p_2/[OR × p2 + (1 − p_2)] = 2 × 0.2/[2 × 0.2 + (1 − 0.2)] = 0.4/(1.2) = 0.33
p^* = (0.2 + 0.33)/2 = 0.265
n = 179 per group

Whether you use a formula or a statistical software, you have to report the sample size based on the method used. There will be slight difference between the sample sizes calculated using various software or formulae but that is acceptable.

■ CONCLUSION

This chapter is not intended to transform you into a statistician who is able to calculate all sorts of sample sizes; but is designed to facilitate your communication with the statistician as well as enhance your understanding about sample size estimations. The medical researchers, who usually do not have a mathematical background, can use a software for doing mathematical calculations, but the conceptual understanding is needed for deciding on the assumptions needed to determine the sample size for their research studies. It is advised to take the help of a statistician for sample size determination for your thesis protocol.

KEY MESSAGES

- An appropriate sample size is needed for the results of the research to be valid and reliable.
- Sample size is to be calculated according to the primary objective of the study.
- Calculation of sample size depends upon certain factors such as type of study, estimated statistic of interest such as prevalence, or odds ratio, among others.
- In prevalence studies, only type I error is set, whereas in studies where comparison between two groups is being done, both type I and type II error is set.
- Feasibility and dropout rates should be carefully considered before mentioning the final sample size.
- Various free software such as Epi Info, PS2, G Power, can be used to calculate sample sizes.

■ FURTHER READING

1. Bland JM. The tyranny of power: is there a better way to calculate sample size? BMJ. 2009;339:b3985.
2. Charan J, Biswas T. How to calculate sample size for different study designs in medical research? Indian J Psychol Med. 2013;35(2):121-6.
3. Flight L, Julious SA. Practical guide to sample size calculations: an introduction. Pharm Stat. 2016;15(1):68-74.
4. Florey CD. Sample size for beginners. BMJ. 1993;306(6886):1181-4.
5. Hickey GL, Grant SW, Dunning J, Siepe M. Statistical primer: sample size and power calculations—why, when and how? Eur J Cardiothorac Surg. 2018;54(1):4-9.
6. Sami W, Alrukban MO, Waqas T, Asad MR, Afzal K. Sample size determination in health research. J Ayub Med Coll Abbottabad. 2018;30(2):308-11.
7. Schmidt SAJ, Lo S, Hollestein LM. Research techniques made simple: sample size estimation and power calculation. J Invest Dermatol. 2018;138(8):1678-82.

CHAPTER 14

Ethical Issues in Thesis and Conducting Research

Kirtisudha Mishra

■ INTRODUCTION

The word "ethics" is derived from the ancient Greek word *"ēthikós,"* meaning "relating to one's character", which itself comes from the root word *"êthos"* meaning "character, moral nature." It involves systematizing and recommending rules of right and wrong conduct to govern professional interactions. Ethics are a codified set of rules customized for people in different fields.

While morals relate to personal values, which may be different for different people, ethics are moral codes which every person must adhere to. Both "morality" and "ethics" loosely refer to the difference between "good and bad" or "right and wrong." Morals may be influenced by religion and culture. Thus, what is considered right in one religion may be considered as wrong in another religion. For example, eating meat is considered immoral in some cultures, but in some other cultures, it is acceptable.

Law is where violation leads to punishment, while ethics and morals do not have any such punitive measure.

■ PRINCIPLES OF ETHICS

As a researcher, you are responsible for protecting the dignity, rights, safety and well-being of the participants enrolled in your study. There are four basic ethical principles which must be taken in account while designing a study:
1. Respect for autonomy
2. Beneficence
3. Nonmaleficence
4. Justice

Respect for Autonomy

This refers to respecting the decision-making capacities of individuals, thereby upholding the fundamental principle of respecting the dignity of the individual. Accordingly, the researcher must take a voluntary and informed consent before enrolling any individual in the study.

Beneficence and Nonmaleficence

The word *"beneficence"* has its origin from Latin meaning "to do good." *"Nonmaleficence"* is derived from the Latin phrase *"primum non nocere"*, meaning "first, do no harm." The conduct of the research should be such that it ensures a favorable balance of benefits and risks. If any risk/discomfort to the participant is inevitable, the social and scientific value of the research should be able to justify the risk.

Distributive Justice

Participants must be recruited in an impartial manner. Vulnerable individuals/groups should not be included in research, just because they are easy to enroll. Care must be taken to ensure that the individuals enrolled in the research are selected in such a way that the benefits and burdens of research are equitably distributed among them.

The four basic principles mentioned above have been expanded into twelve general principles:

1. *Principle of essentiality*: Whereby, the use of human participants is considered to be essential for the proposed research.
2. *Principle of voluntariness*: Whereby the decision-making capacity of the participant is respected. After explaining the research protocol to the participant, the latter should have the right to agree or not to agree to participate in research, as also to withdraw from research at any time.
3. *Principle of nonexploitation*: Whereby the recruitment of research participants is impartial and the benefits and burdens of the research are distributed fairly without discrimination.
4. *Principle of social responsibility*: Whereby the research is planned and conducted without disturbing social harmony in community relationships.
5. *Principle of ensuring privacy and confidentiality*: Privacy is the right of an individual to control the information that can be collected, stored, shared, or disclosed. Confidentiality is the obligation of the researcher to safeguard the entrusted information, protecting against unauthorized access, use, disclosure or modification.
6. *Principle of risk minimization*: Whereby, efforts are taken by the researcher, at all stages of the research, to ensure that the risks are minimized.
7. *Principle of professional competence*: Whereby the research is planned, conducted, evaluated, and monitored throughout by persons who are competent and have the appropriate experience and/or training.
8. *Principle of maximization of benefit*: Whereby efforts are taken to design and conduct the research in such a way as to maximize the benefits to the research participants and/or to the society.
9. *Principle of institutional arrangements*: Whereby institutions where the research is being conducted, have policies for appropriate research governance.
10. *Principle of transparency and accountability*: Whereby data generated from the research must be recorded in a fair, honest, impartial and transparent manner. The records should be available for possible external scrutiny.
11. *Principle of totality of responsibility*: Whereby all stakeholders involved in the research are responsible for all actions taken for the purpose of research.
12. *Principle of environmental protection*: Whereby researchers are accountable for ensuring protection of the environment and resources, complying to national guidelines and regulations.

INFORMED CONSENT

Written, informed, voluntary consent safeguards the individual's autonomy to make a free and voluntary decision whether to participate in the research.

The process involves three essential components:
1. Provide relevant information to potential participants.
2. Ensure that the information is comprehended by them.
3. Ensure voluntariness of participation.

Essentials of Informed Consent

- This communication process between the researcher and the participant should not

- only be before enrollment, but also continued throughout the duration of the study.
- The consent should be obtained voluntarily and not under threat or coercion of any kind or by offering any undue incentives.
- Detailed information regarding the research, including all the expected benefits and harms/discomfort must be disclosed to the proposed participant in simple terms, in the language in which the participant understands.
- If an individual is not capable of giving voluntary, informed consent, the consent of the legally acceptable/authorized representative (LAR) should be obtained. If a participant or LAR is illiterate, a literate impartial witness, who is neither a relative of the participant nor involved in the research, should also be present during the informed consent process. The witness should be a literate person who can read the patient information sheet (PIS) and consent form and understand the language of the participant.
- The informed consent document (ICD) has two parts: (1) Patient/participant information sheet (PIS) (**Box 14.1**) and the (2) Certificate of participation (**Box 14.2**). Information about the research is included in the PIS, followed by the consent form in which the participant acknowledges that she/he has understood the information given in the PIS and is volunteering to be included in that research. The ICD, i.e., PIS and certificate of consent, should have the required elements (given below) and should be reviewed and approved by the ethics committee (EC) before enrollment of the participants.
- Adequate time should be given to the participant to read the consent form and clarify her/his doubts from the investigator before deciding to enroll in the research.
- The researcher who administers the consent must also sign and date the consent form.
- A copy of the PIS should be given to the participant for his/her record.
- Young children do not have the cognitive ability to comprehend the details of the study and make decisions and hence are considered vulnerable because their autonomy is compromised. Older children, even with cognitive ability to understand the research, lack legal capacity to consent. Thus, the decision regarding participation and withdrawal of a child in research must be taken by the parents/LAR.

Most importantly, the ICD (shown in **Boxes 14.1** and **14.2** in English) should be prepared in the language understood by the enrolled participant/caregiver.

ASSENT

A child's agreement to participate in research is called assent. In addition to consent from parents/LARs, assent should be obtained from children of 7–18 years of age. If the child objects, this wish must be respected. If a child is above 7 years of age, the researcher has to explain the proposed research in a very simple manner, in a language which the child understands. Content of the assent form has to be in accordance with the developmental level and maturity of the children to be enrolled.

Important Points about Assent

- There is no need to document assent for children below 7 years of age.
- For children between 7 and 12 years, verbal assent must be obtained in the presence of the parents/LAR and should be recorded.
- For children between 12 and 18 years, written assent must be obtained. This assent form also must be signed by the parents/LAR.

PARTICIPANT/PATIENT INFORMATION SHEET

All the participants of the study must be provided a written document (PIS) containing the following information:

Box 14.1: Informed Consent Form: Part 1: Patient Information Sheet

Patient Information Sheet
Title: "Daily versus Depot Oral Vitamin D3 for Treating Nutritional Rickets"
Name of Principal Investigator: Dr ABC
Name of Supervisor: Dr XYZ
Name of Organization: UCMS and GTB Hospital, Delhi

- **Introduction**
  - I am Dr ABC working as postgraduate student in University College of Medical Sciences and Guru Teg Bahadur Hospital, Delhi
  - I am doing research on "daily *versus* depot oral vitamin D3 for treating nutritional rickets" wherein children participating in the study will receive oral vitamin D3 and calcium for treatment of rickets in accordance with global recommendations on treatment of this disease
  - You may discuss anything in this form with anyone else you feel comfortable talking to. You can decide whether to participate or not after you have talked it over. You do not have to decide immediately
  - There may be some words you do not understand or things that you want me to explain more about because you are interested or concerned. Please ask me to stop at anytime and I will take time to explain
- **Purpose of the research**
  The recent recommendations on treatment of nutritional rickets in children advocate the use of lower doses of vitamin D3, given orally, either as daily doses or as a one-time mega dose. The scientific evidence for these recommendations are derived from studies conducted in children who are fair-skinned. Vitamin D deficiency is greater in dark skinned populations and these recommendations need to be tested in these children
- **Type of research intervention**
  This study is a comparative study involving treatment of nutritional rickets in children who have previously never received any form of vitamin D3 or calcium medications
- **Participant selection**
  We are inviting children with nutritional rickets, attending the outpatient/emergency/inpatient areas of the pediatrics department of GTB hospital
- **Voluntary participation**
  Your participation in this research is entirely voluntary. If you choose not to participate all the services you receive at this center will continue and nothing will change. The choice that you make will have no bearing on any work-related evaluations or reports
- **Procedures**
  - During this study, the selected children will undergo detailed history and examination. Participants will be divided in two groups. The groups are selected by chance, and both groups will receive the standard treatment. One group will receive single oral vitamin D3 (60,000 IU in children 3–12 months, 150,000 IU in children >12 months to 5 years) on day 1 as vitamin D granules under direct supervision. Other group will receive daily oral vitamin D3 (2,000 IU in children 3–12 months and 4,000 IU in children >12 months to 5 years) as vitamin D3 drops for 3 months duration. Children in both groups will receive oral calcium supplementation (250 mg/day for infants and 500 mg/day for children 12 months to 5 years) for 3 months duration
  - 3 mL blood sample will be taken from your child at time of enrollment and on day 90 in all children. 2 mL venous blood will be drawn at 4 weeks. X-rays of both wrist and knee will be done at beginning of study and 12th week to assess severity of disease and response to treatment respectively
  - The research will take place over 3 months. During that time, it will be necessary for you to come to the hospital on three occasions

Contd…

Contd...

- **Risks**
  There will be minor discomfort while drawing the blood samples. We will try to make it as painless as possible. There may also be a risk of low or high calcium in blood which will mostly cause no problem but sometimes can result in symptoms which we will manage by appropriate treatment
- **Benefits**
  The child will be benefitted by treatment and close follow-up. The community will be benefitted as and when these results get published and are provide robust scientific evidence for these recommendations
- **Reimbursements**
  You will not be provided any incentive or any travel expenses to take part in the research
- **Confidentiality**
  We will not be sharing information about you to anyone outside of the research team. Any information about you will have a number on it instead of your name and only the researchers will have access to the information. Relevant information about investigations of your child will be shared with you
- **Sharing the results**
  Nothing that you tell us today will be shared with anybody outside the research team, and nothing will be attributed to you by name. It is likely that results of this study get published later but all data will be anonymized
- **Right to refuse or withdraw**
  You do not have to take part in this research if you do not wish to do so. You may stop participating in the research at any time that you wish without your job being affected. I will give you an opportunity at the end of the interview/discussion to review your remarks, and you can ask to modify or remove portions of those, if you do not agree with my notes or if I did not understand you correctly
- **Who to contact**
  If you have any questions, you can ask them now or later. If you wish to ask questions later, you may contact any of the following: (Dr ABC1234567890 email at drabc@hotmail.com) and (Dr XYZ 0987654321, email at drxyz@gmail.com)
  You can ask me any more questions about any part of the research study, if you wish to. Do you have any questions?
  This study has been approved the Institutional Ethics Committee for Human Research, University College of Medical Sciences, Delhi

Essential Elements of Patient Information Sheet

- Title of the research project.
- Statement mentioning that it is a research.
- Purpose and methods of the research in simple language.
- Estimated number of participants to be enrolled.
- Expected duration of the participation, frequency of contact, and types of data to be collected.
- Expected benefits to the participant or community from the research. It is important to convert medical terminology into simple, easily understandable words. Translation into local language must be done very carefully as often the online translation results in bizarre and meaningless sentences.
- Any foreseeable risks, discomfort or inconvenience to the participant resulting from participation in the study.
- Extent to which confidentiality of records would be maintained.
- Payment/reimbursement for participation and incidental expenses depending on the type of study.
- Free treatment and/or compensation of participants for research-related injury and/or harm.

> **Box 14.2: Certificate of Consent: Part II of Informed Consent Form.**
>
> **Certificate of Consent**
> I have been invited to participate on research about "daily *versus* depot oral vitamin D3 for treating nutritional rickets" I have read the foregoing information, or it has been read to me. I have had the opportunity to ask questions about it and any questions that I have asked have been answered to my satisfaction.
> I agree to take part in the research and allow my child to be included in this study.
> Print name of child   _____
> Print name of parent/caregiver   _____
> Signature of parent/caregiver   _____
> Date   _____ (Day/month/year)
>
> *If illiterate*
> I have witnessed the accurate reading of the consent form to the parent, and the individual has had the opportunity to ask questions. I confirm that the individual has given consent freely.
> Print name of witness (not a parent)_____Thumb print of participant
> Signature of witness _____
> Date _____ Day/month/year
>
> **Statement by the researcher/person taking consent**
> I have accurately read out the information sheet to the potential participant and to the best of my ability made sure that the participant understands that the following will be done:
> 1. Detailed clinical history and examination.
> 2. Treatment of child with daily low dose or single high dose oral vitamin D determined by lottery.
> 3. Collection of blood samples and X-rays.
>
> I confirm that the participant was given an opportunity to ask questions about the study and all the questions asked by the participant have been answered correctly and to the best of my ability. I confirm that the individual has not been coerced into giving consent and the consent has been given freely and voluntarily.
> A copy of this ICF has been provided to the participant.
> Name of Researcher/person taking the consent _____
> Signature of Researcher/person taking the consent _____

- Freedom of the individual to participate and/or withdraw from research at any time without penalty or loss of benefits to which the participant would otherwise be entitled.
- The identity of the research team and contact persons with addresses and phone numbers, (e.g., PI/Co, PI for queries related to the research and chairperson/member secretary/or helpline for appeal against violations of ethical principles and human rights)

Additional Elements which may be Included in Patient Information Sheet

- Any alternative procedures or courses of treatment that is available to the participant, other than the one in research mode.
- If the research could lead to any stigmatizing condition, such as HIV and genetic disorders, provision for pretest and post test counseling.

- Insurance coverage if any, for research-related adverse events.
- Information on possible current and future uses of the biological material including:
  - Period of storage.
  - Participant's right to prevent use of her/his biological sample, such as DNA.
  - Provisions to ensure confidentiality of biologically sensitive information which might be discovered from participant's biological material.
  - Post-research benefit sharing, if research on biological material and/or data leads to commercialization.
  - Publication plan, if any, including photographs and pedigree charts.

RESPONSIBLE CONDUCT OF RESEARCH

Responsible conduct of research (RCR) includes the following components:
- Values
- Policies
- Planning and conducting research.
- Reviewing and reporting research.
- Responsible authorship and publication.

The first four elements are discussed below. Authorship issues are discussed in Chapter 23.

Values

Values of a RCR include honesty, accuracy, efficiency, fairness, objectivity, reliability, accountability, transparency, personal integrity, and knowledge of current best practices. Lack of integrity of the researchers and unethical behavior in scientific research not only nullifies the meaning of the outcomes, but also destroys the public's faith in science.

Policies

Protection of human participants: This responsibility rests with the institution, the EC and the researchers. Also, policies must be in place for monitoring research regarding method of data capture, management, conflicts of interest, reporting of scientific misconduct, and serious adverse events.

Planning and Conducting Research

Quality research requires that every step is planned and designed thoroughly. Protocols need to be made with robust methodology.

Data acquisition, management, sharing, and ownership: The integrity of research is valid only when data are collected by appropriate, fool-proof methods. Data are useful, only when it is recorded accurately and stored carefully. Data may be recorded in hard copy, soft or electronic copy. Researchers should ensure clarity about data ownership, publication rights, and obligations following data collection.

After collection, it is of utmost importance that the data be properly stored, protecting against damage, loss or theft, as it may be needed at a later stage to confirm research findings, or to be re-analyzed. Back-up data of computer files should be saved in a secure place at a site that is different from the original data storage site.

Reporting Research

Once a research is completed, it must be published, irrespective of the results. Otherwise, it would be most unethical to expose another set of participants to the same risks to obtain the same results.

GUIDELINES ON ETHICS IN PATIENT CARE AND RESEARCH

The Nuremberg Code of 1947 was the first international treatise emphasizing the essentiality of obtaining voluntary consent, whenever a research is done involving human beings. This was followed by the Declaration of Helsinki guidelines in 1964, by the World Medical Association, the latest version being issued in October 2013. In 1979, the Belmont Report, for the first time, stated the three basic ethical principles while doing research in human subjects: Respect for persons, beneficence, and justice.

The International Conference on Harmonization (ICH) brought out the Good Clinical Practice Guidelines E6 (R1) in 1996, with revised version as E6 (R2) in 2016. UNESCO's Universal Declaration on Bioethics and Human Rights (2005) also defined the Universal Codes of Ethics to be adopted by the member countries. The Indian Council of Medical Research (ICMR) has brought out revised National Guidelines for Biomedical and Health Research in 2017, which is adapted from the international guidelines.

■ DATA SAFETY MONITORING BOARD

Data collected and stored in a clinical trial requires continuous monitoring to ensure that the rights of the trial participants are safeguarded. Data Safety Monitoring Board (DSMB) is a group of independent experts, external to the trial, who regularly review the accumulated data from ongoing clinical trials and advise the sponsor about the continued safety of the trial participants, validity, and scientific merit of the trial.

Not all clinical trials require a DSMB. It is particularly required in trials dealing with the objectives of saving lives or to reduce the risk of a major adverse health outcome. DSMB should also be established in case of long-term trials even in non-life-threatening diseases, in order to do interim analysis.

The DSMB is authorized to stop a study midway, if it finds any harm/potential of harm to the participants, based on interim data evaluation.

■ REGISTRATION OF TRIAL

It is now mandatory to register all clinical trials with the Clinical Trials Registry of India (CTRI) maintained by the ICMR. Registration with CTRI is voluntary for other types of biomedical and health research. Only the trials which are registered in any of the public databases are considered for publication by most major biomedical journals of India.

■ INSTITUTIONAL ETHICS COMMITTEE

Every research proposal must be reviewed by an Institutional Ethics Committee (IEC), and only after approval by the IEC, the investigator can proceed with the research. The institute is responsible for establishing an IEC for ethical review and monitoring of the research projects.

Composition of Ethics Committee

The composition of IEC is such that it has a balance between medical and nonmedical members, with experience, robust knowledge and training in research ethics. The committee is chaired by a senior, well-respected person, not affiliated to the institute, who is accountable for independent and efficient functioning of the committee. The Member Secretary is responsible for organizing and conducting the meetings. Other members of the committee include clinicians, basic medical scientist, lay person, legal expert, and social scientist.

Roles and Responsibilities

- Institutional Ethics Committee is entrusted with the responsibility of ensuring protection of the dignity, rights, safety and well-being of the research participants.
- The IEC must ensure ethical conduct of research by the investigator team.
- The IEC must ensure that universal ethical values and international scientific standards are followed.
- The IEC should assist in the development and education of researchers, clinicians, students, and others in the institute.
- The IEC should ensure that the privacy of the individual and confidentiality of data are protected.
- The IEC should review progress reports, final reports, and adverse events/serious adverse events.
- The IEC should recommend appropriate compensation for research-related injury, if any.

CONCLUSION

Any research done on human participants must be conducted within the boundaries of four ethical principles, namely, respect for autonomy, beneficience, nonmaleficence, and justice. However scientific a research may be, transgression of the rights and safety of the participants devalues the study and degrades the respect of the researchers. As a postgraduate student, it is important that ethics of research be ingrained in you, right from this early stage of your scientific career.

KEY MESSAGES

- There are four basic ethical principles to be followed in any research study: (1) autonomy, (2) Beneficence, (3) nonmaleficence, and (4) justice.
- A patient information sheet, giving explicit details, written in a lucid language, understandable by the participant, is a *sine qua non* of any research study.
- After comprehending the research procedure, voluntariness of participation must be ensured, without any kind of coercion or incentive.
- Before commencing any research, the protocol must be reviewed and approved by an independent ethics committee, functioning within the scope of national or international standards.

FURTHER READING

1. EUPATI. (2016). Clinical Trial Data Safety Monitoring Board (DSMB). [online] Available fromhttps://www.eupati.eu/clinical-development-and-trials/clinical-trial-data-safety-monitoring-board-dsmb/[Last accessed April 30, 2020].
2. Horner J. Morality, ethics, and law: introductory concepts. Semin Speech Lang. 2003;24(4):263-74.
3. ICMR. (2017). National Ethical Guidelines for Biomedical and Health Research Involving Human Participants.[online] Available from https://www.icmr.nic.in/sites/default/files/guidelines/ICMR_Ethical_Guidelines_2017.pdf [Last accessed April 30, 2020].
4. World Medical Association. (2018). WMA Declaration of Helsinki: ethical principles for medical research involving human subjects. Available from https://www.wma-declaration-of-helsinki-ethical-principles-for-medical-research-involving-human-subjects.pdf [Last accessed April 30, 2020].

CHAPTER 15

Preparing a Case Record Form: Get, Set, and Go

Pankaj Kumar Garg

■ INTRODUCTION

What is a Case Record Form (CRF)?

- A CRF is a printed or electronic document used in a study to collect and record the required information as per the protocol.
- Although the thesis protocol provides the detailed methodology for conducting the trial, the case record form (CRF) is the main day-to-day tool that enables the correct information to be captured at the right time.
- Case record form forms an integral part of the thesis protocol, and must be attached before submission of protocol for approval. CRF should ensure that there is no discrepancy between the "specified methodology" and "what is actually being recorded".

Purpose of the Case Record Form

- Collects relevant data in a *specific format* in accordance with the objectives.
- Facilitates the uniform recording of the data by different observers through standardization.
- Allows for efficient and complete data transfer to the excel sheet or to the SPSS sheet for processing, analyzing, and reporting.

■ ATTRIBUTES OF A GOOD CASE-RECORD FORM

Identifying Details

Obviously, you will have the identifying details of the patients; however, you must enter the identifying details in the header section of the word file of CRF and always number the pages. It will help to correctly identify and relocate the detached CRF pages.

Layout Style

You have to adhere to the general principles of good design while making CRF for your thesis project. Obviously, you have to make it look good. Your CRF should not look wordy and complicated. You need to remember time and again that your CRF should be so simple and clear that any of your friends can also fill it, if need arises, without making errors.

Font style does influence the readability of the CRF. Times New Roman or Arial font is good for text articles. You should not select very small or big font-sized text. Text smaller than 10 points is too small for easy reading while larger than 12 points is too large and will occupy a lot of space of CRF. A 12-point-sized font seems fit for text questions. You also need to adhere to the same font style and size throughout your CRF to have uniformity and familiarity.

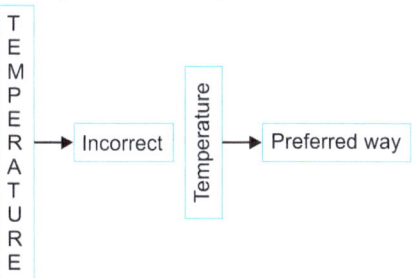

If the text needs to be turned 90°, e.g., for column headers, you must turn the texts as complete words and not as individual letters stacked on top of each other.

Contents of Case Record Form

1. Avoid open questions unless your study design specifically demands it.

   ```
   Site of involvement on intestinal tuberculosis:....
                           OR
   Site of involvement in intestine tuberculosis:
   Duodenum ☐    Jejunum ☐    Ileum ☐
   Colon ☐                        (Preferred way)
   ```

2. You must try to collect the value of a variable in the form of continuous data and not categorical data. A continuous data can always be converted into categorical data while the reverse is not possible. See the box below.

   ```
   Duration of cough:
   <4 weeks ☐   4–8 weeks ☐   8–12 weeks ☐
                >12 weeks ☐

   Duration of cough: ........(in weeks) (Preferred way)
   ```

3. If a few variables are to be measured repeatedly, you must clearly record them in tabular form specifying the time. See **Table 15.1**.
4. Always remember to write the measurement of units in the CRF. See the Box below.

   ```
   Height...... OR Height (in cm)...... (Preferred way)
   Temp...... OR Temp. (in °C)...... (Preferred way)
   ```

TABLE 15.1: Format for repeated recording of a variable.

Time	Pulse rate	Respiratory rate
At admission		
6 hours		
12 hours		

Format of the Questions

Use simple and short sentences. Asking two questions together (known as double-barreled questions) may create erroneous answers— "have you had fever and loose stools?" Positive answer may mean he had fever or loose stools, or both fever and loose stools.

Try to word all the questions in a manner so that their answers cannot be changed. See the example below.

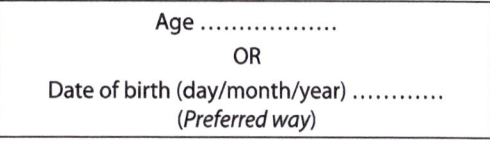

You must refrain from framing double negative questions. For example, "Don't you have any pain for the last 24 hours?" Instead asking "Are you pain-free for the last 24 hours?" would be better.

Coding of Options

Coding of options is very important when there are multiple answers for a single question (**Fig. 15.1**).

Coding will help you in transferring the data from CRF to master sheet. So, you are advised to discuss with your guide and statistician in length while designing the CRF. A model CRF is provided as (**Annexure**) to this Book.

Pre-study Checking of Case Record Form

It is advisable to fill a few CRFs (around 10) with hypothetical data and analyze this data to check

```
                                    (Preferred way)
Gender          Male          ☐   OR  Gender          Male (1)      ☐
                Female                                Female (2)
Site involved   Duodenum      ☐   OR  Site involved   Duodenum (1)  ☐
                Jejunum       ☐                       Jejunum (2)
                Ileum         ☐                       Ileum (3)
                Colon         ☐                       Colon (4)
```

Fig 15.1: Example of coding of options.

if the objectives of the study are being fulfilled or not. This exercise would straightaway bring out any error in the CRF which must be revised again. Remember, any error detected in the CRF after the study is complete, cannot be corrected.

Electronic Case Record Form

It is increasingly becoming common to design an electronic CRF in a computer software—Microsoft access or in SPSS. The researcher can carry it in a palmtop or in a tablet and quickly fill it. This also provides a quick analysis of the data which is already recorded in an analyzable form.

■ CONCLUSION

A well-designed CRF is an essential step in the conduct of a study and makes your life easy when you perform meaningful analysis of the data at the completion of the study. Enough time must be spent in designing the CRF.

KEY MESSAGES

- A CRF is the soul of a research project and due diligence must be given in its design and content.
- A case record must be made objective, simple, and easy to fill.
- You must always fill a few CRFs with hypothetical data at the beginning of the study to check whether it is able to address all the stated objectives in the study.

■ FURTHER READING

1. Lu Z, su J. Clinical data management: Current status, challenges, and future directions from industry perspectives. Open Access J Clin Trials 2010;2:93-105.
2. Bellary S, Krishnankutty B, Latha MS. Basics of case report form designing in clinical research. Perspect Clin Res. 2014 Oct;5(4):159-66.

CHAPTER 16

Planning the Statistical Analysis

Pankaj Kumar Garg

INTRODUCTION

This chapter is not intended to make you understand the complex formulae or calculate various statistical values, but to enable you interpret the common statistical terms. This chapter will also help you in deciding which statistical tests are applicable to your research question.

POPULATION VERSUS SAMPLE

If your mom asks you to go to the market and buy 5 kg rice, you would go to a rice shop and ask the shopkeeper to show you a variety of rice. The shopkeeper would show you a number of rice bags. What would you do? You would, then, pick a handful of rice from a bag and assess the quality of whole of the rice in that particular bag. You would do the same thing repeatedly for all the bags and would select the one you feel is of best quality. Let us come back to statistics: What you would be doing is exactly the same what the sampling means. Actually, you would be selecting a "sample" of rice from the bag of rice "population" to decide the quality of rice in various bags. And, you assume that a handful of rice, the sample, would truly represent the quality of rice in the bag, the population (**Fig. 16.1**).

- A *population* is a total collection of anything about which inferences are to be made in any study.
- A *sample* is a small part of the population; it is selected to represent the population from which it is drawn, in order to carry out a study or research.

The question arises as to why we should really sample the population. Why cannot we consider the entire population for the purpose of the study or investigation; this will really provide us the true results about the population, without any assumption. But, is it feasible? Perhaps not.

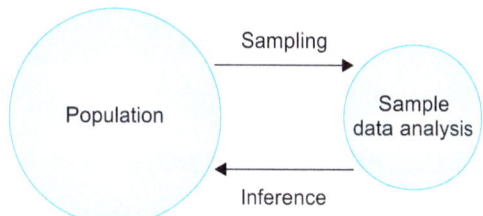

Fig. 16.1: An ideal sample should be representative of the population, and inferences drawn by studying the "sample" should be applicable to the "population."

There are many reasons that necessitate sampling. The first and foremost is the size of the population which may not be manageable. A sample has a size which is feasible for you. Sample size is dictated by many factors that include the overall size of the population and available resources at hand, such as time and money. One cannot study an unlimited population; however, study on a subset (sample) is definitely possible. However, the subset has to be representative of the population. Following are the examples of scenarios where the sample is not representative of the population:

Population	Sample
All medical students in India	Medical students in Delhi
All adults (above 21 years of age) in India	Adults in East Delhi
All patients suffering from tuberculosis in India	Hospitalized tuberculosis patients in AIIMS
All medical teachers in India	Medical teachers in University of Delhi

In case of taking Census, any form of sampling would not give us the exact number, unless we study the population in totality. Census is a classical example where the whole population is included.

You must have seen a lot of discussion on exit polls during election times over television. Exit poll is a post-voting poll which is conducted just after a voter walks out after casting his or her vote to predict the actual result (of the population) on the basis of the information collected from a few hundred or thousand voters (sample).

■ VARIABLES AND DATA

- A *variable* is something whose value can vary. For example, age, gender, and ethnicity are variables.
- *Data* are the values you get when you measure a variable. For example, 22 years (for the variable age), male (for the variable sex), or Aryan (for the variable ethnicity).

Categorical versus Continuous Data

There are broadly two types of data:
1. Categorical or continuous data
2. Numerical or continuous data

1. Categorical data is one which can be placed into categories or groups. Examples:
   a. Result: Pass, fail
   b. Blood groups: O, A, B, AB
   c. Severity of disease: Mild, Moderate, Severe
2. Continuous (numerical) data is the one which can be measured in whole numbers and fractions. Examples:
   a. Height: in exact cm or in inches
   b. Weight: in exact grams or kg
   c. Blood pressure: in exact mm Hg

When you analyze continuous data, you would sometimes wish to group the numerical values into categories. For example, you may want to analyze age data in age groups (<20 years, 20–40 years, >40 years), even though the respondents were asked to enter their age as a numerical value. So, a numerical or continuous data can easily be converted and expressed as a categorical data.

Paired versus Unpaired Data

Two measurements or values of a variable in the same subject before and after an intervention are called *paired data*. Two measurements are said to be paired when they come from the same observational unit (subject/patient/person). Measurements are also considered paired when a variable is measured in a case and a matched control. Measurements or values of a variable that are not related to each other are called *unpaired data*; this means that two measurements are said to be unpaired when they come from the different observational units. A few examples follow:

Paired data	Unpaired data
Blood pressure of an individual before and after taking a drug	Blood pressure in two different persons after taking a drug
Helicobacter pylori sensitivity before and after proton pump inhibitor treatment	*Helicobacter pylori* sensitivity in gastric cancer and duodenal patients
Blood sugar in an individual before and after lactose ingestion	Blood sugar in diabetics and nondiabetics after lactose ingestion

Dependent versus Independent Variables

In a study, the *independent variable* is one that is varied or manipulated or controlled by the researcher. In contrast, *dependent variables* are not controlled or manipulated in any way but instead are simply measured or recorded; they vary in relation to the independent variables. For example, a good crop yield will depend upon water irrigation, fertilizers, and pesticides. So, crop yield is a dependent variable while water irrigation, fertilizers, and pesticides are independent variables.

CENTRAL TENDENCY AND DISPERSION
Measures of Central Tendency

Central tendency is defined as middle value of data which represents the whole data. Let us put this in another way: The value around which all the observations in the data set appear to concentrate. There are several ways in which the central tendency for a particular data may be represented. You will soon realize that this depends upon the type of data, whether continuous or categorical.

For continuous data: Three common measures of central tendency are—mean, median, and mode.
- Mean:
  - Sum of all values divided by the number of values.
  - Most common measure of centrality.
  - Most useful when data follow normal or Gaussian distribution (bell-shaped curve). We will soon discuss this.
- Median:
  - "Middle" value when observations are arranged in either ascending or descending manner. It can be simply put as: Median is the value such that half of all the observed values are above and half of the values are below it.
  - Most useful measure when data is nonuniform.
- Mode:
  - Most frequently observed value.
  - Rarely used.

For *categorical data*, we use proportions or its percentage.

Measures of Spread or Dispersion

Measures of spread or dispersion of a data provides an idea of the extent to which the values are clustered or spread out. The most common measures to describe variability are *standard deviation* (SD) and *interquartile range* (IQR).

Standard deviation: It provides information about how the data is spread out or scattered around the mean. Let us take an example of age of five individuals 23, 25, 27, 29, and 31. Here SD will tell how the rest of the values are spread out around 27, the mean. Statistically, SD is a function of the squared differences of each observation from the mean. One SD includes 68% of values while two SDs include 95% of values around the mean (**Fig. 16.2A**). You should note that this presumes a normal or Gaussian distribution.

Interquartile range: It provides information about how much the data vary around the median when observations are arranged in either ascending or descending manner. It includes middle 50% of values from 1st quartile (25th percentile) to 3rd quartile (75th percentile) (**Fig. 16.2B**).

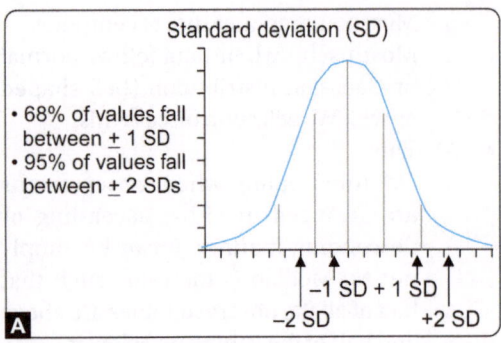

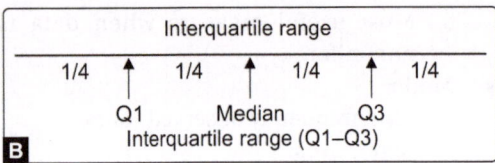

Figs. 16.2A and B: Standard deviation and Interquartile of dispersion.

Choosing the Appropriate Central Value and Measures of Dispersion

To select the appropriate measure of central tendency and dispersion, you would need to identify whether the distribution of your data is uniform (Normal) or not (Skewed). Uniform data do not have extreme values and frequency distribution graph is symmetrical. Nonuniform data has outlier values and frequency distribution graph is asymmetrical. This may be better appreciated with graphs as given in **Figure 16.3**.

Let us see an example:
Riya wants to know whether the students in her class are obese or not. So, she records the weight of all 20 students of her class. She gets a data set of 20 observations (weight) that looks like: 50, 52, 53, 54, 55, 58, 60, 64, 64, 64, 65, 65, 66, 67, 67, 69, 70, 70, 71, and 72. In this case, the mean weight is the sum of all the weight scores divided by 20. This turns out to be 1256/20 = 62.8 kg. Now see another scenario. If two obese students of weight 140 and 152 kg, respectively, are added to the class, the mean weight would become 1548/20 = 70.3 kg. Even though 70.3 kg

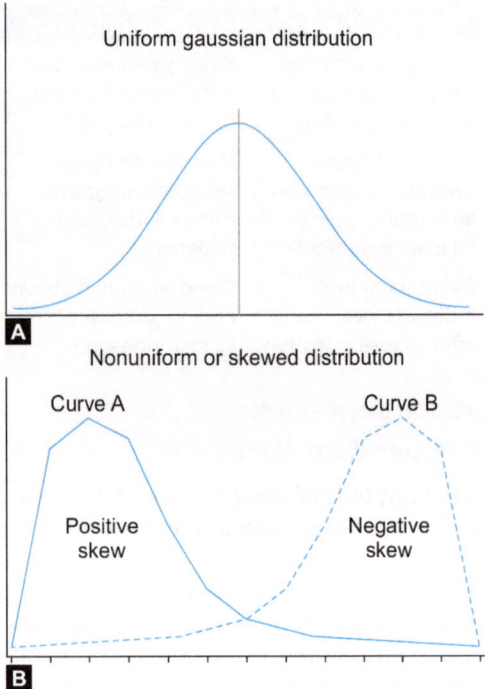

Figs. 16.3A and B: (A) Uniform and (B) Skewed distribution.

is mean weight, it is greatly exaggerated by the unusually high weight values of two obese students of 140 and 152 kg, respectively, compared to other weights. Though most of the students' weights are below the average of 70.3 kg, they all look overweight if we see arithmetic mean only. Clearly, mean does not express the centrality in this case. Remember, median is a better tool to show centrality in these scenarios where there are outlier values. In other words, median is better symbolic of centrality, if data is nonuniform. So, in the given example, the median is 65, which represents central weight of the students better, as it is not affected by the outlier values, the weight of two obese students. The same holds true when we describe the dispersion or spread of the data. SD is affected by the extremes of the data while IQR is relatively immune to this. **Flowchart 16.1** will help you in deciding how available data should be presented.

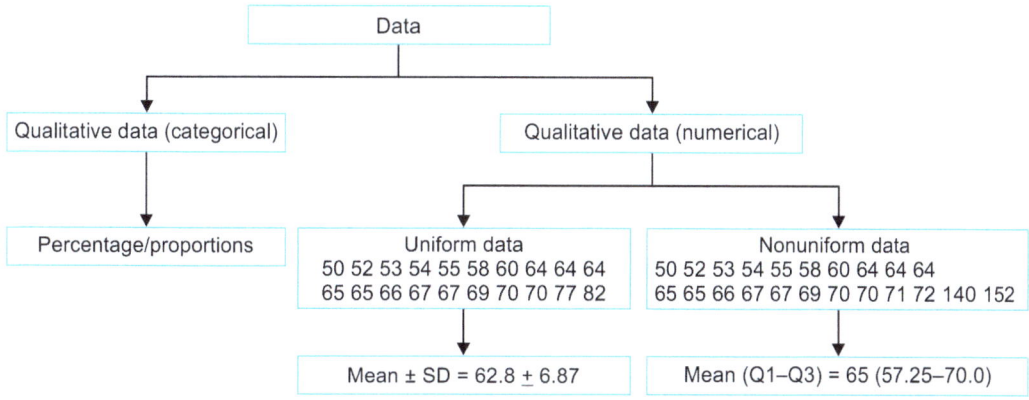

(SD: standard deviation)
Flowchart 16.1: Mean versus median in uniform and nonuniform data.

RELATIONSHIP BETWEEN THE VARIABLES

Correlation

Till now, we were discussing a data set produced by measuring a single variable. In the real-time scenario, we must be dealing with a data set produced by measuring a number of variables.

Example:
Riya records age and height of 30 students. Here, she will have two data sets of two variables, namely age and height.

Let us discuss the concept of correlation. It is a statistical tool which measures the relationship between two variables. Two variables are said to be in correlation if the alteration in one variable will result in alteration in the other variable. It is important to note that correlation can be assessed only if both dependent and independent variables are numerical (continuous) in nature.

Types of Correlation

- Positive and negative correlation
- Linear and nonlinear correlation

A *positive correlation* means that as one variable increases, the value of the other variable also increases. Two variables are said to be *negatively correlated* if the value of one variable goes up and the value of other variable comes down.

Examples:
- Positive correlation:
    - Age and height
    - Rainfall and crop yield
- Negative correlation:
    - Reading hours and concentration
    - Car mileage and resale value

Correlation Coefficient (Box 16.1)

- Correlation coefficient denotes the strength of correlation.
- The correlation coefficient is represented by the letter "r." The value of correlation coefficient varies from −1.0 to +1.0.

You must realize that the correlation does not represent causation. In other words, effect and cause conclusions cannot be derived from the correlation. Let us see why we cannot do so.
- We cannot predict the direction of the cause just based on correlation. Whether A causes B or *vice versa*? Suppose you consider two variables: Crop yield and rainfall. While correlation analysis would show a high degree of association between these two variables, it would not tell you whether increase in rainfall will cause increase in crop yield or whether an increase in crop yield will cause an increase in rainfall; however, you know crop yield is dependent

> **Box 16.1: Correlation coefficient.**
> - Range: −1 to +1
> - The closer to 0: The weaker the linear relationship
> - The closer to −1: The stronger the negative linear relationship
> - The closer to +1: The stronger the positive linear relationship
> - A correlation coefficient value of 0.8 means a stronger correlation than a correlation coefficient of 0.3. A correlation coefficient value of 0 means no correlation
> - Correlation coefficient values of −2.8, 4.5, 1.9, and 10.7 cannot exist. (Range: −1 to +1)
> - Correlation can only be seen if both the variables (dependent and independent) are numerical or continuous

on rainfall and not the other way round according to the theoretical background.
- One must never confuse correlation with causation. All that correlation represents is that the two variables are associated. There may be a third variable, a confounding variable that is related to both of them.

Examples:
- There is a positive correlation between ice cream sales and drowning deaths per month. However, it would be absolutely inappropriate to infer a causal relationship: *Ice cream causes drowning.* It is likely that a third variable "summer weather" is associated with both: People buy more ice creams and go for swimming in summer.
- A teacher's salary and price of vodka over the years may be highly positively correlated. It does not mean that as the teacher's salary increases over the years, price of vodka also goes up. Price inflation is the third variable which may have determined this association.
- A high positive correlation may be observed between the shoe size of school children and their reading skills; however, we know the growing vocabulary of children with age cannot make their feet get bigger. In fact, "Age" is the third factor involved here. As the children get older, they learn to read better and, at the same time, they outgrow their shoes.

Regression Analysis

Regression analysis is a statistical tool which helps us predict the value of one variable from the other known variables, and also identifies the association between the variables at the same time. In regression analysis, there is a dependent variable, which is the one you are trying to explain, and one or more independent variables that are related to it. You need to decide, based on your theoretical knowledge, what should be the dependent and independent variables. It is possible to predict the value of dependent variable from the value of independent variables if there is some association between the dependent and independent variables and there is some theoretical basis for that association.

Example:
Riya does an analysis to find a positive correlation of 0.7 between duration of surgery and the duration of hospital stay. She knows, from her medical knowledge, that surgery will precede the stay and not the other way round; her theoretical knowledge also says, "longer the duration of surgery, greater would be the hospital stay." So, Riya knows, hospital stay is the dependent variable while duration of surgery is an independent variable. Regression analysis will help her predict the hospital stay based on duration of surgery. Regression can be simple, multiple, or logistic.

Simple Regression

Simple regression allows you to investigate the role of "one predictor at a time" (and its effect on the response), so you have one independent variable and one dependent variable. If you wish to predict blood pressure based on the age of a person, you will use simple regression analysis.

Multiple Regression

Multiple regression allows you to investigate the role of "more than one predictor at a time" (and its effect on the response). Therefore, you can have many independent variables and one dependent variable. Most of the time you will find many variables which will be used to predict one dependent variable. Blood pressure does not depend upon age only; there are many other factors also such as lipid profile, weight, and gender. So, you will use multiple regression analysis if you wish to predict blood pressure based on many independent variables.

Logistic Regression

You use logistic regression analysis when dependent variable is a categorical one, and you want to predict it based on many independent variables. The independent variables could be categorical or continuous. If the dependent variable has two categories (male/female, dead/alive, etc.), it is known as *binary logistic regression analysis*. If the dependent variable has more than two categories (mild/moderate/severe, live/dead/lost to follow-up, etc.), it is known as *multinomial regression analysis* (**Box 16.2**).

■ RELATIVE RISKS AND ODDS RATIOS

Odds Ratio

Odds compare events with non events. If India wins three out of every five cricket matches against Pakistan, its odds of winning are 3 to 2 (expressed as 3:2). Thus, odds look at both sides of the coin: Win versus lose, present versus absent, improvement versus deterioration. We can thus summarize that odds express probability of one side of the coin (winning, for example) in the numerator and probability of the other side of the coin (losing, in this example) in the denominator.

> **Box 16.2: Correlation and regression.**
>
> **Goal of correlation analysis:**
> Quantify the strength of the correlation between two numerical or continuous variables
>
> **Goal of regression analysis:**
> Predict the value of a dependent variable from the values of at least one independent variable (also known as predictors). The independent variables can be continuous or categorical
> - *One independent variable*: Simple regression analysis
> - *More than one independent variable*: Multiple regression analysis
> - *Categorical dependent variable, two categories*: Binary logistic regression analysis
> - *Categorical dependent variable, > two outcomes*: Multinomial logistic regression analysis

Example:
Let us say, 20% of the patients suffering from myocardial infarction in the treatment group died. That means 80% of the patients survived in the treatment group. So, what are odds of death in the treatment group? Odds of death would be calculated by keeping the chances of death in the numerator (20%) and chances of survival (80%) in the denominator. So, odds would be 20%/80%. This is equal to ¼. Now, if 25% of the patients in the control group died; 75% of the patients survived. So, odds of death in the control group would be 25%/75% (1/3).

Please note that odds ratio (OR) can be defined as a ratio of ratios. OR expresses the odds of occurrence of a particular outcome in the presence or absence of a specific exposure. In the above-mentioned example, it can be described as odds of death in the treatment group as the numerator versus odds of death in the control group as denominator. The OR would be equal to (1/4)/(1/3) = 3/4 or 0.75. As 0.75 is <1, we can say probability of dying in the treatment group is more as compared to probability of dying in the control group. Had the odds ratio been >1, let us say 1.5, it would have meant odds of dying in the treatment group is 1.5 times more as compared to odds of dying in the control group.

Relative Risk

Risk is the probability of happening of an event in relation to all the possible events. If India wins three out of every five cricket matches against Pakistan, its probability of winning is 3/5 (60%).

Relative risk (RR) is a comparison between risk levels in two different groups. In other words, RR compares the risk (incidence) of an event in a group with a specific exposure with that of another group without specific exposure, e.g., lung cancer in smokers versus nonsmokers.

It must be reiterated here that RR is based upon the incidence of an event in two groups, one group with exposure and another without exposure of a risk factor. So it is advisable to use RR for prospective cohort studies.

Relative Risk versus Odds Ratio

You will see many a times OR and RR are used interchangeably; however, you must understand the difference between the two.

Example 1:
Let us assume, isolated isoniazid intake causes peripheral neuropathy in 10 of 1,000 patients while combination of isoniazid and ethambutol causes peripheral neuropathy in 20 of the 1,000 patients. The RR of peripheral neuropathy following combination drug intake would be 20/1000 ÷ 10/1000 = 2 while OR would also be 20/980 ÷ 10/980 = 2.

Example 2:
Let us again assume, isolated isoniazid intake causes hepatitis in 10 out of 100 patients while combination of isoniazid and rifampicin causes hepatitis in 40 out of 100 patients. The RR of hepatitis following combination drug intake would be 40/100 ÷ 10/100 = 4 while OR would also be 40/60 ÷ 10/90 = 6.

You must have realized that the OR is approximately the same as the RR if the outcome of interest is rare. For common events however, they can be quite different.

Relative risk is used in cohort studies where one measures development of an event in the exposed and nonexposed groups (development of lung cancer in smokers and nonsmokers). However, RR cannot be used in case–control studies where the event has already occurred, and one measures frequency of exposure in the study group (frequency of smoking in lung cancer patients). So, OR is used in case–control studies.

■ CONCEPT OF HYPOTHESIS TESTING

Let us explain the concept of hypothesis testing by giving an example. Suppose your friend Raju says I am a very good batsman; he claims to score the runs at an average of 90/match. You will be very glad to know and will include him in your team. He plays three matches as your team member and scores runs at a dismal average of 20/match. Can you accept his claim anymore, perhaps not. But, we must also remember this may be just a chance finding. There may be several reasons for his low scoring: Maybe he had a bad day, maybe the opposition ballers were extremely good, maybe the weather was poor or maybe he was not in form that day. Suppose had he scored runs at an average of 70/match in three matches, you would have believed his claim of scoring runs of 90/match more easily; or, in other words, chances of his claim being true would have been higher. So, there should be a cutoff of average runs in three matches he played as a member of your team, below which you are likely to reject his claim, and above which you are likely to accept his claim. Let us say it is 50; it means if he scores runs at or above 50/match in three matches, you are likely to accept his claim. This is what we do in hypothesis testing. Here, the claim made by Raju is a hypothesis. The cutoff value is the critical value or level of significance that you set to accept or reject the claim. Here, the level of significance is 50. The scores he might get in three matches is 20 or 70. We can thus say that 20 is below the level of significance. So, it is different from 90. On the other hand, value 70 is seen as comparable to 90 (because it is >50, the presumed level of significance).

Null Hypothesis

Traditionally, we have always been trained to reject all the new ideas at first go. There comes the concept of "null hypothesis." Raju conducts a clinical trial for testing a new drug A for reduction in blood pressure. And, he would start with the assumption that this new drug A will not decrease the blood pressure. This will be his null hypothesis. His actual claim "new drug A will decrease blood pressure" will be called alternate hypothesis. Now Raju has to decide a level of significance which will help him in rejecting or not rejecting the null hypothesis or, in other words, accepting or rejecting his claim or alternate hypothesis. Suppose he chooses level of significance to be 5% below which he will reject the null hypothesis. That means, if P value in his trial comes out to be <5%, he will reject the null hypothesis and accept his claim or alternate hypothesis and will say "Drug A will decrease blood pressure. If the P value in his trial comes out to be >5%, he will not reject the null hypothesis and not accept his claim or alternate hypothesis and will say "there is no evidence that Drug A will decrease the blood pressure."

You see that this level of significance is arbitrary. Raju might have chosen any value as level of significance; maybe 1%, 2%, or 4%. Lesser the level of significance, more we are sure or confident of rejecting the null hypothesis. Conventionally, we set a level of significance as 5%.

P Value

The P value gives the probability of occurrence of any event by chance. If you toss a coin, the probability of getting tails or heads is 50%. So the P value is 0.5. The lesser the P value, lesser is the probability of occurrence of an event by chance.

- $P = 0.5$ means that the probability of the occurrence of an event by chance is 0.5 in 1 (50%), or 50 : 50.
- $P = 0.05$ means that the probability of the occurrence of an event by chance is 0.05 in 1 (5%), i.e., 1 in 20. $P < 0.05$, thus, usually implies that the occurrence of an event by chance is unlikely or remote.
- $P = 0.01$ means that the event would occur by chance 1 in 100 times only, very unlikely.
- $P = 0.001$ means the event would occur by chance 1 in 1,000 times, very unlikely.

In biostatistics, we denote P value as the probability of the null hypothesis being actually true. Conventionally, if the P value for a null hypothesis comes out to be <0.05 (5%), we assume that the probability of null hypothesis being true is only <5% and, so, we can safely reject the null hypothesis.

Steps of Hypothesis Testing

Step 1: Formulate the Null Hypothesis

The null hypothesis is that there is no difference, on an average, between two groups, or no relationship between two variables. If the null hypothesis is rejected, we would conclude that "the observed difference or relationship in the data is not due to chance alone." In Raju's case, null hypothesis is "Drug A will not decrease blood pressure" while alternate hypothesis is "Drug A will decrease blood pressure."

Step 2: Estimate the *P* Value

As described above, P value gives the probability of null hypothesis being true. You will use various statistical tests to find the P value.

Step 3: Draw your Conclusions

The lower the P value, lesser are the chances of null hypothesis being true, and so the more plausible it is that alternate hypothesis is true. In Raju's case, if P value is 0.02 (2%), the likelihood of the null hypothesis being true is lower and alternate hypothesis (Raju's claim) being true is higher. In contrast, if P value is 0.40 (40%), the likelihood of the null hypothesis being true is higher and alternate hypothesis (Raju's claim) being true is lower.

> Conventionally, we reject null hypothesis when the probability of it being true is <5% or P value <0.05. In other words, we set the level of significance as 5% or (0.05); however, a researcher is free to set P value for his research based on the hypothesis.

Example:
Examination marks and gender of 10 students are as follows:

Marks (%)	Gender
34	F
54	F
48	F
47	F
74	F
48	M
69	M
79	M
38	M
48	M

The average percentage of marks of the female (F) students is 51.4%, while the average percentage of marks of the male (M) students is 56.4%. The difference is 5.0%. It appears that the males have done 5% better. Remember, this inference is based on a group of 10 students only (5 male and 5 female students). If we take another group of 10 students, we may get an entirely different answer. So, how can we be sure that males really performed better?

Let us now do a hypothesis testing. The null hypothesis is that "the gender of the student has no relationship with the marks obtained in the examination." The actual difference in the average marks in our small sample of 10 students is 5.0%. We will now apply appropriate statistical test to find out the P value to ascertain the probability of our null hypothesis being true. The P value comes out to be 0.58. What does it mean? It means that the probability of our null hypothesis being true is 58%. As this probability is quite high (more than our conventional level of significance of 5% or 0.05), we will not reject our null hypothesis; we will conclude that there is no evidence for relationships between gender of the students and their examination marks.

■ CHOOSING THE APPROPRIATE STATISTICAL TEST

Choice of different tests will depend upon the following factors:
- Whether the variable is categorical or continuous?
- Whether the data in that variable is normally distributed or not?
- Whether the data is paired or unpaired?

Algorithm in **Flowchart 16.2** shows how an appropriate statistical test may be selected based on the above parameters.

■ CONCEPTS OF TYPE I AND TYPE II ERRORS

You must have understood by now that you reject the null hypothesis when probability of its being true is <5% (P <0.05); this cutoff of 5% is purely by convention. Please think, when we choose this cutoff of 5% or P value of 0.05, we are actually accepting that there is 5% chance (1 in 20) of rejecting the null hypothesis when it is, in fact, correct; and we will accept the incorrect alternate hypothesis. This error is called **type I error**. You can make error the other way round also; you may fail to reject the null hypothesis when it is, in fact, wrong. This error is called **type II error**. A type I error is expressed by the Greek letter alpha (α) while the type II error by the Greek letter beta (β) (**Table 16.1**).

In simple words, you make a type I error when you tell a gentleman that he is pregnant

Planning the Statistical Analysis | 119

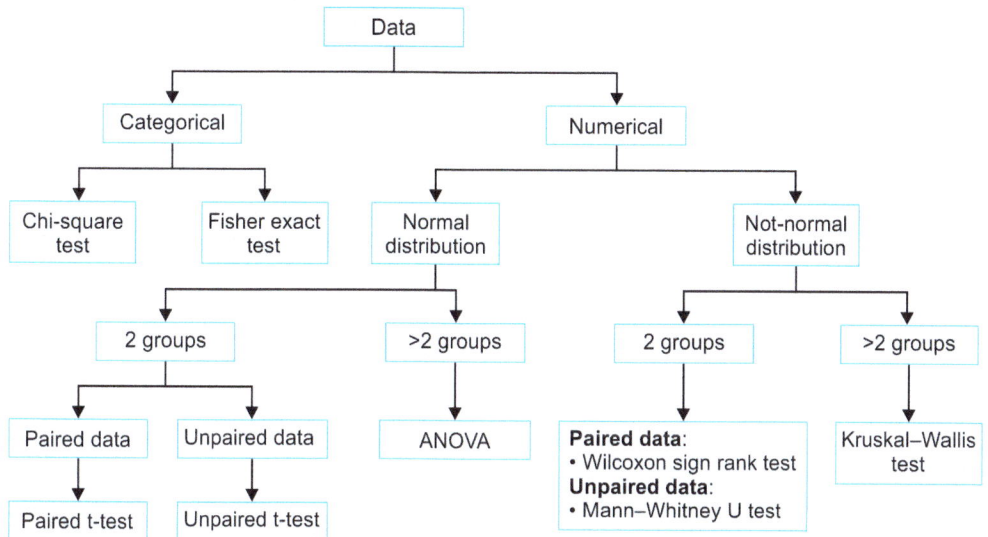

Flowchart 16.2: Choosing a statistical test based on the type of data.

TABLE 16.1: Type I and type II errors.

Decision of hypothesis testing	Null hypothesis is actually true	Null hypothesis is actually false
Do not reject null hypothesis	Correct decision	Erroneous decision (**type II error**)
Reject null hypothesis	Erroneous decision (**type I error**)	Correct decision (**power**)

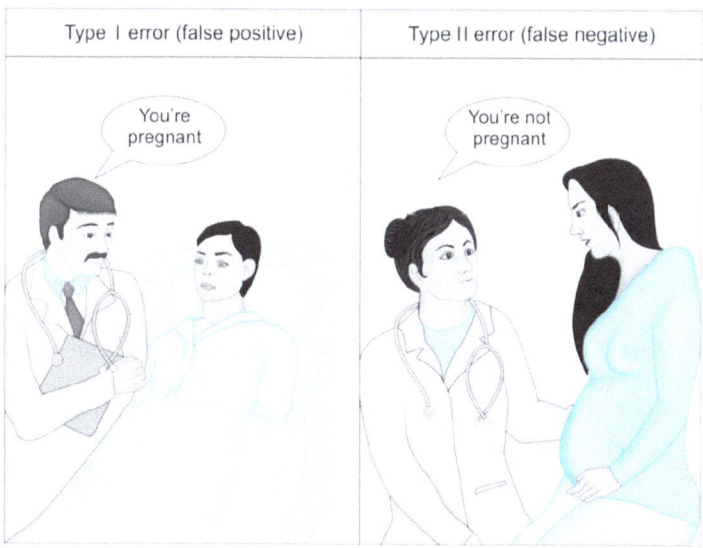

Fig. 16.4: Type 1 versus type II error.

(false positive); you make a type II error when you tell a pregnant lady that she is not pregnant (false negative) (**Fig. 16.4**).

Type I error is more dangerous than type II error as type I error will lead to rejection of a null hypothesis when it is true. Concluding that a drug A is effective when it is really not (type I) now becomes an extremely serious error, you will prescribe ineffective new drug A instead of an old effective drug to the patients. Type II error will result in declaring the drug A ineffective when it is actually effective. This will result in denying patients a useful drug A; however, this is less serious than prescribing them an ineffective drug (type I error). So, conventionally we set type I error lower than type II error in a research design.

Concept of Power

The power of a statistical hypothesis test measures the test ability to reject the false null hypothesis, i.e., to make a correct decision.

So, power of a test = $1 - \beta$ (type II error)

The power of a test can be any value from 0 to 100%. Ideally we want a test to have power of 1 (100%). The more the sample size, higher is the value of power. Conventionally, we set power of a test as 0.8 or 80%, or, in other words, we accept 20% type II error in our research design. However, a researcher is free to decide the value of power for his study design based on his research question

■ CONFIDENCE INTERVAL

If I ask you what percentage of people in India like to watch cricket, you might say almost 60–70%, and you can further add that you are 90% sure. You are actually making a 90% confidence interval of 60–70% people in India who like to watch cricket.

Confidence interval provides a range of values which includes true parameter with a probability defined in advance (coverage probability, confidence probability, or confidence level). The confidence level of 95% is usually selected. This means that the confidence interval covers the true value in 95 out of 100 times the study is performed.

Here is an example. Suppose a researcher wants to know how much are the average marks secured by the MBBS students in their final professional examination. There are 250 students in the class. In order to save time and resources, the researcher talks to 20 students to record their marks. So, the class of 250 is the population and the group of 20 students, who shared their marks with him, becomes the sample. He calculates the average marks of these 20 students and it turns out to be 80. Can he assume that the average marks of 250 students would also be 78. Perhaps not! If he takes another 20 students, the average marks are likely to different. In this way, can we ever extrapolate the average marks of a sample of 20 students to the whole population 250 students as the repeated sampling with a different group of 20 students would yield a different result every time. Here comes the importance of the confidence interval which is a statistical tool to extrapolate the results of the sample to the population with a margin of error.

If the researcher calculates a range of average marks (76–84) based on the discussion with 20 students and extrapolates that the average marks of the whole population of 250 students would lie in this range with some degree of surety, this range is known as *confidence interval* and the degree of surety is known as *confidence level*. The confidence interval is calculated on either side of the sample mean.

Traditionally, we take a confidence level of 95%, it means that if the study is repeated 100 times, the result would fall in the confidence interval 95 out of 100 times. Again, if the researcher claims that the average marks of the 20 students are 80 with 95% confidence interval of 76–84, it means that if he keeps on calculating average marks of 20 different students, he would get average marks between 76 and 84 in 95 out 100 times. In other words, he would get average marks of <76 or >84 in only 5 out 100 times.

If I say mean IQ score of 50 students of IIT Delhi is 90 (95% CI 80–100), it means I am 95% confident that mean IQ of IIT students will lie somewhere between 80 and 100, it may be 81 or 92 or 99). In other words, you repeatedly take a sample of 50 different students, 95 out of 100 times, your measured mean IQ score will fall between 80 and 100.

Shorter is the confidence interval, more relevant are the results. Ramesh finds the literacy rate in Delhi as 50% with a 95% confidence interval of 20–80% from his study. Suresh also conducts a similar study and calculates the literacy rate in Delhi to be 50% with a 95% confidence interval of 40–60%. Whose results are more reliable and make sense? Obviously, the results of the study conducted by Suresh are more reliable compared to the study conducted by Ramesh, and provides a better picture of true literacy rates in Delhi.

The width of confidence interval is inversely proportional to the sample size. Remember, larger is the sample size, shorter is the confidence interval and more reliable results are.

EVALUATION OF A DIAGNOSTIC TEST

A diagnostic test is supposed to correctly identify the persons who have the disease from the people who do not have the disease. In other words, the diagnostic test should give us positive results in the persons who have the disease, and should give us negative results in the persons who do not have the disease. No diagnostic test is ideal; any diagnostic test may give you positive result in healthy people or negative result in diseased people.

Now, you must understand four terms which will be frequently used in this section.
1. *True positive:* Diagnostic test gives a positive result in a person who has the disease.
2. *True negative:* Diagnostic test gives a negative result in a person who does not have the disease.
3. *False positive:* Diagnostic test gives a positive result in a person who does not have the disease.
4. *False negative:* Diagnostic test gives a negative result in a person who has the disease.

Sensitivity and Specificity

There are two basic measures of the inherent accuracy of a diagnostic test: Sensitivity and Specificity. They are equally important and none of them can replace the other one—both should be reported simultaneously.

Sensitivity of the test is the ability of the test to correctly identify those who have the disease, i.e., true positives.

$$\text{Sensitivity} = TP/(TP + FN)$$

Specificity of the test is the ability of the test to correctly identify those who do not have the disease, i.e., true negatives.

$$\text{Specificity} = TN/(TN + FP)$$

Sensitivity and Specificity are inversely proportional; it means as the sensitivity increases, the specificity decreases and *vice versa*. What do we mean by this? Let us say that a blood glucose level >140 mg/dL is test positive for diabetes while <140 mg/dL is test negative for diabetes. This has a sensitivity of 90% and specificity of 80%. What does it mean? 90% sensitivity means we would be missing 10% of the patients who actually have diabetes but are test negative (blood sugar <140); 80% specificity means 20% of the persons would be labeled as diabetic falsely as their blood sugar is >140. Now, if we raise the cutoff value of 140 to 160 mg/dL, what will happen? Almost no normal person would be having blood sugar of >160. Hence, false positive results would decrease; or, in other words, specificity would increase. Think what would happen to sensitivity? Sensitivity would decrease as many diabetic patients who have blood sugar 140–160 would be missed by raising the cutoff to 160.

When would you minimize false positives; in other words, would you like to have a test with high specificity?

Minimizing false positives is important when the costs or risks of follow-up therapy are high and the disease itself is not life-threatening. The prostate cancer in elderly men is one example; routine screening with prostate-specific antigen (PSA) has not proved beneficial considering slow and protracted course of the disease. Similarly, obstetricians must consider the potential harm from a false positive maternal serum alpha-fetoprotein (AFP) test (which may be followed up with amniocentesis, ultrasonography and increased fetal surveillance as well as producing anxiety for the parents and labeling of the unborn child) against potential benefit.

When would you minimize false negatives; in other words, would you like to have a test with high sensitivity?

We do not want to have many false negative if the disease is serious, progresses quickly, and can be treated more effectively at early stages or easily spreads from one person to another.

Positive and Negative Predictive Values

The rapid advancement in the biochemical and radiological investigations has created new challenges for the clinicians to decide the appropriate management strategies for their patients; however, we also know that no investigation is perfect. The clinician's dilemma lies in the following questions: "What is the probability of the patient having the disease when the test result comes back as positive?" and "What is the probability of the patient not having the disease when the test result comes back as negative?" The answers to these two questions are called the positive and negative predictive values, respectively.

Positive predictive value (PPV) is the proportion of patients who tests positive and actually have the disease. In other words, PPV will tell you the probability of the person having the disease, if he turns positive.

$$PPV = TP/(TP + FP)$$

Negative predictive value (NPV) is the proportion of patients who tests negative and are actually free of the disease. In other words, NPV will tell you the probability of the persons not having the disease, if he turns negative.

$$NPV = TN/(TN + FN)$$

Example:
The D-dimer sign has been described as an important indicator of deep vein thrombosis (DVT). Suppose you evaluate 285 suspected patients of DVT with D-dimer and confirm your diagnosis with venogram.

D-dimer	DVT present	DVT absent
Positive	100	15
Negative	10	160

(DVT: deep vein thrombosis)

The sensitivity of the d-dimer to diagnose DVT is 100/110 = 0.909 or 90.9% while specificity is 160/175 = 0.914 or 91.4%. The PPV is 100/115 = 0.869 or 86.9% while NPP is 160/170 = 0.941 or 94.1%. The sensitivity (90.9%) indicates the probability of the D-dimer being positive among patients with DVT while the PPV (86.9%) indicates the probability of a person to have DVT following positive d-dimer. In other words, sensitivity is a property of the diagnostic test and it helps the clinician decide which test to use; however, PPV indicates the presence of disease and guides the clinician to initiate the treatment after the diagnostic test shows a positive result. Specificity (91.4%) tells us the probability that the D-dimer will be negative among patients without DVT. NPV (94.1%) indicates the probability of the absence of the DVT in the patients if the D-dimer test is negative. In other words, high NPV will help the clinician to rule out a particular disease if the diagnostic test is negative, and will allow him to consider other probable diagnoses.

Please ponder: PPV and NPV are not fixed characteristics of a diagnostic test and are influenced by the disease prevalence. In contrast, both sensitivity and specificity are fixed characteristics of a diagnostic test.

Example:
Suppose we apply a diagnostic test to different population having different disease prevalence. Let us see how PPV and NPV differ in these scenarios.

1. **Disease prevalence: 25%**

	Disease present	Disease absent
Test positive	900	300
Test negative	100	2700

Sensitivity: 90%
Specificity: 90%
PPV: 75%
NPV: 96%

2. **Disease prevalence: 90%**

	Disease present	Disease absent
Test positive	3240	40
Test negative	360	360

Sensitivity: 90%
Specificity: 90%
PPV: 99%
NPV: 50%

Hence, positive and negative predictive values are influenced by the prevalence of disease in the population that is being tested. If we test in a population with high prevalence of disease, it is more likely that the persons who test positive have the disease than if the test is performed in a population with low prevalence.

CONCLUSION

Statistics is an indispensable and unavoidable part of your thesis project. Understanding of and proficiency in basic statistical methodology will help you communicate with your statistician to plan relevant statistical analysis for your thesis project. The knowledge of statistics guides you to use appropriate methods to collect data, employ correct statistical tools for analysis, and present the data assiduously. You may feel that the depth of knowledge of basic statistics that you have acquired now is little and superficial; however, it would increase gradually as you stay in research longer and imbibe more difficult statistical concepts.

KEY MESSAGES

- Use mean (standard deviation) and median (interquartile range) to represent central tendency of parametric and nonparametric data, respectively.
- Correlation does not represent causation.
- Relative risk is used in cohort studies while odds ratio is calculated in case–control studies.
- Select proper statistical tests in testing hypothesis as they are different for parametric and non-parametric data.
- Statistical significance is not always equivalent to biological equivalence.

FURTHER READING

1. Choudhary D, Garg PK. 95 % confidence interval: a misunderstood statistical tool. Indian J Surg. 2013;75(5):410.
2. du Prel JB, Hommel G, Röhrig B, Blettner M. confidence interval or p-value?: Part 4 of a series on evaluation of scientific publications. Dtsch Arztebl Int. 2009;106(19):335-9.
3. Indrayan A. Simple Biostatistics for MBBS, PG Entrance and USMLE, 4th edition. India: Academa Publishers; 2013.
4. Lee JJ. Demystify statistical significance—time to move on from the P value to Bayesian analysis. J Natl cancer Inst. 2011;103(1):2-3.
5. Garg PK. Large standard deviation: think before you write. World J Surg. 2015;39(3):808-9.
6. Garg PK, Mohanty D. Mean (standard deviation) or mean (standard error of mean): time to ponder. World J Surg. 2013;37(4):932.
7. Prasad K. What are relative risk, number needed to treat and odds ratio? Ann Indian Acad Neurol. 2007;10:225-30.
8. Weinstein S, Obuchowski NA, Lieber ML. Clinical evaluation of diagnostic tests. AJR Am J Roentgenol. 2005;184(1):14-9.

CHAPTER 17

Results: Fruits of the Labor

Rehan Ul Haq

"If I could, I would always work in silence and obscurity, and let my efforts be known by their results."
—Emile Bronte

■ INTRODUCTION

The Oxford dictionary defines "Results" as "an item of information obtained by experiment or some other scientific method". In the context of your thesis, "Results" refer to the observations that have been made by you during your research based on the data you have collected. The "Results" section is a vital link between the Material and Methods section and the Discussion section. It is the section where observations pertaining to the primary and secondary outcomes are presented. Hypotheses are either accepted or rejected on the basis of results. The main purpose of this section is to present your observations in a comprehensive and systematic manner, so that others can understand them.

This section has to be a balanced mix of narration, tables, figures, and graphs.

■ WHAT DATA ARE AVAILABLE AND HOW TO PRESENT THEM

At the end of data analysis, the biostatistician would usually provide you with a large volume of data and observations. Determining how much to present and how to present are the key decisions which you have to take.

Most of the available data can be categorized as follows:
- *Participant data*: Baseline data and participant flow data.
- *Outcome data*: Data about the primary and secondary outcome measures.
- *Ancillary data*: Significant findings other than the primary and secondary outcome measures.
- *Other data*: Any other findings including complications.

Participant Data

Participant data includes (1) The baseline data and (2) The participant flow data.

Baseline Data

The baseline data provides descriptive statistics about the characteristics of the study participants which includes the following information:
1. *Demographic data*: Age, sex, and its distribution.

2. *Clinical data*: Baseline health indicators, comorbidities, and relevant confounding factors.
3. *Social data*: Education, income, and family size.
4. *Other parameters* which are directly or indirectly relevant to the study topic.

These data are important because they help the clinicians and researchers to judge how relevant the results are for individual patients. While presenting this data, take care of the following:

- Categorical variables such as sex must be presented as proportion or percentage. It is a must to include numbers, whenever percentages are reported.
- Continuous variables such as age and weight must be summarized as mean. Whenever mean is given, standard deviation and/or range must also be provided.
  The mean (SD) age was 65 (±10) years.
- When continuous data have a skewed distribution, present the median and interquartile range (25-75 percentile).
  The median (IQR) duration of the therapy was 75 (40-100) hours.
- Variables with small number of ordered categories should not be treated as continuous variable; instead number and proportion must be reported in each category. This can usually be best done with the help of a table (**Table 17.1**).

Note that, in the above example, sex is a categorical variable and age is a continuous variable, while daily alcohol intake is a variable with small number of ordered categories.

- For randomized control trials, a table comparing the demographic, clinical, and social characteristics of the group should be provided (**Table 17.2**). This is because although proper random assignment prevents selection bias, it does not guarantee that the groups are equivalent at baseline. However, one must understand that any difference in the baseline characteristics is because of chance rather than bias. Therefore, using tests of significance like P value to highlight these differences in descriptive tables is illogical and should be avoided.

It is sometimes observed that students go overboard describing and comparing the baseline participant data, a temptation which must be strictly avoided because this is not the main aim of the study. Participant data are important only because they allow the reader to analyze how important the results of the study would be for individual patients.

TABLE 17.1: Baseline data of a single group.

Parameter	Data (n = 1,458)
Sex (%)	
Male	936 (64%)
Female	522 (36%)
Age at enrollment mean (+SD)	45.7 (±10.5) years
Daily alcohol intake (%)	
None	250 (17%)
Moderate	853 (59%)
Excessive	355 (24%)

TABLE 17.2: Baseline data of two groups.

Study group		Group A (n = 150)	Group B (n = 150)
Age in years. mean (SD)		55.6 (17.1)	54.0 (14.7)
Sex	Male	80 (53.3%)	70 (46.6%)
	Female	70 (46.6%)	80 (53.3%)
ASA Grade	I	60 (40%)	70 (46.6%)
	II	60 (40%)	60 (40.0%)
	III	30 (20%)	20 (13.3%)
Quality of bone (Singh's index)	≤3	90 (60%)	100 (66.6%)
	>3	60 (40%)	50 (33.3%)

Participant Flow

This refers to the information about the number of individuals at each stage of study:
1. Number of potentially eligible patients (those *available*).

2. Number of patients examined for eligibility (those *approached*).
3. Number of patients confirmed eligible (those *fulfilling inclusion criteria*).
4. Number of patients included in the study (those fulfilling inclusion and exclusion criteria).
5. Number of patients who completed follow-up.
6. Number of patients finally analyzed

Losses and exclusion from all groups together with records must be given. This can usually be best represented with a *participant flowchart* (**Flowchart 17.1**).

Outcome Data

This is the most important part of the Results section. For each primary and secondary outcome variable, you must present the results precisely as a summary. Remember the following important points:

A. If There is Only One Group

i. The summary data about categorical variables must be represented as percentage, proportion, or rate along with the actual (absolute) numbers. Ideally, the results should be presented as n/N (%) (**Table 17.3**).

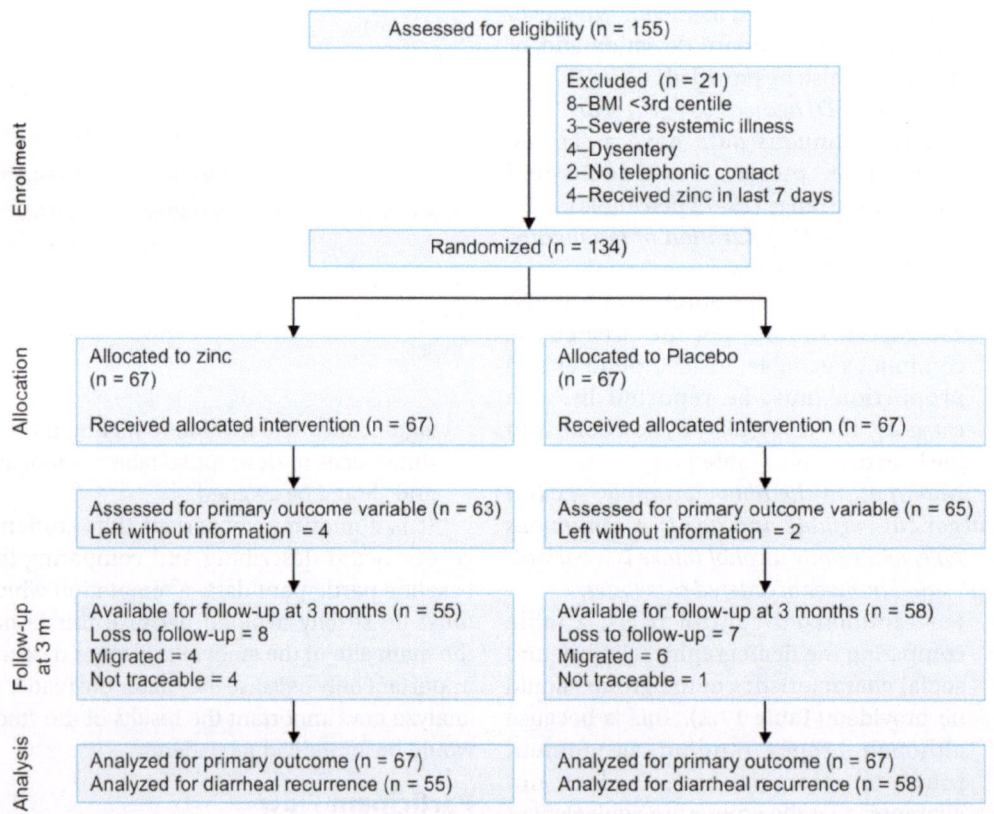

Flowchart 17.1: Trial profile of a randomized, placebo-controlled trial of zinc supplementation for acute dehydrating diarrhea in children aged 5–12 years.
(*Source*: Negi R, Dewan P, Shah D, Das S, Bhatnagar S, Gupta P. Oral zinc supplements are ineffective for treating acute dehydrating diarrhoea in 5–12-year-olds. Acta Paediatrica. 2014;104(8):e367-71.)

i. For categorical variables, the effect size must be represented in the form of both relative effect [risk ratio/relative risk (RR) or odds ratio (OR)] and absolute effect (risk difference) (**Table 17.4**); neither the relative measure nor the absolute measure alone indicates a complete picture of the effect and its implications.

Example of categorical variables: Early administration versus delayed selective administration of surfactant in preterm babies with high risk of developing respiratory distress syndrome (RDS) (**Table 17.4**).

ii. For continuous variables, the effect size is usually the "difference in the means" (**Table 17.5**).

ii. The summary data about continuous variables must be presented as mean with standard deviation (**Table 17.3**) and/or range (if the data follows Gaussian distribution); or as median with interquartile range (if the variable does not follow a normal distribution).

Example: *Functional outcome and union rates following fractured neck femur (n = 350) at 6 and 12 months* (**Table 17.3**).

B. If There are More Than One Group

Besides the summary data, the contrast between the two groups (known as *effect size*) must be provided.

TABLE 17.3: Outcome data of a single group.

Variable	Outcome at 6 months n = 315	Outcome at 12 months n = 290
Functional outcome score (0–100) mean (SD)	65.5 (13.9)	55.5 (10.9)
Pain at rest score (0–100) mean (SD)	11.5 (2.5)	10.5 (2.3)
Pain at walking score (0–100) mean (SD)	15.5 (3.5)	12.5 (3.0)
Fracture union rate (%)	80% (252/315)	90% (261/290)

TABLE 17.4: Outcome data for categorical variable (of 2 groups)

Primary outcome	Number		Risk ratio (95% CI)	Risk difference (95% CI)
	Early administration (n = 1,344)	Delayed selective (n – 1,346)		
Oxygen dependence	429 (31.9)	514 (38.2)	0.84 (0.75–0.93)	–6.3 (–9.9 to –2.7)

In the above example, number and percentages are depicted in column 2 for the two groups (early versus late). The next two columns display the risk ratio and risk difference between the two groups.

TABLE 17.5: Outcome data for continuous variables of 2 groups.

Score	Nail group (n = 150)	Plate group (n = 150)	Adjusted difference between means (95% CI)
Function score (0–100) [mean (SD)]	83.2 (14.8)	79.8 (17.5)	4.52 (–0.73 to 9.76)
Pain at rest (0–100) score [mean (SD)]	1.43 (2.2)	2.61 (2.9)	–1.29 (–2.16 to –0.42)
Pain on activity (0–100) score [mean (SD)]	2.57 (2.9)	3.54 (3.38)	–1.19 (–2.22 to –0.16)

Values in columns are in mean (SD) for continuous variables

Example of continuous variables: *Randomized control trial comparing functional outcome at 6 months in patients with intertrochanteric fractures managed with "nail" versus "plate"* (**Table 17.5**).

iii. For both categorical and continuous variables besides the point estimate, (e.g., population mean and population proportion), one must also present the confidence interval (CI) estimate, because it represents the range of likely values for the population parameter. Usually, a 95% confidence interval is conventional but other levels can be used.

To summarize, depending upon the type of data and the nature of the study, one must present the outcome data as shown in **Table 17.6**.

P-Values

When tests of significance are used, the result must be represented as the P values. Whenever P values are given, the exact value must be provided. One must remember that P values summarize the *statistical significance* and do not address clinical significance. This is because P values depend upon both the magnitude of association and the precision of the estimate (the sample size).

When the sample size is large, results can reach statistical significance ($P<0.05$) even when the effect is small and clinically unimportant. Conversely, with small sample size, results can fail to reach statistical significance, yet the effect is large and potentially clinically important. It is extremely important to assess both statistical and clinical significance of results.

Example:
In a randomized control trial comparing intraoperative blood loss in patients with intertrochanteric fractures managed with "nail" versus "plate", the difference in the mean blood was 20 mL and the P value was less than $P<0.05$ hence, statistically significant. However, from experience, we know that a difference of 20 mL blood loss is usually not clinically significant. Thus, in this case, the statistically significant difference is not clinically relevant.

Ancillary Data

Ancillary data usually involve reporting of significant findings other than the primary and secondary outcome variables. This includes subgroup analysis, adjusted analysis, etc. This also includes *post hoc analysis*, i.e., analysis of data after the experiment has concluded for patterns that were not specified initially. However, there is a possibility that multiple analysis of the same data would result in false positive findings. Therefore, one must resist the temptation of multiple subgroup analysis.

Other Data

Any other important observation must also be reported. Description of all important harms, unintended effects, adverse effects, and complications must be enumerated. Brief statement about how these were managed and final outcome of these patients must also be included.

TABLE 17.6: What should be presented in the outcome data.

	Categorical variable	Continuous variable
One group	Percentage, proportion or rate, etc.	Mean with standard deviation and/or range
Two groups	Difference in proportions or rates, relative effect (risk ratio or odds ratio) and absolute effect (risk difference)	Difference in means

■ SEQUENCE IN WHICH RESULTS SHOULD BE PRESENTED

There are various logical sequences in which the results can be presented. The most widely acceptable sequence for biomedical thesis is moving from a general overview to more specific issues.

Participant Data

At the beginning of the Results section, you must give a brief description about the population from which the sample has been taken. This can be done by defining the place of work, the duration of study period, and information about patient population catered by the mentioned place of work.

"The study was done at the Department of Orthopedics, University College of Medical Sciences and GTB Hospital, Delhi which caters to a large underprivileged urban population of Delhi, from December 2018 to December 2019."

This gives the readers and other researchers an idea about the population from which the sample population has been derived.

Following this, the baseline data and participant flow data (represented by a participant flow diagram) must be presented.

Outcome Data

The data about the primary and secondary outcomes should be presented after this. The outcome data should be presented in the same sequence in which the primary and secondary outcomes have been listed in the aim and objectives section. However, sometimes it can be presented from most significant to least significant, or in chronological order.

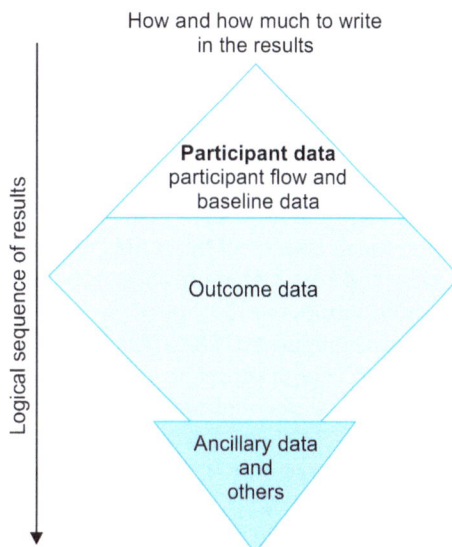

Fig. 17.1: Presentation of Results.

Ancillary Data

Results of post hoc analysis, subgroup analysis, etc., must then be presented.

Other Data

Finally, toward the end of the Results section, a description of all important harms, unintended effects, adverse effects and complications must be enumerated. A statement about how and when the results were assessed must also be included. One must not exclude the findings which do not support the hypothesis because this would make the results biased, which is against the spirit of the research.

Figure 17.1 provides a diagrammatic depiction of logical sequence of presentation of Results and relative length of each of these components.

Curtailing the Presentable Values

When reporting the mean or other measured or calculated values, an appropriate number of decimal places must be reported. The values should reflect the degree of precision of the original measurement. A few examples follow:
- The mean and SD of heart rate, respiratory rate, and blood pressure to be reported in whole numbers only (mean heart rate 82 beats per minute, NOT 82.3 beats per minute)
- The mean age of adults needs to be reported only to one decimal place, not four (e.g., 68.1 years, NOT 68.1276 years).
- For summary statistics (e.g., mean and standard deviation), report one digit more than presented in the raw data.
- For percentages, the nearest whole percent, (e.g., 35%) is usually adequate, although sometimes to the nearest tenth of a percent can be done, (e.g., 35.4%).
- Report exact *P* values for all main analyses.

CONCLUSION

The purpose of the results section is to present the key observations of your research without interpreting their meaning. So, do not include your own interpretations, views, and opinions in this section. When summarizing your data, do not include raw data or intermediate calculations in this section. Use appendix for providing the master chart. Ensure that your data is accurate and consistent throughout the manuscript. Do not cook up data. Data in text and tables need to be consistent.

KEY MESSAGES

- Present those results first which are relevant to the question(s) presented in the Introduction, irrespective of whether or not the results support the hypothesis.
- Use a judicious mix of text, tables, and graphs. Avoid overuse and abuse of tables and figures.
- Organize the data in the Results section in a logical order.
- Use the past tense when you refer to your results.
- Write with accuracy, brevity, and clarity.

FURTHER READING

1. Bahadoran Z, Mirmiran P, Zadeh-Vakili A, Hosseinpanah F, Ghasemi A. The principles of biomedical scientific writing: Results. Int J Endocrinol Metab. 2019;17(2):e92113.
2. Enarson DA, Kennedy SM, Miller DL, Bakke P. Interpreting and reporting results. Int J Tuberc Lung Dis. 2004;8(12):1506-9.
3. Moher D, Hopewell S, Schulz KF, Montori V, Gøtzsche PC, Devereaux PJ, et al. CONSORT 2010 Explanation and Elaboration: updated guidelines for reporting parallel group randomised trial. BMJ. 2010;340:c869.
4. Ng KH, Peh WC. Presenting the statistical results. Singapore Med J. 2009;50(1):11-4.
5. Ng KH, Peh WC. Writing the results. Singapore Med J. 2008;49(12):967-9.
6. Snyder N, Foltz C, Lendner M, Vaccaro AR. How to write an effective results section. Clin Spine Surg. 2019;32(7):295-6.
7. Tuncel A, Atan A. How to clearly articulate results and construct tables and figures in a scientific paper? Turk J Urol. 2013;39:16-9.

CHAPTER 18

Converting Results to Text, Tables, and Graphs: Represent the Findings

Amir Maroof Khan

■ INTRODUCTION

When I finished collecting my results, my dad asked me, "what did you find in your study?" I had the filled case record forms, the data spreadsheet, and the statistical analysis reports, all in front of me, but, I was confused at that time and started wondering, "how would I describe and present my findings? And what would my results look like?"

What are Results?

The Results section is the blandest, but, the juiciest section of the whole research document. It is bland because it consists of statements of the findings in a very straightforward, noninterpretative manner, and juicy, because it has got the extracted findings from your study. Here you summarize the data collected in the form of actual statements of the observations, using tables, graphs, and statistics.

> "The compulsion to include everything, leaving nothing out, does not prove that one has unlimited information; it proves that one lacks discrimination"(Aaronson,1977).

■ GETTING STARTED

What to Include in the Results Section; and What to Exclude?

When you have all the findings of your analyses, it is an uphill task deciding what to include and what to exclude in the Results section. It is not necessary to include each and everything you got in your analyses. For deciding this, you should first go through your analyses and review what all you have got. Then, have a relook at the research question and the objectives stated in your research protocol. Being focused on the research question, the objectives of the study and your methods section, which have already been predefined, will smoothly guide you into what to include and what to exclude.

> Usually the order of arrangement of the Results section is from general overview to specific issues.

Do not exclude a finding because it does not support your hypothesis. This will make a biased report and is against the spirit of research. Only exclude those things which are not a part of the research question and the objectives of the study. The Results section may be very short, but this is alright, if it meets the objectives of the study that you set out.

What should you Start with?

As mentioned earlier, the sequence of arrangement of the Results section is from general overview to specific issues. Thus, the first part of the Results section is usually descriptive which gives an overview or a big picture of what you did, without repeating the methods section.

This can be different for different types of studies. In a randomized controlled trial (RCT), a short descriptive account about the number of cases and controls and whether there is a similarity between the cases and controls can be a starting point. Even in a cross-sectional survey, the first section should consist of a mention of sociodemographic characteristics of the surveyed subjects. Thus, the reader gets to know the context on which to base the specifics of the main results, which will follow.

Do not present complex statistical analysis findings in the beginning of the result section. Results obtained by simple statistical methods such as descriptive analysis, bivariate analysis should be mentioned before moving on to complex analysis such as regression models and others.

Example

Of the 1,000 people who initially expressed interest in participating, 948 (94.8%) were enrolled; 488 participants were randomly assigned to the intervention group and 460 to the control group. **Figure 18.1** *shows the numbers of subjects who were screened and who participated in the study intervention and follow-up. Demographic characteristics and smoking behavior were similar in the incentive and control groups (***Table 18.1***).*

■ WHICH IS THE BEST WAY TO PRESENT YOUR FINDINGS?

The answer to this question is not a set of specific rules but some general considerations

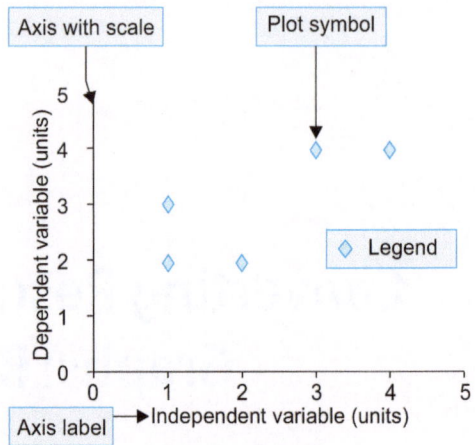

Fig. 18.1: Components of a graph.

that can help you in deciding it. The foremost rule being that it should facilitate the reader in understanding the findings; without confusing and burdening the reader in grasping the contents of the results.

The four ways of presenting any finding are as follows:
1. Text
2. Tables
3. Graphs
4. Photographs/photomicrographs

Text

Text refers to words in writing, arranged in paragraphs. This form is most used to describe your findings. As a standalone form, it is used to convey most of the findings in the Results section. Even when a table, graph, or photograph is depicted, some textual matter is necessary to support these illustrative materials. The associated textual matter should not be a complete repetition of the matter presented in the table or the graph but just highlight the main point/s you want to convey through it.

Always use past tense in writing the results because the study has already been done and the results have been achieved, e.g., *"a total of 30 patients were studied."*

TABLE 18.1: Proportion of individuals with hypertension among nonsmokers, former smokers, and current smokers.

Smoking status	N	Blood pressure		
		*Normal	Mild hypertension	Moderate/severe hypertension
Nonsmoker	580	464 (80.0)	60 (10.4)	56 (9.6)
Former smoker	400	306 (76.4)	60 (15.0)	34 (8.6)
Current smoker	484	333 (68.8)	122 (25.2)	29 (6.0)

Data in parentheses indicate percentages.
*Normal, <140 mm Hg systolic blood pressure or <90 mm Hg diastolic blood pressure; Mild, 140 to <160 mm Hg systolic blood pressure or 90 to <100 mm Hg diastolic blood pressure. Moderate/severe, ≥160 mm Hg systolic blood pressure or ≥100 mm Hg diastolic blood pressure.

Do not be verbose in citing your findings. For example, "*It is very clearly shown in Table 18.1 that drug A inhibits the growth of species X very effectively.*" Instead, it should be written as: "***Table 18.1** shows that drug A inhibits the growth of species X.*"

Also, write in active voice.
- It has been shown by **Table 18.1** *that drug X is more effective than drug Y* (passive voice).
- **Table 18.1** *shows that drug X is more effective than drug Y* (active voice, preferred).

Text descriptions of the comparisons should clearly mention the magnitude, the direction, and the statistical significance of the difference. Magnitude of the difference is the amount of difference found and direction tells us whether the difference is because of an increase or decrease in the observed measurements. The statistical significance will tell the reader about chance playing a role in the observed difference. A statement such as "*X had a significant positive relationship with Y ($r^2 = 0.80$, $P = 0.025$)*" has all the three attributes, i.e., magnitude (r^2), direction (positive), and statistical significance (P value).

Mentioning Statistics in the Text

Statistical results are one of the evidences and not the only evidence in proving a hypothesis. Statistical test values along with their *P* values should be mentioned in the text. There is no need to describe the statistical theories here. Report exact *P* values and not just as "significant" or "nonsignificant". Technical terms such as "normal", "random", "significant", etc., should be used in the correct context and not in a layman fashion.

Do not confuse clinical significance with statistical significance when writing the statistical results. Certain differences may be statistically significant but clinically nonsignificant and even *vice versa*. You may find a 2 mm decrease in systolic blood pressure as statistically significant, but clinically it may be irrelevant and *vice versa*. A decrease or an increase in the values is important, and needs to be reported as such, even if the statistical significance is not reached.

When expressing the differences between proportions or percentages, you should make it clear whether it is percent change or percentage point change. A change from 50% to 25% can be expressed as a 50% change or a change of 25 percentage points.

Variation in the data should always be mentioned. A measure of central tendency such as "mean" or "median" should be accompanied by a measure of dispersion such as "standard deviation" or "interquartile range" in order to represent the complete data. "Standard error" should be avoided generally, as it speaks about the whole population whereas your findings are restricted to the sample that you have studied.

Example 1

The mean (SD) systolic blood pressure in the two groups were 107 (5.7) and 133 (10.9) mm Hg, respectively. Student's t-test revealed a highly significant difference (P <0.001).

In this case, the statistical package provided a *P* value of zero. Remember NOT to report a *P* value of zero because it is highly improbable that an event can never occur, even by chance. In such cases, report *P* value as <0.001.

Example 2
The percentage of smokers was 66.2% (62/94) in the hypertensive group, and 50% (47/94) in the nonhypertensive group. Chi-square analysis revealed that this was a significant difference (P = 0.023), suggesting that there was a relationship between smoking and hyperten-sion.

Tables and Graphs

When the amount of data to be presented is huge, tables, and graphs are helpful. Tables and graphs should be complete in themselves. Any person not familiar with the study should be able to understand the table and graph presented. They should be properly numbered. And yes, always cite the table and graph in a consecutive manner in the Results section. Highlight the main finding of the table/graph without repeating the whole thing again.

> Tables and graphs should be complete in themselves.

- Use a table when exact numbers are important.
- Use a figure when visual display of trends/comparisons is more important than exact numbers.

Specific Considerations for Tables

When should a tabular form be preferred? If the data can be presented in a text format and can be easily comprehended, then tables should be avoided. Mentioning too many numbers in the text format would make the reading and interpretation of the results cumbersome, and it is better to opt for a tabular form in such cases. To some extent, tables are also helpful in depicting a relationship between two or more variables in the Results section, as it can show the relationship of the variables in the rows and the variables in the columns.

Every table should be cited in the text. When a table is cited in the text, it is not abbreviated as Tab 1 or Tab 2, but mentioned in full, i.e., *Table 1 shows that....* As soon as a table is cited, it should be placed/embedded in the text. Another alternative (as is used for preparing manuscripts for publication in a journal), is to place all the tables at the end of the "Results" section. A table should be complete in itself with all its components in place.

> Always check the numbers and percentages in the rows and whether their total and other calculations are accurate.

Components of a Table
- *Rows:* Rows should be arranged in a logical fashion from top to bottom, e.g., ascending order of income categories.
- *Columns:* Columns should be arranged in a logical order from left to right, e.g., increasing dose categories of the drug in different groups.
- *Heading:* Caption/legend/heading should be mentioned on the top of the table with proper numbering.
- *Column titles:* Appropriate column titles should be mentioned in the table itself.
- *Body of the table:* The body of the table is the data mentioned in the rows/columns.
- *Footnote:* If something more needs to be explained about a certain item in the table, put some symbol in front of that item. Then you can place a footnote explaining those terms.

See **Table 18.1** for example of above description.

Specific Considerations for Graphs/Figures

When should you use a graph/figure? When the need is to have an effective and clear visual display of comparisons or relationships and exact numbers in it does not hold much relevance, it is better to have a graph instead of text/table. Graphs are referred to as figures in the Results section. All figures should be referenced in the text as "Fig. 1" or "Figure 1".

Simple and easy-to-understand graphs are the most powerful ones.

In a figure, you first decide about the X- and Y-axis, and where the origin is from the bottom (in contrast to a table where there are column headings at the top). And that is why the legend/caption of the figures is situated below the figure (in contrast to a table where there is a caption/legend/heading at the top of the table). Simple graphs are the most powerful ones. Using too many colors, 3D types, background shadings, etc., make the figures very distracting to the reader.

Components of a Graph (Fig. 18.1)

- *Axis*: The axis (x and y) should be labeled with proper units specified. Conventionally, the independent variable is plated on x-axis and the dependent variable is placed on the y-axis.
- *Axis labels*: Appropriate axis labels with units specified should be mentioned.
- *Scales*: The scales of the axes should be specified depending on the range of data represented in that figure.
- *Legends*: The point types or bar areas or line types in the plot area should be specified as legends in a side box in the chart area.
- *Caption*: Also the figure should be sequentially numbered in front of the caption of the figure.

After you have decided that a graph is a better way to represent certain data, you have to further decide which type of graph is the most appropriate for that particular data.

Which type of graph is appropriate to depict your variables?

Very often, an inappropriate graph distorts the data. The type of graph depends on the type of variables that are going to be presented on the X- and Y-axis. A guide for selecting an appropriate graph is provided in **Figure 18.2**.

Example 1: Plot the age (in months) of the studied children by sex.

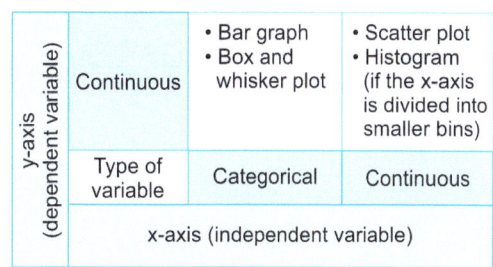

Fig. 18.2: Decision-making matrix for selecting an appropriate graph based on the types of variables to be presented.

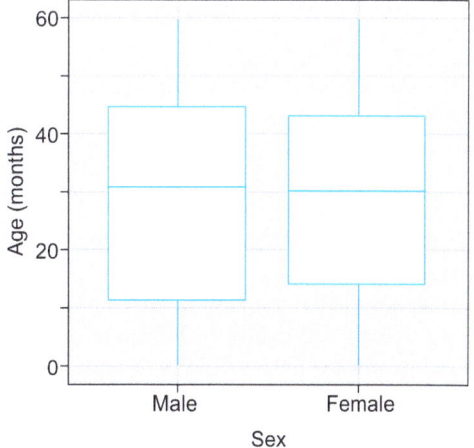

Fig. 18.3: Box plot of age in months of the studied children according to sex.

You have to present the distribution of age in months with respect to the sex of the studied children. Decide first on the axis as follows:
- Sex → categorical variable → x-axis
- Age in months → continuous variable → y-axis

Taking help from **Figure 18.2**, you will find that a bar chart or a box plot is appropriate for depicting this information. The box plot of age in months of the studied children with respect to sex is shown in **Figure 18.3**. Box plots help us to compare the distribution of the continuous data with respect to the various categories of the categorical variable. The middle band in the box is the median of the data.

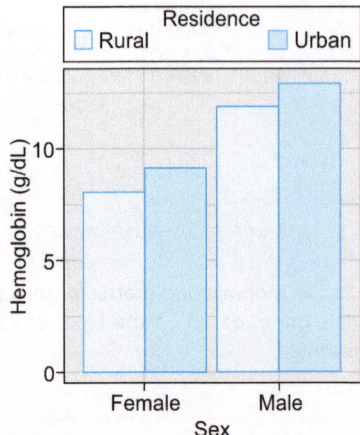

Fig. 18.4: Bar chart depicting hemoglobin values of the studied subjects according to sex and place of residence.

Example 2: *Plot the hemoglobin values of the studied subjects with respect to sex and place of residence.*

Because the hemoglobin values depend on the sex (male or female) and place of residence (rural or urban) both, you will have to plot the hemoglobin values (dependent and continuous variable) on the y-axis and sex and place of residence (independent and categorical variables) on the x-axis. As suggested by **Figure 18.2**, a bar chart or box plot can be used. We have drawn a single bar chart to depict the complete information (**Fig. 18.4**).

Example 3: *Plot the relationship of y-var (dependent and continuous variable) and x-var (independent and continuous variable) with respect to a factor (categorical variable).*

Using **Figure 18.2**, a scatter plot or a histogram can be made. **Figure 18.5** shows a scatter plot for depicting this information.

Example 4: *Plot the distribution of hemoglobin in the studied population.*

You must plot the number of subjects (count variable) on the y-axis with respect to the hemoglobin values (continuous variable) on the x-axis. Here you will have to divide the hemoglobin values into small groups (x-axis) and see that how many individuals have that

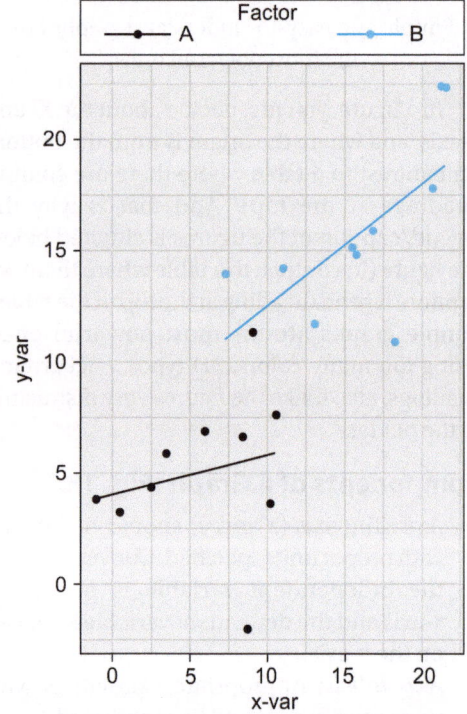

Fig. 18.5: Scatter plot depicting the relationship between x-var and y-var with respect to factor.

much hemoglobin level (y-axis). **Figure 18.6** depicts the histogram for depicting this information.

Photographs/Photomicrographs

If you are presenting some pathological, radiological, or microbiological findings, a photomicrograph/photograph becomes essential. Even in certain clinical cases, describing the signs and photographs becomes indispensable.

Care should be taken when documenting photographs, especially of the face where risk of breaching patient confidentiality is very high. The identity of the patient should be hidden, either by blurring, cutting, or hiding a part of the photograph. Also, patient's consent needs to be obtained for publishing the photo in thesis.

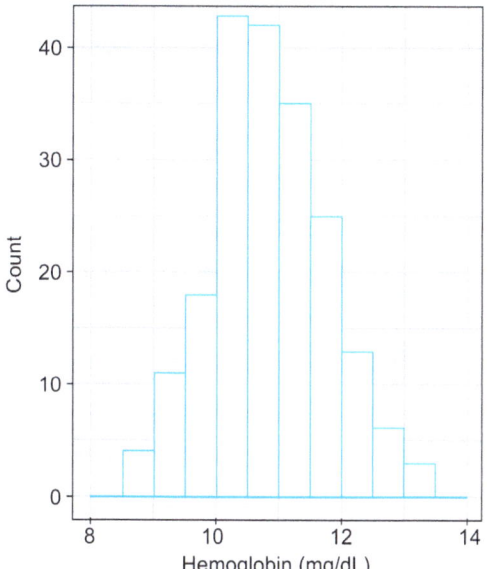

Fig. 18.6: Distribution of hemoglobin values in the studied population.

Any such photograph/photomicrograph, where dimensional measurements are required, an internal scale marker should be attached. The color of the background of the photograph and even the text, symbols or arrows should be such that clarity is not compromised.

CONCLUSION

The Results section of your thesis helps the reader to know what you found in your study. The Results section should therefore, mirror the findings with respect to the *a priori* stated research objectives. Do not avoid mentioning a finding because it does not fit your assumption. Any finding, other than your stated objectives should be mentioned as "additional analysis" at the end of the results section. The order of mentioning your findings must be from simple analytical findings to more complex ones. Text, tables, and graphs are the common ways to depict your results. Usually, the text mode is preferred, but tables are better if too many numbers are to be mentioned, and graphs are preferable if you want to show a trend. The tables and figures should be complete in all respects to the extent that they can be understood independently. The tables and figures should be cited in the text. Do not interpret your findings in the results section.

KEY MESSAGES
- Do not interpret results in the Result section. Just present them.
- Make sure that the data are accurate.
- Avoid repetitions of the same findings in text, table, and figure.
- Present the findings relevant to your research question.
- Mention the findings even if they fail to support your hypotheses.
- Use SI units throughout.
- Raw data should not be included in Result.

FURTHER READING

1. Bahadoran Z, Mirmiran P, Zadeh-Vakili A, Hosseinpanah F, Ghasemi A. The principles of biomedical scientific writing: results. Int J Endocrinol Metabol. 2019;17:e92113.
2. Campbell MJ, Swinscow TDV. Statistics at square one, 11th edition. Chichester: John Wiley and Sons;2011.
3. Cole TJ. Too many digits: The presentation of numerical data. Arch Dis Child. 2015;100:608-9.
4. Diong J, Butler AA, Gandevia SC, Heroux ME. Poor statistical reporting, inadequate data presentation and spin persist despite editorial advice. PLoS One 2018. 13(8): e0202121. [online] Available fromhttps://doi.org/10.1371/journal.pone.0202121 [Last accessed April, 2020].
5. Khan AM, Ramji S. Reporting statistics in biomedical research literature: the numbers say it all. Indian Pediatr. 2016;53:811-4.
6. Mukherjee A, Lodha R. Writing the results. Indian Pediatr. 2016;53:409-15.
7. Ng KH, Peh WC. Presenting the statistical results. Singapore Med J.2009;50(1):11-4. [online] Available from http://www.crc.gov.my/pdf/guide_medical/1_8_Presenting_the_statistical_results.pdf [Last accessed April, 2020].
8. Ng KH, Peh WC. Writing the results. Singapore Med J. 2008;49(12):967-8. [online] Available from http://www.crc.gov.my/pdf/guide_medical/1_6_1_Writing_the_results.pdf [Last accessed April, 2020].

CHAPTER 19

Discussion: The Most Read Part of the Thesis

SV Madhu, Dheeraj Shah

▪ INTRODUCTION

Discussion is the most critical portion of your thesis. You have conducted your research, analyzed your findings, and written your results. Now is the time to revisit and take a fresh look at your work. Writing a good Discussion usually requires several writing attempts.

▪ PURPOSE OF DISCUSSION

In the Introduction section, you would have logically underscored the significance and need for your work. So, carefully re-read your Introduction before writing Discussion.

Attempt to answer the questions you raised in the Introduction, explain how your results support the answers and how your answers fit in with existing knowledge on the topic. All this requires careful evaluation of the results you have obtained in your research, which, therefore, become the main purpose of the Discussion.

While the Introduction starts generally and narrows down to the specific hypothesis, the Discussion starts with specific interpretation of the results and then moves outward toward generalizations and applicability of what has been found to a broader context.

The purpose of writing Discussion is fourfold:
1. To answer your research question or hypothesis.
2. To justify your approach.
3. To critically evaluate the strengths and weaknesses of your methods.
4. To interpret and explain your results.

▪ STRUCTURE AND CONTENTS OF DISCUSSION

In the Discussion section, you state your interpretations and opinions, explain the implications of your findings, and make suggestions for future research.

The Results and the Discussion sections of your thesis are very closely related. But while the Results section is a factual statement of your observations and allows for no personal opinion, the Discussion is the right place to state your interpretations and opinions. You should now think through your observations carefully and provide credible and logical explanations. Discussion is the place for critical reasoning and critical writing rather than merely restating the results.

> **Box 19.1: Key elements of a good discussion.**
> - Summarize your results (avoid data)
> - Discuss strengths, limitations, possible sources of bias and how they might affect generalizability of results
> - Place your results in the context of published literature
> - Provide implications for clinical practice and directions for future research

There are four elements of a good Discussion, as outlined in **Box 19.1**. These should be written in sequential order.

1. Summarize your Results

Your Discussion should begin with a one-page summary of the study's key findings written concisely. This should include a mention of your research question and how much your findings have answered the question.

Do
- Highlight the most significant findings.
- Emphasize on the main objectives and outcome.

Don'ts
- Don't repeat detailed descriptions of data and results.
- Don't introduce new results.
- Don't give a detailed "statement of problem".

2. Discuss Strengths, Limitations, Possible Sources of Bias, and How they Might Affect Generalizability of Results

It is always good to discuss the methodology of your study, especially its strengths and weaknesses, immediately after the summary of your findings. Discuss how your methodology is better suited to answer the research question. Also discuss the various limitations of your study and how these could affect your conclusions.

Do
- Always include limitations of your study.

Don'ts
- Don't start with limitations.
- Don't harp too much on limitations resulting in your work being undermined.
- Don't fail to acknowledge limitations altogether.
- Don't end with limitations.

3. Place your Results in the Context of Published Literature

Compare your results and relate them with other studies to support their validity. For every result that you want to discuss, you should find results from other publications that have a bearing on your work. Set-up a dialog between your results and those of previous workers. Note the similarities, differences, common or different trends. Show how your study either corroborates, extends, refines or conflicts with the previous findings. If your results differ from others' findings, you should try to explain why. Explain how the new data you have generated is positioned in the context of what is already known.

For this, you must revisit your review of literature and try to understand what your findings imply, including how they fit in with previous work. It is your review of the literature which will provide all the necessary background information. Effective utilization of your review will help you refine and give direction to your discussion. A comprehensive and updated review of literature is the key to a good discussion.

Do's
- Read the whole articles, not just abstracts.
- Focus on the main objectives and outcome.
- Compare all the relevant outcomes.
- Discuss studies on both sides of the issue.
- Mention study setting and numbers.
- Critically analyze the results explaining the possible reasons for any differences.

Don'ts

- Don't discuss every possible issue, flaw, and concept.
- Don't compare outcomes not relevant to objectives.
- Don't repeat data and restate results without interpretation.
- Don't simply present results of other studies without critical analysis.
- Don't be critical of authors of other studies for their results.
- Don't repeat the introduction.

4. Provide Implications for Clinical Practice and Directions for Future Research

State the major conclusions from your study and present the theoretical and practical implications of your observations. Discuss the clinical and public health implications where relevant. For example, the conclusion that smoking increases the prevalence of diabetes has obvious implications for the prevention of diabetes. Discuss the implications of your study for future research and be specific about the next logical step for future researchers. For example, in the above case, the next logical step would be to plan an intervention study with cessation of smoking.

Do's

- Include clinical and public health (not statistical) implications of your study.
- Mention significance of your findings.
- Mention the circumstances/conditions where results do not apply.
- Differentiate between strong and weak results while drawing conclusions.

Don'ts

- Don't inflate the importance of findings of the study.
- Don't make strong claims about weak results.
- Don't speculate unnecessarily and guess beyond what can be supported by your data.
- Don't attribute relationships as "causal" when your data supports only "associations" or "correlations".
- Don't fail to give concluding statements.
- Don't overstate your conclusions.
- Don't give conclusions not assessed in study findings (e.g., cost effective, feasible).

■ HOW TO ORGANIZE YOUR DISCUSSION: 10 POINTS

The organization of the discussion is important. Before starting, you should try to develop an outline to organize your thoughts in a logical sequence. Follow these steps:

1. Organize the discussion from the specific to the general; your findings to the literature, to theory, to practice.
2. Begin by addressing your hypothesis and answering questions you asked in the introduction using the same key terms.
3. Support the answers with the results. Explain how your results relate to the questions raised and why they are valid. Also explain how your results relate to the literature and how they fit in with previously published knowledge on the topic.
4. Address all the results relating to the questions, regardless of whether or not the findings were statistically significant.
5. Describe the trends and relationships that emerge from the interpretation of each major finding and put them in context. The sequencing of providing this information is important: First state the answer, then the relevant results and then cite the work of others.
6. Defend your answers by explaining why your explanation is better and more logical than others by discussing both sides of the argument to add strength to what you have to say. If there are more than one possible explanation for your results, discuss all of them even if these are conflicting.

7. Discuss any unexpected findings. Begin the paragraph with this finding and then describe it.
8. Identify the possible limitations and weaknesses and comment on their relative importance to your interpretation of the results and how they may affect the validity of the findings.
9. Summarize concisely the principal implications of the findings, regardless of statistical significance. Provide one or two recommendations for further research.
10. Explain how the results and conclusions of this study add to our knowledge or understanding of the problem being investigated.

HOW TO CONNECT ALL THE ELEMENTS AND PROVIDE A FLOWING TEXT IN DISCUSSION

To make your message clear, the Discussion should be kept as short as possible while clearly stating your interpretations and defending your explanations. Side issues should not be included, as these tend to undermine the main message. So, be brief, concise, specific, and focused.

Write your Discussion in short paragraphs. Use subheadings, if necessary.

Your Discussion should tell a story with a clear message. Hence, you should carefully sequence the order of the findings that you wish to discuss in a manner that the link between each of the answers and explanations is not broken and there is a smooth flow of text. Never lose sight of the underlying theme of your message.

CHECKLIST

Once you have written your discussion, make sure you have included all the vital ingredients of this section. You should use the following checklist as a guide to ensure that nothing is missed out.

In your discussion, you should have:
- Summarized your main results.
- Interpreted (not described) your results.
- Discussed the significance of your results.
- Explained whether your results prove or disprove your hypothesis.
- Discussed your results in the light of previous research (confirmed or refuted previous studies).
- Explained the wider implications (importance) of your work.
- Discussed any problems with, or limitations of, your study.
- Made suggestions for improvements.
- Suggested directions for future research.

CONCLUSION

A well-organized Discussion section shows how well you have interpreted your work and how well you have answered your research question. You should therefore, spend enough time writing Discussion and carefully structure the content keeping in mind all the important elements and ingredients as well as all the do's and don'ts. A well-written Discussion gives the right perspective to your research and is the key to its proper understanding.

KEY MESSAGES
- Write "Discussion" in a sequential way.
- Avoid repetition of results (data).
- Focus of comparison should be on the main study objectives and outcome.
- Critically analyze your study in the context of existing literature and for implications.
- Discussion should be based directly on study findings.

■ FURTHER READING

1. Bagga A. Discussion: The heart of the paper. Indian Pediatr. 2016;53(10):901-4.
2. Bresson L. [How to write the "Discussion" part of your article, master's essay or thesis]. Gynecol Obstet Fertil. 2009;37(4):372-3.
3. Cals JW, Kotz D. Effective writing and publishing scientific papers, part VI: Discussion. J Clin Epidemiol. 2013;66(10):1064.
4. Foote M. The proof of the pudding: how to report results and write a good discussion. Chest. 2009;135(3):866-8.
5. Hess DR. How to write an effective discussion. Respir Care. 2004;49(10):1238-41.
6. Höfler M, Venz J, Trautmann S, Miller R. Writing a discussion section: how to integrate substantive and statistical expertise. BMC Med Res Methodol. 2018;18(1):34.
7. Makar G, Foltz C, Lendner M, Vaccaro AR. How to write effective discussion and conclusion sections. Clin Spine Surg. 2018;31(8):345-6.
8. Masic I. How to write an efficient discussion? Med Arch. 2018;72(4):306-7.

CHAPTER 20

Writing the Conclusion: Bringing Down the Curtains in Style

Nidhi Bedi, Pooja Dewan

■ INTRODUCTION

The Conclusion section of a thesis aims to provide a synthesis of the key points of your research. The objective is to make the readers understand the relevance, results, and implications of your research. This section is sandwiched between the Discussion and References section of your thesis and you will get down to writing this part usually as you get ready to wind up your thesis.

The "Conclusion" section serves two main functions. The first is to summarize and bring together the main areas covered in the research, which might be called "looking back"; and the second is to give a final comment or judgment on this which may be called "looking ahead." The Conclusion section should thus provide succinct answers to the research questions and also raise new questions for future.

While the Introduction section proceeds from general information to more specific issues of your research, the Conclusion intends to move over from the more specific points of your research to provide a general overview (or implications) of your research.

■ ELEMENTS OF THE CONCLUSION SECTION

The Conclusion section is usually brief, not exceeding 300–400 words. You may write it in a maximum of two paragraphs, or sometimes in bulleted text. The Conclusion needs to cover the following aspects of your research:
- Key results or findings in context of the objectives.
- General implications of your findings.

The first part of the structure is "the looking back" part. Herein you will synthesize your key findings and provide answers to your research questions. You need to begin by clearly stating the key results in context of your objectives. It is important to frame this part using the PICO format, i.e., describe the *p*articipants, the *i*ntervention you used, *c*omparator (or control) group if any, and the *o*utcome variables. It is important to briefly mention the study design as well. Remember that you do not go into statistical details but only provide a broader result of your research. This part conveys the inference you have drawn from your research. An example is given in **Box 20.1**.

> **Box 20.1: Stating the key findings in context of objectives using PICO format.**
>
> In this placebo-controlled randomized controlled trial conducted on 120 children, we did not find any beneficial role of short-term oral vitamin D supplementation (1,000 IU in children aged <1 year and 1,500 IU for children aged ≥1 year for 5 days duration) in hospitalized under-five children with severe pneumonia as per the WHO definition.
>
> We found no significant difference in the median duration of resolution of severe pneumonia in interventional group versus control group. Also, the duration of hospitalization, time to resolution of tachypnea, chest retractions, and hypoxia, and time to initiation of feeds were comparable in the two groups. Vitamin D supplementation was well tolerated in all age groups without showing any major side effects.

> **Box 20.2: Implications of the study considering its strengths and limitations.**
>
> Short-term supplementation of oral vitamin D has no beneficial effect on resolution of severe pneumonia in under-five children, as is evident in our study. However, the results of this study are limited by the lack of estimation of serum vitamin D levels in the study participants which could guide on the adequate dose of vitamin D to be used in these children. It may be useful to take note of the fact that the low dose of vitamin D supplement used in our study was planned keeping in mind the LOAEL and NOAEL, with no previous studies available to support higher doses. Also, there was no clear demarcation between bacterial and viral acute LRTI in our study. The strength of our study includes its randomized placebo-controlled design and the adequate sample size.

The next part should highlight the implications of your findings for practitioners. It may be useful to spell the strengths and limitations of your work again but do not go overboard. **Box 20.2** exemplifies this section. You need to close this section with a clear statement on recommendations for policy/practice. It may be useful to provide a direction for future research as well (**Box 20.3**).

> **Box 20.3: Looking ahead: future directions and recommendations.**
>
> Further studies are required wherein the role of higher doses of vitamin D supplementation needs to be assessed. Also, the effect of longer duration of vitamin D supplementation in these children should be evaluated for its therapeutic effect in childhood pneumonia. Concomitant estimation of vitamin D levels will also help in providing a clear understanding of the impact of vitamin D supplementation on severe pneumonia in children. Till more research is available, we do not recommend routine oral vitamin D supplementation in childhood pneumonia.

■ DO'S AND DON'TS OF WRITING THE CONCLUSION

Writing the Conclusion section can be pretty daunting, as often this section holds the key to success. It is therefore important to re-read the Introduction, Objectives, Results, and Discussion section before we write the conclusion. You need to consider the following points as you write this section.

Do's

- Remember to answer your research question.
- It is important to synthesize your findings. You need to analyze what is available evidence and how your research corroborates or contradicts the evidence.
- You need to present your findings like an expert and convince the readers of the contribution of your research to the body of science.
- Your research may have contributed with a new technique, a new treatment, a contradiction of the prevalent policy, or a novel finding; it is important to spell it out in this section once again. While doing so, relate your research to the evidence that is available, and elaborate on what your research adds.
- You may use a mix of tenses (past, present, and future) when you write this section. You

may use the present tense to explain your findings and to make it evident that your statements still hold at the time of reading. You will use the future *tense* while making recommendations for further work. Refer to **Table 20.1** to see the use of tenses in this section.

Don'ts

- Avoid restating the results in numbers.
- Do not add statistical values but provide an inference of your results.
- Refrain from focusing your results on unimportant issues or adding any new objectives which were not part of your original study plan.
- The Conclusion section needs to be brief but a painfully short Conclusion section will only bring out the "writer's block" and will not push forward any new ideas.
- An over-simplification and repetition of all findings is also unnecessary.
- Do not include conclusions that do not emerge from evidence in the present study.

■ COMMON ERRORS IN WRITING THE CONCLUSION

You should avoid using an emotional tone like apologizing for the small sample size, as this may not convince the readers of your findings. It is important to convey your opinion without being too pompous or authoritative. It is also important to avoid over-generalization and portraying that your thesis did more than it actually did. Do not shy away from focusing on the specific (but maybe small) contribution your research made. **Table 20.2** illustrates the common errors in writing the conclusion.

TABLE 20.1: **Use of tenses while writing the various elements of the conclusion.**

Element	Tense/verb form	Example
Looking back	Simple past tense	This study *was conducted* with the purpose of ascertaining the role of routine antifungal prophylaxis in preterm babies
Restating the findings of your research	Simple past tense	We *found* that the pattern of sleep is different in various phases of menstrual cycle
Explaining the findings	Present tense	This work *shows* the existence of autonomic imbalances in acute and chronic pain states which affect not only the cardiovascular system but also the pulmonary profile, bringing about alterations in the ventilation
Limitations	Simple past	Since the sample size of our study *was* small, these results may not be directly extrapolated to the general population
Implications for practice/policy	Use verbs such as likely, it is possible, may, might, seems, etc.	Three-dose vaccination with recombinant hepatitis B vaccine *may* prove as beneficial as a four-dose vaccination schedule
Future directions	Future	Effect of viral load on immune response to vaccination *needs to be* evaluated in more studies with a larger sample size
Recommendations	Simple present	We *do not advocate* any change in the current policy regarding hepatitis B vaccination in the healthy preterm newborns

TABLE 20.2: Avoidable styles of writing the conclusion.

Style	Example
Sherlock Holmes conclusion: Adding new objectives	*Objective*: To compare the pulmonary function tests (PFTs) in prepubertal and postpubertal adolescents *Conclusion*: We found that the pattern of PFT is different in various phases of menstrual cycle. PFTs are better in prepubertal adolescents compared to postpubertal adolescents
'Grab bag' conclusion: Focusing on minor points	*Objective*: To compare the efficacy of ferrous sulfate with ferrous carbonate in improving hemoglobin in under-five children *Conclusion*: Ferrous sulfate is more cost-effective compared to ferrous carbonate in increasing hemoglobin level. Both drugs showed a comparable increase in hemoglobin
That is my story and I am sticking to it: Too authoritative	*Objective*: To compare seroprotection rates following primary immunization with double dose (20 mcg) recombinant hepatitis B vaccine (rHBV) administered at 0, 1, and 6 months versus 0, 1, 2, and 6 months in HIV-infected children receiving antiretroviral therapy *Calculated sample size:* 198 per group *Studied sample size:* 25 per group *Conclusion*: We found that in comparison to the three-dose schedule of rHBV, four-dose schedule had significantly higher titers 1 month after completion of vaccination schedule. HIV-infected children must be offered four doses of rHBV for primary immunization
We shall overcome: Overly emotional	*Objective*: To assess the effect of exercise on stress in medical students *Conclusion*: This study was conducted in a limited time on limited sample. We could only compare before and after values and could deduce changes only between these values. If the study was of longer duration, multiple time assessments would have been possible and then the trends of changes could have been determined. Better results may have been obtained with larger sample size. Information extracted from a small sample size is often highly skewed. Recommendations of this study do not apply on general population

Source: Writing Center: University of North Carolina at Chapel Hill. Conclusions. [online] Available from https://writingcenter.unc.edu/tips-and-tools/conclusions/[Last accessed April 30, 2020].

■ CONCLUSION

The Conclusion section must recap the scientific evidence, highlight your contribution, and provide a future direction to the readers. Also, remember that the examiner will usually read the Conclusion in the end and the impression is likely to carry with him/her. Hence, save the best for last!

> **KEY MESSAGES**
> - Provide succinct answers to the research questions and also raise new questions for future.
> - Include the following elements: (1) key results or findings in context of the objectives and using the PICO format, (2) implications of your findings and directions for future research, (3) recommendations regarding policy/practice.
> - Summarize or wrap up the main points in the conclusion. Remember to highlight any new finding of your study, however, avoid adding new objectives at this point of the study.
> - "Recap not repeat" is the key to a good conclusion.

FURTHER READING

1. Essay-lib.com: Custom Writing Service. (2020). How to write a conclusion for a research paper. [online] Available from https://essay-lib.com/write-conclusion-research-paper/ [Last accessed April 30, 2020].
2. Paperpile: Research and Writing Guides. (2020). How to write an excellent thesis conclusion. [online] Available from https://paperpile.com/g/thesis-conclusion/ [Last accessed April 30, 2020].
3. Writing Center: University of North Carolina at Chapel Hill. Conclusions. [online] Available from https://writingcenter.unc.edu/tips-and-tools/conclusions/ [Last accessed April 30, 2020].

Summary: The Essence of Thesis

Pooja Dewan, Nidhi Bedi

INTRODUCTION

Summary is a concise statement of the major elements of the research undertaken by you in your thesis. The purpose of having a Summary is to give a quick overall impression of the research work undertaken by you.

Why do we need the Summary?

The Summary is *not* like the trailer of a movie, instead it is like a "short film" or a "featurette" wherein the whole story is conveyed in a shorter time. The Summary is intended to give a complete overview of your research work to the reader, in short time. The Summary should be written in a way to reflect the research conducted by you in a nutshell and to persuade the readers to go through the details of your research work. To enable a good comprehension, the Summary must be complete (should not hide anything), clear, concise, and cohesive.

FORMAT FOR WRITING THE SUMMARY

The Summary aims to condense the thesis and should not exceed two pages. You need to cover the four major elements of your research work in the summary, *viz.*, (1) the introduction (including background, justification, and objectives), (2) the methodology undertaken, (3) the key results of your research, and (4) conclusions and recommendations. These elements must be arranged in the above sequence to allow coherent and logical structuring of the thesis. You can present the text of Summary in a structured or unstructured format.

Structured Summary

A structured format, using subheadings, helps ensure completion and prevents omission of key elements. You may opt for a 10-point format or a 4-point format as shown in **Table 21.1**. While opting for a 4-point format, it is important to ensure that the methods section is detailed and covers the necessary information.

Unstructured Summary

You may write the Summary in an unstructured format wherein the information is conveyed in running text, in paragraphs, without the use of subheadings. You can write the Summary in four sequential paragraphs, one each on

TABLE 21.1: Checklist for a 4-point and 10-point Summary/Abstract.

4-point format	10-point format
1. Introduction	1. *Background* (lacunae in literature and justification for the study)
	2. *Objectives* (primary and secondary)
2. Methods	3. *Study design*
	4. *Study duration*
	5. *Study setting*
	6. *Participant* details (sample size, inclusion criteria, exclusion criteria)
	7. *Interventions/methodology*
	8. *Outcome measures*
3. Results	9. *Results*:
	i. Baseline data/details of participants (number, age, sex, etc.)
	ii. Results of primary outcome variables
	iii. Results of secondary outcome variables
	iv. Additional significant findings/results (if any)
4. Conclusions and recommendations	10. *Conclusions and Recommendation*:
	i. Conclusion
	ii. Recommendations for policy, practice, and future research

background and rationale, methods, results, and conclusions. You could also write the Summary in bulleted text. Example of an unstructured summary is given in **Box 21.1**.

ELEMENTS OF SUMMARY

Introduction

Background of the study needs to be presented at the beginning of the Summary. It should include the existing literature relevant to the research, the lacunae in literature, your research question, and the objectives of your research work, in a sequential manner. State clearly the primary and secondary objectives. The aim of introduction is to introduce and justify the topic, followed by stating the aim and objectives of the study. **Box 21.2** is an example of this section.

Methods

Methods section of the research work must include the following subsections namely: study design, duration of the study, place of the study, participants (sample size, inclusion, and exclusion criteria), methods/interventions, and outcome measures (primary and secondary). This is the most crucial part of presentation as it enables the reader to decide the quality of study and thereby the level of evidence. It also allows the readers to validate the claims made by you in your results and conclusions section. An example of methods section is outlined in **Box 21.3**.

Results

The results of the study must address the objectives of your study. Remember to provide results for each of your outcome variables included in the primary and secondary objectives. The summary should also provide the number of patients who completed the study and number of dropouts at various stages of the study. Information of results in numerical values such as mean (standard deviation), median (interquartile range), proportions, relative risk, and odds ratio (95%

> **Box 21.1: Example of unstructured summary.**
>
> *Title of thesis*: **Oral zinc supplementation for acute diarrhea in children older than 5 years—A randomized controlled study.**
>
> **Summary**
>
> The therapeutic role of oral zinc supplementation in acute diarrhea among children <5 years is well established. Despite the preponderance of diarrheal disease as well as zinc deficiency among older children and given the beneficial effects of zinc in diarrhea, no scientific evidence exists for assessing the role of zinc supplementation in older children (>5 years) with acute dehydrating diarrhea. We conducted this study to ascertain whether zinc supplementation in children aged 5–12 years with acute diarrhea is beneficial. The primary objective of this study was to evaluate the effect of oral zinc supplementation on the time taken for resolution of acute dehydrating diarrhea in children older than 5 years of age. Recurrence of acute diarrheal episodes in the next 3 months was the secondary objective.
>
> We conducted this randomized double-blind placebo-controlled study between November 2016 and April 2018. Children aged 5–12 years, presenting to pediatric emergency of a tertiary hospital in Delhi, with acute watery diarrhea (≥3 episodes of loose stools over previous 24 hours) of <72 hours duration, with some or severe dehydration were assessed for inclusion. Children with dysentery, severe systemic illness or those who received any zinc containing multivitamin/mineral supplementation for >7 days in last 3 months were excluded. Participants were randomized to receive 20 mg of elemental zinc twice a day for 14 days (n = 60) or placebo (n = 60) besides the standard WHO treatment of diarrhea and dehydration. The primary outcome of this study was the time taken for clinical resolution of diarrhea and the secondary outcome variable was the recurrence of acute diarrhea in the next 3 months.
>
> We recruited 120 children in this study, 60 each in the zinc and placebo groups. There were 72 boys, 34 in the zinc supplemented group and 38 in the placebo group; the sex distribution was comparable in both groups. All children could be followed up following discharge from the hospital for 3 months duration. The mean (SD) age of participants in both groups was similar [zinc: 7 (2.3) years; placebo 7.1 (2.2) years]. The mean (SD) serum zinc level was 63.5 (19) µg/L in the zinc group and 64 (19.2) µg/L in the placebo group. Seventy-five children (62.5%) were found to be zinc deplete (serum zinc <65 µg/L). The mean (SD) time taken for resolution of diarrhea was similar in the two groups [zinc: 62.1 (17.1) hours; placebo: 63 (16.8) hours]. The two groups were comparable with respect to the mean (SD) duration of hospital stay [zinc: 10.1 (9.2) days; placebo: 11 (9.8) hours]. The risk of having an episode of diarrhea in the subsequent 3 months was reduced by 44% in the zinc group [OR (95% CI); 0.6 (0.23–1.18) $P = 1.18$)]. A subgroup analysis in the zinc depleted group also did not reveal any benefit of zinc supplementation for the above outcome variables.
>
> We conclude that zinc supplementation in acute dehydrating diarrhea in children >5 years does not result in early resolution of illness but there is a trend of fewer diarrheal episodes in subsequent 3 months. We do not recommend zinc supplementation in children >5 years of age with acute diarrhea. There is a need to assess the preventive role of zinc in diarrhea in children >5 years with community-based trials with adequate sample size.

confidence intervals) should be mentioned as it represents the authenticity of results. Any significant positive or negative finding or adverse effect should always be mentioned along with *P* values. There is no need to include any figures or tables. The results should justify your claims. **Box 21.4** illustrates the results section of a thesis.

Conclusions and Recommendations

You need to conclude by summarizing your findings and follow it with recommendations for any change in policy or practice and need for future research (e.g., See **Box 21.5**). Making towering claims not backed by your results will

Box 21.2: Example of "Introduction" in the Summary.

Title of thesis: Oral zinc supplementation for acute diarrhea in children older than 5 years—a randomized controlled study.

Introduction

Background: The therapeutic role of oral zinc supplementation in acute diarrhea among children <5 years is well established.

Justification and lacunae: Despite the preponderance of diarrheal disease as well as zinc deficiency among older children and given the beneficial effects of zinc in diarrhea, no scientific evidence exists for assessing the role of zinc supplementation in older children (>5 years) with acute dehydrating diarrhea.

Objectives: We conducted this study to ascertain whether zinc supplementation in children aged 5–12 years with acute diarrhea is beneficial. The primary objective of this study was to evaluate the effect of oral zinc supplementation on the time taken for resolution of acute dehydrating diarrhea in children older than 5 years of age. Recurrence of acute diarrheal episodes in the next 3 months was the secondary objective.

Box 21.3: Example of Methods in the Summary.

Methods

Study design: Randomized double-blind placebo-controlled study

Study duration: November 2016–April 2018

Place of study: Inpatient and emergency pediatrics ward of a tertiary hospital in Delhi.

Participants: 120 children aged 5–12 years presenting to pediatric emergency with acute watery diarrhea (≥3 episodes of loose stools over previous 24 hours) of <72 hours duration, with some or severe dehydration were included. Children with dysentery, severe systemic illness or those who received any zinc containing multivitamin/mineral supplementation for >7 days in last 3 months were excluded.

Intervention: Participants were randomized to receive 20 mg of elemental zinc twice a day for 14 days (n = 60) or placebo (n = 60) besides the standard WHO treatment of diarrhea and dehydration.

Outcome measures: Primary—time taken for clinical resolution of diarrhea. Secondary—recurrence of acute diarrhea in the next 3 months.

Box 21.4: Example of "Results" in the Summary.

Results

Baseline data: We recruited 120 children in this study, 60 each in the zinc and placebo groups. There were 72 boys, 34 in the zinc supplemented group and 38 in the placebo group; the sex distribution was comparable in both groups. All children could be followed up following discharge from the hospital for 3 months duration. The mean (SD) age of participants in both groups was similar [zinc: 7 (2.3) years; placebo 7.1 (2.2) years]. The mean (SD) serum zinc level was 63.5 (19) µg/L in the zinc group and 64 (19.2) µg/L in the placebo group. Seventy-five children (62.5%) were found to be zinc deplete (serum zinc <65 µg/L).

Results for primary objectives: The mean (SD) time taken for resolution of diarrhea was similar in the two groups [zinc: 62.1 (17.1) hours; placebo: 63 (16.8) hours].

Results for secondary objectives: The two groups were comparable with respect to the mean (SD) duration of hospital stay [zinc: 10.1 (9.2) days; placebo: 11 (9.8) hours]. The risk of having an episode of diarrhea in the subsequent 3 months was reduced by 44% in the zinc group [OR (95% CI); 0.6 (0.23–1.18) P = 1.18)].

Additional analyses: A subgroup analysis in the zinc depleted group also did not reveal any benefit of zinc supplementation for the above outcome variables.

Box 21.5: Example "Conclusions" in the Summary.

Conclusion

We conclude that zinc supplementation in acute dehydrating diarrhea in children >5 years does not result in early resolution of illness but there is a trend of fewer diarrheal episodes in subsequent 3 months. We do not recommend zinc supplementation in children >5 years of age with acute diarrhea. There is a need to assess the preventive role of zinc in diarrhea in children >5 years with community-based trials with adequate sample size.

put off the reader and hence utmost caution is needed while framing this part of the Summary. At times, a line on some additional finding which may be of reader's interest can be added.

■ WHERE TO PLACE THE SUMMARY IN THE THESIS?

Different universities may have different guidelines for writing the Summary, so it is best to check with your department for inserting the Summary at appropriate place in the text. The University of Delhi requires the Summary to be placed towards the end of the thesis, after appendices; some other universities prefer that a thesis summary is placed at the beginning of a thesis (after the title page and the acknowledgments section). Some universities, such as the National Board of Examinations, require the Summary of thesis to be submitted separately and in addition to the thesis document.

■ ATTRIBUTES OF A GOOD SUMMARY

The four essential attributes of a Summary are:
1. *Complete*: It should be complete so as to cover the major parts of the research project and what is new. Tally the elements listed in the checklist (**Table 21.1**) with your Summary to ensure completion.
2. *Concise*: The Summary must be crisp and to the point. A verbose summary with lengthy statements, excessive use of jargon, prepositions or adjectives, will defeat the very purpose of having a summary. Empty statements such as "more research is needed" or "it is interesting to know that" should be avoided.
3. *Cohesive*: The matter must be placed in a logical order and should be cohesive so as to have a continuation with the previous part. The four elements of introduction, methods, results, and conclusions must be placed sequentially.
4. *Clear*: It should be clear, well readable, well organized, and devoid of too many jargons or acronyms.

Do's and Don'ts of Writing the Summary

Do's

- Write the Summary after the research work is completed and the rest of the sections have been written.
- Read the thesis again before writing the Summary and make notes of significant points to be included in summary.
- Highlight the uniqueness of your findings in your conclusions.
- Use the past tense, e.g., "we concluded...."
- You could use the personal tone, e.g. "we think....." or "I/we found that...."
- Title of the Summary should match with the title of thesis.
- Check for spelling mistakes and grammatical errors before you finalize.
- Before you finalize, ensure the 4C's (complete, clear, concise, and cohesive).
- Be honest in presenting/summarizing the results and observation.

Don'ts

- Do not include discussion in your Summary.
- Do not use words which can be disrespectful to human life such as "use of cases or subjects instead of patients, using males/females instead of men/women."
- Do not make claims not based on your own findings.
- Do not include any new information in your conclusions which is not there in the main text.

- Do not include routine assessments done as a part of research or detailed information on statistical tests. For example, "we considered *P* value <0.05 as significant" can be avoided in the summary.
- Do not include any figures, images, or tables in summary.
- Do not include references or cite literature in the summary.

CONCLUSION

A Summary is a succinct section which provides a complete picture of the research work undertaken by you. It may be presented in a structured format using headings and subheadings, or in an unstructured format. It should cover the four major elements of your research work in sequential order, viz., the introduction, the methodology, the key results of your research, and conclusions and recommendations.

KEY MESSAGES

- Summary may be presented in a structured or unstructured format.
- It should be complete, concise, cohesive, and clear.
- Summary should not contain figures, images, or tables, discussion section, or references.
- Summary should be written only after you have completed writing the rest of the thesis.

FURTHER READING

1. Andrade C. How to write a good abstract for a scientific paper or conference presentation. Indian J Psychiatry. 2011;53(2):172-5.
2. Dewan P, Gupta P. Writing the title, abstract and introduction: Looks Matter! Indian Pediatr. 2016;53(3):235-41.
3. Editage Insights. (2017). How can we write a summary of a thesis? [online] Available from: https://www.editage.com/insights/how-can-we-write-a-summary-of-a-thesis [Last accessed April 30, 2020].

CHAPTER 22

Writing References

Piyush Gupta, Amir Maroof Khan

■ INTRODUCTION

References are an integral part of any research paper, including thesis. This chapter mentions all the essential elements which you need to know to write references in your thesis.

■ WHY REFERENCES ARE IMPORTANT

- References lend credibility and precision to your work. If you write an article based on your own thoughts without referring to other people's work on the same topic, it practically has no weightage as those could be just your own ideas without any supporting scientific evidence.
- Referencing helps you emphasize that there are unanswered questions on the subject, based on the current literature and that a particular dimension of the topic is still unexplored.
- To acknowledge the contribution of those who have already done research on the subject.
- To justify a meticulous search of existing literature on the topic of your research.

"References need to be cited and quoted correctly. They are akin to mortar, which not only bind the bricks together in a wall, but also lend it the most vital elements: Strength and durability" (Gupta P, et al. Indian Pediatrics. 2005).

■ KEY TERMS USED IN REFERENCING

Reference list: It consists of a list of references cited in the thesis, arranged in a predefined manner. Only that material can be used as references, which you have quoted in your thesis.

Bibliography: It is the list of all study material consulted, including that which is not cited in your thesis. It amounts to something like "suggested reading" if the reader wishes to learn further.

Cross-reference: It refers to a reference quoted in an article that you have used as a reference.

Citing: This means acknowledging an idea or a concept of another author. A citation tells the readers where the information came from. In your writing, you cite or refer to the source of information. More a research is cited, more creditable that research is thought to be.

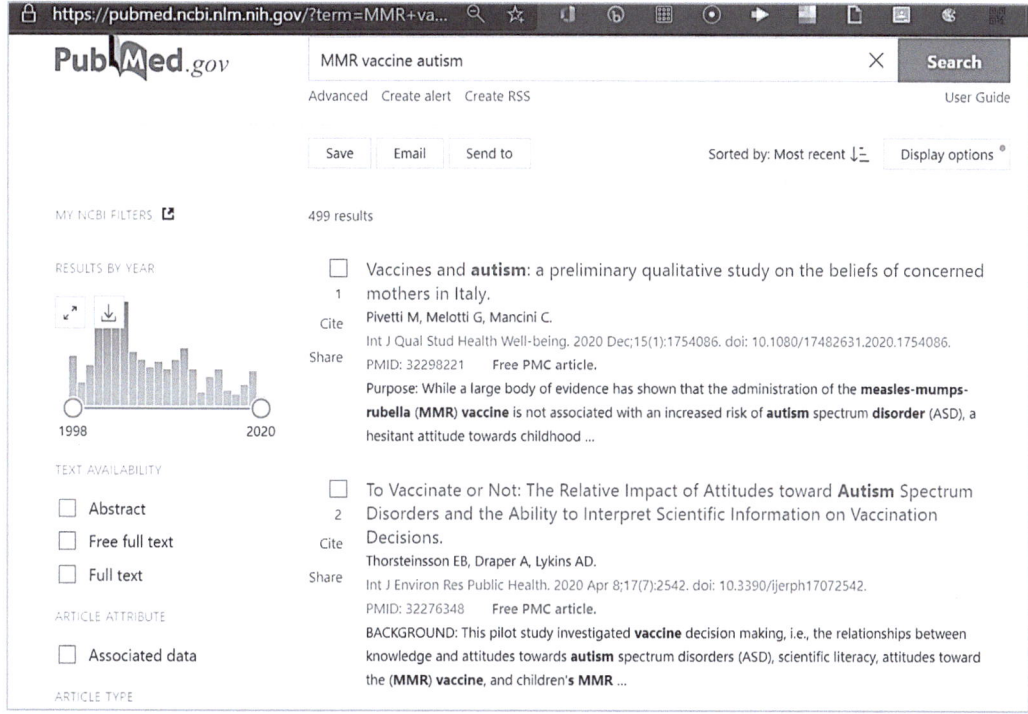

Fig. 22. 1: Searching for literature on measles, mumps, and rubella (MMR) vaccine and autism. *(For color version, see Plate 2)*

WHICH REFERENCES TO INCLUDE IN THESIS

Include only Relevant References

References need to be relevant to the topic/concept that you are referring to. The following example will clarify the concept of relevance. Suppose you have to find reference for the topic "*MMR vaccine and autism in children*". You search for the keywords "MMR vaccine" and "autism" in PubMed. When you will enter these two terms in PubMed browser, you will get score of results.

As you can see in the screenshot in **Figure 22.1,** this gives you 499 results. Now let's see the first 10 results only. These are depicted in **Box 22.1**. You will realize, of these only 1, 6, 8, and 10 (highlighted) appear relevant to our topic of interest. You will thus retrieve and cite only these articles in your thesis.

Include Recent References

Do not miss any recent research on the topic related to your thesis. It is important to be current and cite all articles that have been published related to your topic in last 10 years. There is a gap of usually 18–24 months between submission of your protocol and thesis. It is possible that during this period, more articles have been published related to your topic. Thus, a fresh literature search has to be done when writing the review of literature for thesis. It ensures that you do not miss out on any recent articles published during this period.

Usually, limit the number of references to 25–30 for thesis protocol and maximum 100 for the thesis.

Sources of References

In writing a scientific article, thesis, or book, the information is gathered from various sources

> **Box 22.1: Identify relevant references related to "measles, mumps, and rubella (MMR) vaccine and autism."**
>
> 1. Pivetti M, Melotti G, Mancini C. Vaccines and autism: a preliminary qualitative study on the beliefs of concerned mothers in Italy. Int J Qual Stud Health Well-being. 2020;15(1):1754086.
> 2. Thorsteinsson EB, Draper A, Lykins AD. To vaccinate or not: The relative impact of attitudes toward autism spectrum disorders and the ability to interpret scientific information on vaccination decisions. Int J Environ Res Public Health. 2020;17(7):2542.
> 3. Qian M, Chou SY, Lai EK. Confirmatory bias in health decisions: Evidence from the MMR-autism controversy. J Health Econ. 2020;70:102284.
> 4. Jama A, Lindstrand A, Ali M, Butler R, Kulane A. Nurses' perceptions of MMR vaccine hesitancy in an area with low vaccination coverage. Pediatric Health Med Ther. 2019;10:177-82.
> 5. Kun E, Benedek A, Mészner Z. Védőoltásokkal kapcsolatos kételyek és elkötelezettség a magyarországi egészségügyi alapellátásban dolgozók körében [Vaccine hesitancy among primary healthcare professionals in Hungary]. Orv Hetil. 2019;160:1904-14.
> 6. Madlon-Kay DJ, Smith ER. Interpreters' knowledge and perceptions of childhood vaccines: Effect of an educational session. Vaccine. 2020;38(5):1216-9.
> 7. Koslap-Petraco M. Vaccine hesitancy: Not a new phenomenon, but a new threat. J Am Assoc Nurse Pract. 2019;31(11):624-6.
> 8. Ward JK, Peretti-Watel P, Bocquier A, Seror V, Verger P. Vaccine hesitancy and coercion: all eyes on France. Nat Immunol. 2019;20:1257-9.
> 9. Carrieri V, Madio L, Principe F. Vaccine hesitancy and (fake) news: Quasi-experimental evidence from Italy. Health Econ. 2019;28(11):1377-82.
> 10. Campbell-Scherer D. Evidence from large Danish cohort does not support an association between the MMR vaccine and autism: facts in a post-truth world. BMJ Evid Based Med. 2019;24(5):198-9.

> **Box 22.2: Sources of references.**
> - Journals
> - Books and theses
> - Conference papers and proceedings
> - Internet and other electronic sources including online databases
> - Multimedia material, CD-ROM, software, E-book
> - Newspaper article, monographs, and dictionaries
> - Documents of government, societies, professional organizations, expert groups and other academic bodies
> - Telecasts and broadcasts, video-recordings

which make the reference list. The most common sources are medical journal articles and books. **Box 22.2** provides a comprehensive list of material that can be used as references. As thesis is a scholarly work, most references to be cited in it should be cited from journal articles.

■ HOW TO WRITE REFERENCES AND INSERT CITATIONS

It is of utmost importance to ensure: (1) Accuracy of references, (2) Appropriate selection of references, and (3) Appropriate placement of reference citations. Adhere to the following rules:
- Cite correctly and completely.
- Cite exactly as given by authors.
- Check the references from PubMed.
- Avoid citing cross-references, unless you have read that article yourself.

Selection of References

- Prefer references of articals published in indexed journals.
- Avoid articles published in languages other than English.
- Avoid referencing from abstracts of conferences and papers under submission.
- Avoid using personal communication as references. This cannot be included in the references list, though it can be cited in the text.

- Do not overinflate the thesis with too many references; it does not make the research any better.

Styles for Writing References

We will introduce you to the two most common formats used for citing references and preparing the references list. Choose the one that is preferred by your university. Also, take the help of your supervisor. The two reference styles are as follows:
1. Harvard style (less commonly used)
2. International Committee of Medical Journal Editors (ICMJE) or Vancouver style (mostly used)

Harvard Style

> Depending on the depth, rate and total mass of discharge, and oceanographic conditions as well, deposited cuttings form piles of few centimeters up to 3 m high and spread over distances of >200 m from the outflow (Daan and Mulder, 1993). During the exploratory phase, the deposition of cuttings and the associated fluids is the main cause of environmental changes (Breuer, et al. 2004).
>
> *References*
>
> Breuer, E, Stevenson, AG, Howe, JA, Carroll, J and Shimmield GB (2004). Drill cutting accumulations in the Northern and central North Sea: A review of environmental interactions and chemical fate. Marine pollution bulletin, 48, 12–25.
>
> Daan, R and Mulder, M (2016). Long-term effects of OBM cutting discharges at a drilling site on the Dutch continental shelf. Netherlands Institute for Sea Research (NIOZ) internal report, 1993–15.

Note the following in above example:
- References are cited in the text in parentheses (brackets).
- Text in brackets would include the surname of first author, postfixed by et al., and followed by the year in which the article was published. For example, [(Breuer et al. 2004)] in the above example.
- Note that for two authors, surnames of both authors are cited, while for a paper where number of authors exceeds two, only the first author's surname is cited, followed by et al.
- The references list is prepared in an alphabetical manner, i.e., starting from A to Z. This is irrespective of the sequence in which the citations appear in the text. For the above example, Breuer et al. will be listed first, followed by Daan and Mulder.
- Do not number the references as 1, 2, 3….. in the references list.

ICMJE (Vancouver) Style

The name Vancouver is derived from a meeting of editors of prominent journals at Vancouver, Canada in 1988 where a system of writing references was approved as the standard for international publications. The Vancouver style was, thus, the beginning of accepted standard of writing the reference list. It is also referred to as the "author-number style". This has been further modified by the ICMJE.

> Combining pulse oximetry with clinical examination can enhance the clinician's ability to detect life-threatening heart disease.[1,2]
>
> *References*
>
> 1. Richmond S, Wren C. Early diagnosis of congenital heart disease. Semin Neonatol. 2012;6:27–35.
> 2. Wren C, Reinhardt Z, Khawaja K. Twenty-year trends in diagnosis of life-threatening neonatal cardiovascular malformations. Arch Dis Child Fetal Neonatal Ed. 2016;93:33–5.

Note the following:
- References are cited in the text as superscripts.
- References are designated by Arabic numerals in the text, in a sequential manner only. For example, the first article cited in the text is numbered as 1. This number is unique for this reference and if there is a need to cite the same reference again in the text, the same number is cited.
- The references list is prepared as a numbered list, starting from 1, 2, 3… and so on, and in the same sequence in which these are cited in the text.

- Details of each reference are provided in the references list against its respective assigned number.

INTERNATIONAL COMMITTEE OF MEDICAL JOURNAL EDITORS (ICMJE) OR VANCOUVER STYLE: KEY ELEMENTS

Citing Authors' Names in Thesis

- The work of other authors needs to be quoted in all the chapters of your thesis, except in Summary, Results, and Conclusions.
- When you quote a work in running text of your thesis (e.g., review of literature), references can also be quoted by authors' names. In doing so, quote only the surname of the author from the reference in the text; omit the initials. For example, if the reference author is Pramod Kumar Sharma... write only Sharma, omit the P or PK. *"Sharma[1] has supported this view..."*
- The above example pertains to a single author reference; however, most of the articles have multiple authors. While referencing them in text, write the name of the first author and postfix it with 'et al'. That implies 'and others......' For example, if the authors of the article to be cited are Pramod Kumar Sharma, OP Verma, Piyush Gupta, and BK Jain; quote as:
"Sharma, et al.[1] have supported this view that ...."

Numbering the References

Every reference mentioned in your text must be included in reference list given at the end of the thesis.
- You should prepare this list by the sequence in which the references appear in the thesis. Once a reference has been allotted a number, the same number is used whenever it is quoted again in whole of the thesis. If there is more than one article by the same authors, each article will have a separate reference number.
- The number given in the reference list is to be mentioned in the text where the reference is cited. This is written as a number in a square bracket after the name of the author or as a superscript.
Anderson [5], Kite [9] and Schultzer [21] conducted similar experiments....
OR
Anderson[5], Kite[9], and Schultzer[21] have observed that....
- If the name of the author comes at the end of a sentence or there is a symbol after the name, the reference number comes after that.
The finding has also been confirmed by Gupta, et al. [7].
- In a running discussion or text, sometimes the names of the authors are not mentioned. The references are then mentioned just by their numbers.
Several studies[12,23,34] have been conducted to observe the effect of steroids on.....
- If a statement is supported by references that appear consecutively in the reference list, they are written with a hyphen between the first and the last number.
This finding has also been reported by many authors.[42-49]
- If there are only two authors for an article, let us say Pramod Kumar Sharma and OP Verma, quote both surnames in the text. *"Sharma and Verma[1] postulated that ...."*
- The reference list is composed only after the text of entire thesis is finalized. The order in which the references appear in the text decides the sequence of the reference in the references list.

Writing Reference for an Article Published in a Journal

Name(s) of the Author(s)

A journal reference starts with the name(s) of the author(s); surnames followed by initials;

in the same order as published in the original article. This is followed by the complete title of the article. Abbreviated name of the journal appears next. And finally, there is the year of publication; volume, and issue: and first-last page numbers.

Write surname first for each author followed by a space and then his/her initials. If there are more than one authors, separate author names from each other by a comma and space. If there are more than six authors, write the names of only first six authors, postfixed by et al.

Journal Names

All journals indexed in PubMed have standard abbreviations. For example, *Indian Pediatrics* is abbreviated as *Indian Pediatr* by PubMed. These abbreviations are used uniformly across the globe. It is mandatory to use the same abbreviation in writing a reference from a journal article.

"Journal of Bone and Joint Surgery" is written as *J Bone Joint Surg*.

"Journal of Accident and Emergency Medicine" is written as *J Accid Emerg Med*.

A complete list of abbreviations of indexed journals is available on PubMed.

Journal not indexed in PubMed. For these journals, do not abbreviate their names for references list. Provide the full name. For example, *Indian Journal of Practical Pediatrics* (a journal not indexed by PubMed) has to be written as such and *not* to be abbreviated as *IJPP* or *Indian J Pract Pediatr*.

Article Title

Provide the complete title of the article (as it is) in sentence case. Only the first word is to be capitalized. Do not convert UK English to American (US) English (and vice versa) while writing the references. For example, if the article was published as "Aetiology of diarrhoea in United Kingdom", *do not change* to "Etiology of diarrhea in United Kingdom." This applies irrespective of whichever style (US or UK) you are using for the rest of the text of the thesis.

Publication Year, Volume, and Page Numbers

These elements are the most essential and accuracy is a must, so as to localize the publication and retrieve it.

After the abbreviated journal title, put a period (i.e., a full-stop), then write the year, followed by a semicolon, then write the volume with issue number in bracket, then add a colon, and then write both the first and the last page numbers of the article (separated by a hyphen or dash).

Example

> Francis RL, Achor RWP, Brown AL. Angina pectoris preceding initial myocardial infarction: a clinicopathologic study. Arch Intern Med. 1963;112:226–33.

Writing the Reference for a Chapter from a Book

References can be quoted from monograms and books on a related topic. When you are quoting a book reference, it is written in the reference list in the following standard format:

Author of part, AA. Title of chapter or part. In: Editor A, Editor B, editors. Title: subtitle of Book. Edition (if not the first). Place of publication: Publisher; Year. Pp. Page numbers.

Example

> Argani P, Bexkwith JB. Renal neoplasms of childhood. In: Mills SE (Editor). Sternberg's Surgical Pathology. 4th Ed. Philadelphia: Lippincott Williams and Wilkins; 2004. pp. 2029–30.

Internet Citation

Title of home page. Title URL. Accessed on date.

Example

> American Medical Association. Code of ethics. Appointment changes. Available from: http:/www.ama.assn.org/ama/pub/category/8446.htm. Accessed on Feb. 28th, 2020.

The ICMJE has provided samples of quoting references from various sources. Specific samples are provided further in this Chapter.

■ REFERENCE MANAGERS

Managing references is a tedious task. Storing hundreds of articles and other sources, and retrieval of those sources while writing the thesis, and furthermore changing the order of references while redrafting the thesis consumes a lot of time and energy of the researcher. This can now be avoided by using certain software, popularly known as "reference managers".

Reference managers are software which act as libraries to store various sources of information and retrieve it while writing a thesis/paper. It can manage the numbering of the references and can create a reference list at the end of the thesis. There are many preformatted reference styles which can be selected to write your references. Reference managers store the data online too, which makes it easy for researchers to access their library from anywhere, and this feature also helps researchers to collaborate online.

A few common reference managers used for writing thesis are listed below:
- Mendeley (free, as well as paid version)
- Endnote (paid)
- Zotero (free and paid version, both)

Mendeley

All the software are more or less similar and fulfill the basic tasks of managing references. Let us discuss the Mendeley reference manager in some detail. The advantages of using Mendeley are as follows:
- Mendeley has a desktop version and an online version too. These both work in tandem and are synced when online.
- It can annotate, highlight, or tag each document.
- Online networking with other researchers is easy in Mendeley.
- A folder is created in your computer which stores all your articles and other sources. This makes it easy for you to access your articles just like in any other folder.
- With 2GB of free online storage space, it serves the purpose of most of the researchers, without having to pay.
- You can drag and drop PDFs into the library and extract the relevant information for citations as and when needed.

Steps to use Mendeley

Step 1: Download and install Mendeley from *www.mendeley.com*. It will ask you to create an account and set a login id and password. It will create a desktop icon for you to access it easily.

Step 2: When you open the desktop icon, Mendeley window will open (**Fig. 22.2**). Clicking on the tab named "tools," you will get two options. One is "install web importer' and another is "insert word plug-in".

Step 3: Install web importer, by clicking from the options in tool tab. The web importer can be selected depending upon the browser you use. For example, there are different web importers for Chrome, for Firefox, for Internet explorer, and so on. This will create an icon in your browser (**Fig. 22.3**). When you search an article, you can click this icon to save the article.

Step 4: Install MS Word plugin for Microsoft Word users. For LibreOffice users, you can choose, Install LibreOffice plugin from the tool tab in Mendeley window. In Microsoft Word document, you will find a Mendeley section in "references" tab, once you install the MS Word plugin (**Fig. 22.4**).

Step 5: Insert citations when writing in the Word document. You can do this by clicking on the "insert citations" given in the Mendeley section of the References tab in MS word document (**Fig. 22.4**). This will open the Mendeley library for you to select the relevant article and then "cite".

Writing References | 161

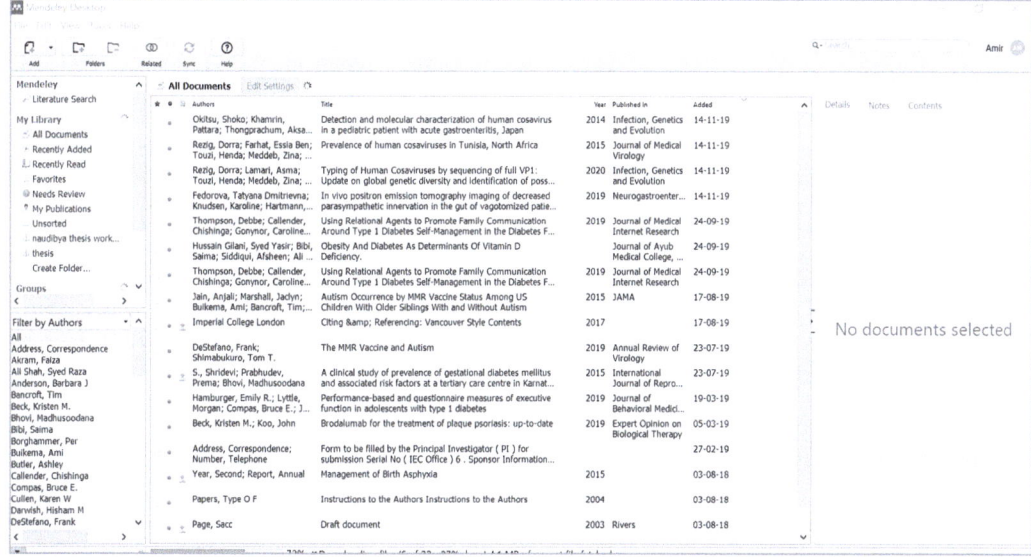

Fig. 22.2: Mendeley window.

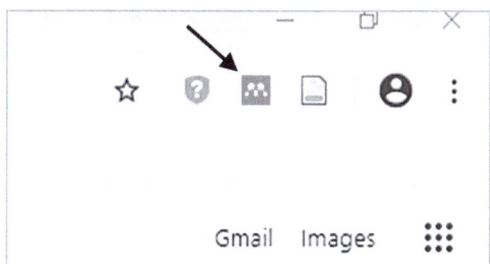

Fig. 22.3: Mendeley web importer icon (indicated by an arrow) as displayed in Google Chrome browser. *(For color version, see Plate 2)*

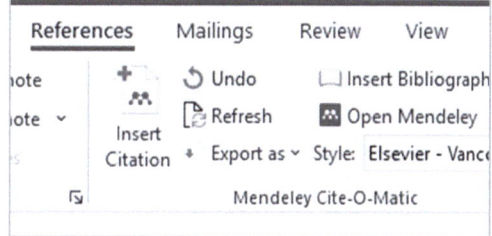

Fig. 22.4: Mendeley section displayed in the references tab of Microsoft Word document. *(For color version, see Plate 2)*

Step 6: Create a "references" list at the end of the thesis or thesis protocol. Use the "insert bibliography" button in the Mendeley section of the references tab in MS word document (**Fig. 22.4**). This will create a list of references for you.

Step 7: If you want to change the style of referencing, you can select from the "styles" options available in the Mendeley section of the references tab in MS word document (**Fig. 22.4**).

Note that the reference managers pull citation-related online data when you import the article by using the Web importer. Sometimes, it may happen that the data is not as per the format in which you want. For example, in some cases the title of the article may be in capital letters or in some other format. You can edit the formatting manually, once you are done with all the citations and creating the reference list. It is important to check all the citations once you complete using the software, to avoid inadvertent errors that might have creeped in.

Even though we have mentioned Mendeley here, this is a personal choice of the authors and there is no conflict of interest. The readers are free to choose whichever reference managers they want to use.

■ ICMJE UNIFORM REQUIREMENTS FOR MANUSCRIPTS SUBMITTED TO BIOMEDICAL JOURNALS: SAMPLE REFERENCES

Sample references typically used by authors of journal articles are provided below. Details are in '*Citing Medicine*'.
Note: Appendix F which covers how citations in MEDLINE/PubMed differ from the advice in *Citing Medicine*.)

Articles in Journals

Standard Journal Article
List the first six authors followed by et al.

| Halpern SD, Ubel PA, Caplan AL. Solid-organ transplantation in HIV-infected patients. N Engl J Med. 2002 Jul 25;347(4):284–7. |

As an option, if a journal carries continuous pagination throughout a volume (as many medical journals do), the month and issue number may be omitted.

| Halpern SD, Ubel PA, Caplan AL. Solid-organ transplantation in HIV-infected patients. N Engl J Med. 2002;347:284–7. |

More than Six Authors

| Rose ME, Huerbin MB, Melick J, Marion DW, Palmer AM, Schiding JK, et al. Regulation of interstitial excitatory amino acid concentrations after cortical contusion injury. Brain Res. 2012;935(1-2):40–6. |

Organization as Author

| Diabetes Prevention Program Research Group. Hypertension, insulin and proinsulin in participants with impaired glucose tolerance. Hypertension. 2016;40(5):679–86. |

Both Personal Authors and Organization as Author

| Vashishtha VM, Bansal CP, Gupta SG; for Indian Academy of Pediatrics. Recommendations of Immunization Committee. Indian Pediatr. 2013;11:999–1012. |

Volume with Supplement

| Geraud G, Spierings EL, Keywood C. Tolerability and safety of frovatriptan with short- and long-term use for treatment of migraine and in comparison with sumatriptan. Headache. 2002;42 Suppl 2:S93–9. |

Pagination in Roman Numerals

| Chadwick R, Schuklenk U. The politics of ethical consensus finding. Bioethics. 2002;16(2):iii–v. |

Article Published Electronically Ahead of the Print Version

| Yu WM, Hawley TS, Hawley RG, Qu CK. Immortalization of yolk sac-derived precursor cells. Blood. 2002 Nov. 15;100(10):3828–31. Epub 2002; Jul 5. |

Books and Other Monographs

Personal Author(s)

| Murray PR, Rosenthal KS, Kobayashi GS, Pfaller MA. Medical Microbiology. 4th ed. St. Louis: Mosby; 2002. |

Editor(s), Compiler(s) as Author

| Gilstrap LC 3rd, Cunningham FG, VanDorsten JP, editors. Operative obstetrics. 2nd ed. New York: McGraw-Hill; 2002. |

Author(s) and Editor(s)

Breedlove GK, Schorfheide AM. Adolescent pregnancy. 2nd ed. Wieczorek RR, editor. White Plains (NY): March of Dimes Education Services; 2001.

Organization(s) as Author
[Edited 12 May, 2009]

Advanced Life Support Group. Acute medical emergencies: the practical approach. London: BMJ Books; 2001. p. 454.

Chapter in a Book

Meltzer PS, Kallioniemi A, Trent JM. Chromosome alterations in human solid tumors. In: Vogelstein B, Kinzler KW, editors. The genetic basis of human cancer. New York: McGraw-Hill; 2002. p. 93–113.

Conference Proceedings

Harnden P, Joffe JK, Jones WG, editors. Germ cell tumours V. Proceedings of the 5th Germ Cell Tumour Conference; 2001 Sep. 13–15; Leeds, UK. New York: Springer; 2002.

Conference Paper

Christensen S, Oppacher F. An analysis of Koza's computational effort statistic for genetic programming. In: Foster JA, Lutton E, Miller J, Ryan C, Tettamanzi AG, editors. Genetic programming. Eurogp 2002: Proceedings of the 5th European Conference on Genetic Programming; 2002 Apr 3–5; Kinsdale, Ireland. Berlin: Springer; 2002. P. 182–91.

Scientific or Technical Report

Issued by Funding/Sponsoring Agency

Yen GG (Oklahoma State University, School of Electrical and computer Engineering, Stillwater, OK). Health monitoring on vibration signatures. Final report. Arlington (VA): Air Force Office of Scientific Research (US), Air Force Research Laboratory; 2002 Feb. Report No.: AFRLSRBLTR020123. Contract No.: F496209810049.

Issued by Performing Agency

Russell ML, Goth-Goldstein R, Apte MG, Fisk WJ. Method for measuring the size distribution of airborne Rhinovirus. Berkeley (CA): Lawrence Berkeley National Laboratory, Environmental Energy Technologies Division; 2002 Jan. Report No.: LBNL49574. Contract No.: DEAc0376SF00098. Sponsored by the Department of Energy.

Dissertation/Thesis

Meena P. Correlation of Sunlight Exposure with Serum 25 OHD Levels in Infants. MD (Pediatrics). Thesis submitted to University of Delhi. 2015.

Patent

Pagedas AC, inventor; Ancel Surgical R&D Inc., assignee. Flexible endoscopic grasping and cutting device and positioning tool assembly. United States patent US 20020103498. 2002, Aug. 1.

Other Published Material

Newspaper Article

Tynan T. Medical improvements lower homicide rate: study sees drop in assault rate. The Washington Post. 2002, Aug 12;Sect. A:2 (col. 4).

Audiovisual Material

Chason KW, Sallustio S. Hospital preparedness for bioterrorism [videocassette]. Secaucus (NJ): Network for continuing Medical Education; 2002.

Legal Material

Veterans Hearing Loss compensation Act of 2002, Pub. L. No. 107–9, 115 Stat. 11 (May 24, 2001).

Dictionary and Similar References

Dorland's illustrated medical dictionary. 29th ed. Philadelphia: WB Saunders; 2000. Filamin; p. 675.

Unpublished Material

In Press or Forthcoming

(Note: NLM prefers "Forthcoming" rather than "In press" because not all items will be printed.)

> Tian D, Araki H, Stahl E, Bergelson J, Kreitman M. Signature of balancing selection in Arabidopsis. Proc Natl Acad Sci USA. Forthcoming 2022.

Electronic Material

CD-ROM

> Anderson SC, Poulsen KB. Anderson's electronic atlas of hematology [CD-ROM]. Philadelphia: Lippincott Williams & Wilkins; 2010.

Website

- World Health Organization. Fact Sheet on Malaria. Available from www.who.int/en/malaria.pdf. Accessed on March 1, 2020.
- American Medical Association [Internet]. Chicago: The Association; c1995–2002 [updated 2001, Aug 23; cited 2002, Aug 12]. AMA Office of Group Practice Liaison; [about 2 screens]. Available from: http://www.ama-assn.org/ama/pub/category/1736.html.

■ CONCLUSION

References are an integral part of a research protocol and thesis. They are essential to provide validity to what you are saying, to document what all is known and to identify the lacunae in existing literature. References should be relevant to the topic of your thesis. Use ICMJE style to cite and list them. You can maintain your references manually or by using a reference manager software. References are cited in the introduction, methods, and discussion section of the thesis. References are not needed for Results, Summary, and Conclusions sections. Maintain consistency in citing the references in the list. The reference list is usually limited to 25–30 for the protocol and 100 for the thesis. Of these, maximum references should be citing the journal articles (at least 70%). The rest can be from books, electronic material, or websites. Do not cite references without going through the full text of the article. Avoid cross referencing as it may lead to vital errors. Every reference mentioned in your text must be included in reference list given at the end of the thesis.

KEY MESSAGES

- References are mostly written in ICMJE (Vancouver) style; wherein the references are cited as Arabic numbers in the text in a chronological manner and listed in the same sequence in a numbered list at the end of the document.
- Use relevant and recent references, preferably from peer reviewed journals. Limit total number to 25–30 in the protocol and 100 for the final thesis.
- Reference list is not the same as bibliography. Avoid using the term bibliography in thesis for listing the references.
- Reference managers are useful software that may help you to compile, cite and list references in the desired format. Mendeley, Endnote and Zotero are common examples.

■ FURTHER READING

1. Indian Pediatrics. (2020). Instruction to Authors. [online] Available from https://www.indianpediatrics.net/author1.htm. [Last accessed 30 April, 2020].
2. Bavdekar SB. Enhance the Value of a Research Paper: Choosing the Right References and Writing them Accurately. J Assoc Physicians India. 2016;64(3):66-70.
3. Cals JW, Kotz D. Effective writing and publishing scientific papers, part VIII: references. J Clin Epidemiol. 2013;66(11):1198.
4. Cals JW, Kotz D. Literature review in biomedical research: useful search engines beyond PubMed. J Clin Epidemiol. 2016;71:115-7.
5. Francavilla ML. Learning, teaching and writing with reference managers. Pediatr Radiol. 2018;48(10):1393-8.
6. Glick M. You are what you cite: the role of references in scientific publishing. J Am Dent Assoc. 2007;138(1):12,14.
7. ICMJE. International committee of Medical Journal Editors (ICMJE) Recommendations ("The Uniform Requirements"). [online] Available from http://www.icmje.org/about-icmje/faqs/icmje-recommendations/ [Last accessed 30 April, 2020].
8. Masic I. The importance of proper citation of references in biomedical articles. Acta Inform Med. 2013;21(3):148-55.
9. Riordan L. Modern-day considerations for references in scientific writing. J Am Osteopath Assoc. 2012;112(8):567-9.

CHAPTER 23

Publication Misconduct and How to Avoid it

Sharmila Banerjee Mukherjee

■ INTRODUCTION

You have reached the point when you are ready to finish writing your thesis after crossing several important milestones; completion of collection of data, statistical analysis, and discussion of your results with your supervisor. You have now been asked to write the Results, Discussion and Conclusions, and put it all in the expected "thesis" format and submit the end product to the university.

What have you done so far?
You have already done an exhaustive literature search. You have gone through each article that you saved, sifted through them, categorized them as relevant and non-relevant, and highlighted the important paragraphs in the relevant ones. You have identified the portions that you think will be useful because they contain definitions, explanations, presentation of methods, and discussion of results of similar studies. You have also probably discovered your intrinsic ability to synthesize facts and arrive at a reasonable scientific conclusion.

What are the challenges now?
You know that you are expected to write each section in a crisp, logical, and sequential manner in a way that it will make sense to anybody who reads your work.

- *Challenge* 1: It has probably been ages since you have literally written something beyond prescriptions or clinical case sheets (maybe it was the final professional examinations?).
- *Challenge* 2: You may find writing in English difficult because your command over the language may not be good or you studied in a different medium.
- *Challenge* 3: You may not fully understand the advanced scientific or extremely technical aspects of the paper that you are expected to summarize.
- *Challenge* 4: In today's world of social media, you are accustomed to using short phrases that mostly consist of abbreviations, mnemonics, and mis-spelt words.

As a result of all these issues and maybe more, you find yourself struggling with putting your thoughts into words.

What do you do?
There are three paths you may end up taking: Writing the paragraph yourself (now that the concept has become clearer in your own mind); rewriting each sentence in a different way (*paraphrasing*); or copying and pasting the paragraph just as it is (with or without

remembering to add a citation). And we all know what happens most of the time! With a deadline to meet, you hurriedly pick up paragraphs/sentences from published articles and copy and paste them into your draft.

Is this the correct approach? Is it ethical? And if not, how should one go about it? In this chapter, I will try to help you understand what "writing malpractice" or "publication misconduct" is, with reference to writing your thesis.

■ ETHICAL WRITING AND PUBLICATION MISCONDUCT

Ethical Writing

"Each of our written works represents an implicit contract between us and our readers in which the reader assumes that, unless otherwise noted, we are the sole authors of the work, the words and ideas are our own, and the ideas, concepts and theories described are accurately and objectively represented to the best of our ability" (Kolin). Thus, the use and misuse of words (by the author) may have serious implications and consequences for the sanctity of his/her work.

Some common errors committed by students like you (as per the guide by the American Office of Research Integrity) while writing, are listed below:
- Inadvertently failing to give credit.
- Borrowing heavily without citing the reference.
- Failing to present an idea that is contrary to the author's observations.
- Presenting an idea as theirs, when it has already been expressed and published elsewhere (rediscovery of ideas).
- Using an idea (that you had read before, but forgotten) as your own; because you think it is your original concept (cryptomnesia).
- Ignorance of how to include citation and references according to standard protocol.

Publication Misconduct

Unethical writing or publication misconduct comprises of an author intentionally indulging in any of Kolin's (2009) *three M's*: Misquotation, Misrepresentation, and/or Manipulation. I like to remember these as *three Misdemeanors* or wrongful activities.

A critical aspect that distinguishes the three M's from error or negligence is the *underlying intent to deceive*. Since the medical profession is considered to be a societal contract, willful deception not only violates fundamental research standards with implications on patient care, but it also debases basic societal values and the trust with which the general public regards medical research [IOM, 2009].

■ TYPES OF PUBLICATION MISCONDUCT

Plagiarism

This term is derived from the latin word *"plagarius"* which literally means kidnapper, robber, misleader, or literary thief. It is one of the most common publication misconducts. The American Association of University Professors defines plagiarism as *"Taking over the ideas, methods, or written words of another, without acknowledgment and with the intention that they be taken as the work of the deceiver"*. This is applicable not only to written text, but also to figures, diagrams, graphs, and even ideas.

Plagiarism covers multiple disciplines: literary, academic, the arts, and science. It is not just restricted to the written format. Presenting other people's ideas or slides without proper acknowledgement is also considered to be plagiarism. Besides obvious sources such as papers and books, ideas, concepts, explanations, etc., are often obtained from casual encounters, lectures, peer reviews, etc. Irrespective of source, if you use someone else's intellectual property in your work, the source needs to be mentioned appropriately.

With relation to theses/dissertations and scientific papers, the sections in which plagiarism occurs the most are the "review of literature", and "discussion".

Types of Plagiarism

The different types and variable extents of plagiarism are described in **Table 23.1**. You have probably already noted a lot of overlap in the language used in the several papers that you have read related to your thesis. Now it will be easier for you to appreciate which author is guilty of plagiarism and the type. What is always difficult to determine is the intent of the author.

There are certain "gray areas" where words, phrases and/or sentences may be replicated and still be considered acceptable. A few examples are being cited here.

- *Use of common knowledge:* This comprises of information that is considered widely known or easily verified. When you use these kinds of facts, references may not be required. However, you must remember that what comprises common knowledge depends upon the detailing and the target audience/readers. When in doubt about whether any fact that has been written in the thesis is common knowledge or not, using citations and references is safer.
- *Use of standard definitions, terminologies or procedures:* Paraphrasing these may not convey the intended meaning as effectively as the original verbatim language. The essence may get lost. If your thesis is on genetics and you want to define an "allele" (described as an alternative form of a gene that occurs at the same locus on homologous chromosomes), it would be extremely difficult for you to rewrite this in your own words. Or suppose your study requires flow cytometry and you want to elaborate upon the underlying principle, imagine how challenging it would be to rephrase a statement like, "Fluorescent molecules get activated and emit light that is filtered and detected by sensitive light detectors in photomultiplier tubes"? These

TABLE 23.1: Types of plagiarism.

Type	Description
Complete plagiarism/intellectual theft	When a researcher submits somebody else's complete work as his/her own
Source-based plagiarism	Misleading citation (incorrect or false reference) or using second hand information, but citing the primary source without actually reading it (i.e., from cross references)
Direct plagiarism	When a section of somebody else's work is copied word to word without using quotation marks and citing the source.
Auto or self-plagiarism	When an author uses his/her own previously published work without attribution. Remember once published the work no longer belongs to the author, but to the journal
Paraphrasing without credit	Making some minor changes in sentences that someone else has written and treating them as your own
Mosaic paraphrasing/patch writing	When phrases or bits of a different source are inserted into one's own work without citation
Misattribution	Attributing a different source rather than the actual source that is used
Translation plagiarism	When scientific work in another language is translated and passed off as your own without acknowledgement

examples are referred to as "boiler plate language", in which portions of text are routinely reused in documents to convey a specific, standard meaning. This practice is considered acceptable if you provide a citation and reference. However, even if you do have to copy these sections, do not do it blindly. Read through each word carefully and check whether it is suitable to the context in which you are inserting it in, and whether the tense (past, present or future) or voice (active/passive) is compatible with the style in which you are writing. A very common mistake that students do is self-plagiarism from their protocol, when they copy-paste sections of "methodology" to their thesis without converting verbs written in future tense to past tense.

- *Fair use:* In cases of literary work that has a copyright, small segments, few sentences, or quotations may be used in the sections that require critical analyses like review of literature or discussion without requiring permission from the copyright holder, provided proper citation and referencing is done. This applies to academic work which is not being used for commercial purpose. For example, in the aforementioned example, if you use a figure from a textbook to depict the principle of flow cytometry in your thesis and give the proper citation and reference, you need not take permission from the copyright owner, since it is for an individual academic purpose, it will be viewed by very limited people and there are no financial implications. However, you cannot use it when you write your paper and send it for publication, even if you have added the reference. In these circumstances you have to obtain permission, though it is still being used for academic purposes.

Fabrication

Fabrication is the corrupt practice of making up data or results or other information without having actually performed the relevant

> **Box 23.1: International and Indian cases of fabrication.**
> - A former professor of ophthalmology at the Massachusetts Eye and Ear Infirmary and Harvard Medical School admitted to having fabricated 21 chromatograms for a National Institute of Health grant application in 2003
> - In 2007, faculty members of the department of Zoology, University of Pune were suspected of publishing papers in prestigious journals by reusing Western Blot data from other studies as their own. These contained photographs with similar bands as well as background signals. Ironically, though the institute where they worked found no substance in the allegations, the papers were retracted from the journals as the journal committees found evidence of falsification beyond reasonable doubt

procedures. This may be followed by principal investigators, research students, research assistants, and non-scientist field workers (interestingly described as "data from under a tree" where the forms are filled up!). It involves making up information at various levels; obtaining informed consent, filling up false clinical details in your case record form, filling in missing data in incomplete forms or making up data without even having conducted the particular activity. Examples of professionals who were caught and exposed in public are given in **Box 23.1**.

This has serious implications way beyond cheating yourself, your supervisor, and your university. If you publish a paper based on these results, you are misleading fellow medical professionals who may change their practice in good faith and result in patient mismanagement. This applies to the following category of falsification as well.

Falsification

Falsification in research is the intentional manipulation (misrepresentation, alteration or omission) of materials, equipment, processes, data, and/or results in such a way that the

> **Box 23.2: International and Indian examples of falsification.**
> - In 2019, the American Office of Research Integrity reported a former visiting fellow at the National Cancer Institute (NCI), who was conducting an Intramural Research study on microRNA expression levels in human cancer cell lines, which was supported by the National Institute of Health. It was found that the researcher altered, reused, and relabeled data related to quantitative real-time polymerase chain reaction, and other assay images
> - Scientists from the Centre for Science & Environment, New Delhi and Indian Institute of Technology, Kanpur (2003–2004) were found to have falsified data in their paper entitled "Analysis of Pesticide Residues in Fruits and Vegetables from different Mandis of Delhi", as well as having in a large degree of plagiarism

> **Box 23.3: Definition of authorship according to the International Committee of Medical Journal Editors (ICMJE) guidelines.**
> Authorship credit should be based on following criteria:
> - Substantial contributions made to conception and design of the study, acquisition, and interpretation of data
> - Drafting the article or revising it critically for intellectual content
> - Approving the final version to be published
> - Being accountable for all aspects of the work; questions related to accuracy or integrity are to be properly resolved

research is not represented the way it was actually conducted, resulting in misleading conclusions being drawn. A few examples are given in **Box 23.2.** Though theoretically different, both fabrication and falsification have some degree of overlap as many authors indulge in both acts "intentionally, knowingly, and/or recklessly" (as described by the American Office of Research Integrity).

Ghost Authorship

This comprises of using professional writers/manuscript writing services instead of writing the thesis yourself. All of you must have seen the touts and pamphlets that are frequently distributed in medical campuses and maybe a few of you were tempted to employ their services. This is academic dishonesty at its worst, equivalent to getting somebody to sit for you in the examination. I take this opportunity to point out to both students and faculty members that this also includes supervisors writing or dictating sections of the thesis for the student, instead of correcting their errors, telling them how to write it properly, and letting them do it themselves. This is considered as unethical as helping the student cheat in his/her theory examinations. It is my personal perception that students do not really view themselves seriously as authors. Let me clear your misconception by referring to the guidelines for claim of authorship listed in **Box 23.3**.

PREVALENCE OF PUBLICATION MISCONDUCT

Let us see what the situation is like in our own country. I am sure you can arrive at a fair estimate based on self-reflection and awareness of the situation among your peers and in your own institute.

In a study conducted by Dhingra et al. on the prevalence of professional misconduct in medical professionals, data were collected from 155 senior residents (within 3 years of obtaining their MD/MS degree) and young faculty members (within 10 years of joining) of 9 institutes across India by anonymous questionnaires. The results revealed that 91% participants claimed some degree of awareness (though 71% felt it was inadequate), 65% had observed gift authorship, 56% data alteration, 53% plagiarism, and 33.5% felt a colleague's name being excluded despite significant contribution.

I would also like to draw your attention to an article in the British Medical Journal (White,

> **Box 23.4: Reasons for publication misconduct.**
> - Easy access to electronic material
> - Ease of copying and pasting text from papers irrespective of format
> - Laxity of supervisor or university to unethical writing
> - Minimal actual interest in research and low levels of motivation
> - Lack of personal investment or commitment to their own education
> - Lack or ignorance of research skills
> - Lack of time
> - *Carelessness:* You think to yourself, "If I do not put in the reference, who is even going to notice?"

2005) which named and shamed an Indian private practitioner based in Moradabad for suspected fabrication and falsification. This author had registered and subsequently published eight randomized controlled trials between 1992 and 1996 in several reputed international journals. The papers were on the risk of cardiovascular disease with various aspects of nutrition. At the onset, these were considered classics with frequent citations by other authors. However, when the papers started getting churned out so rapidly, suspicions were raised and the matter investigated. The immediate aftermath of this scandal was that original papers by other Indian researchers were also viewed with suspicion by the international scientific community.

The usual reasons for publication misconduct during thesis writing are listed in **Box 23.4.**

■ HOW TO AVOID PLAGIARISM

While making notes during the process of synthesis of and/or summarizing existing literature, always write down the source of the information that you intend to use. This will ensure that you do not forget or get mixed-up with another paper when you use that information in your thesis. The important decision to take is whether you want to write it yourself or use verbatim phrases with quotation marks. Irrespective of what you decide, the contribution of the other author must always be acknowledged in your work by proper citation and inclusion of the source in the reference list.

Option 1: I want to write it in my own words
Read and understand the contents of the paper completely. When you write, do not keep the original text in front of you or you may find that you have subconsciously used words or phrases from the paper. After finishing, always inspect your version with the original source to look for any similarity. Either you can do it or you can ask a friend to do it (It is like a calculation error that you may fail to identify, however many times you go through it, but an uninvolved party can detect it immediately).

For example, if I want to include Shakespeare's lines (see below) in an article that I am writing on "Leadership in the medical profession", I may write: *Shakespeare's famous quotation implies that some leaders are considered great by virtue of birth like a crowned prince, some eventually become great by the deeds they perform during the course of their careers, while some suddenly find themselves placed in a position of responsibility and authority and manage to attain great success [Shakespeare]. Leaders in the medical sciences belong to the second and third categories and prove that leadership is a skill that can be learnt and honed.*

Option 2: I want to use it as it is (verbatim)
When you use any information word by word it must be presented properly. That means the use of quotation marks from the start to the end of the segment followed by the appropriate citation. For example, if I want to use Shakespeare's famous words verbatim in my aforementioned article, it will be presented like this: *Shakespeare's famous quotation states, "Be not afraid of greatness: Some are born great, some achieve greatness and some have greatness thrust upon them" [Shakespeare]. The second*

and third examples are applicable to leaders in the medical sciences, which prove that leadership is a skill that can be learnt and honed.

Paraphrasing

Paraphrasing is allowed, "inappropriate paraphrasing" is not. This is most commonly observed in the "review of literature" and "discussion" sections, when you are expected to appraise all the studies that you have included, synthesize the contents, and pen down your views. Here you are supposed to express your understanding of what the author is conveying, in your own words, sentences, and syntax. Remember that changing the voice, or tense, or sequence or adding a few of your own words within the original source does not override the issue of plagiarism. **Box 23.5** gives examples of "inappropriate" and "appropriate paraphrasing".

It may be difficult to completely paraphrase description of methods without altering the meaning, especially if the procedure being described is extremely technical. In these instances, it is safer to use quotation marks, citation, footnotes, and/or if required, block quotation.

Plagiarism can be Detected

Software have been designed to detect text plagiarism based on percentage of textual similarity (based on keywords and sentence alignment) with context to certain sections. Acknowledgments and References are usually excluded from the plagiarism check. Common plagiarism check software includes Turnitin, iThenticate, CrossCheck, HelioBLAST (previously eTBLAST), Copygator, Google Scholar Plagiarism Check, and Viper. Some of them are paid sites while others are free (bur restrict the amount of content that will be checked per day). Alternatively, you can copy and paste text or image that needs to be tested for plagiarism in the Google search bar and press enter. The browser will display any similar content on web, if any.

Box 23.5: Appropriate and inappropriate paraphrasing.

Original paragraph

In India, there are multiple challenges to practice of universal developmental surveillance and screening. Parents are unaware of the existence and need of these services. Healthcare seeking is prioritized for acute illnesses which are not appropriate opportunities for screening. A heterogeneous population of doctors with variable proficiency caters to the health needs of Indian children. If parents' express concerns, they are often given false assurances without proper appraisal. Well-child visits are primarily for immunization with a few perfunctory questions asked about development, if at all (Mukherjee et al. 2014).

Inappropriate paraphrasing

There are multiple challenges to the practice of universal developmental surveillance and screening in India. Parents do not know about these services. Healthcare seeking is for acute illnesses which are not appropriate for screening. A variety of doctors with different capabilities look after the health of Indian children. When concerns are expressed by their parents they are reassured without an evaluation. Well-child visits are mainly for vaccination and occasionally some cursory questions are asked about milestones.

Appropriate paraphrasing

In their narrative review on developmental screening and surveillance, Mukherjee et al. identified several barriers to routine implementation of this practice in Indian children. Parental factors included lack of parental awareness regarding the importance of these practices, health seeking behavior mainly restricted to illness and immunization. The barriers identified among doctors were lack of awareness of the importance of screening as evident by unstructured elicitation of developmental milestones and the practice of not acting on parental concerns and sending their children for further evaluation. These issues were also commented upon in a systematic by Marlow et al. [5]. In addition, they…

The drawbacks of these systems are that they are unable to identify intent, detect plagiarism of idea, translational plagiarism or heavily disguised "inappropriate paraphrasing". Ultimately, the results have to be scrutinized by an expert eye before conclusions are drawn.

Publication misconduct can harm your reputation and career

It is a misconception that since publication misconduct is common, nothing will happen. Remember, authors do get caught and may have to pay heavy penalties in terms of their career and reputation.

INDIAN REGULATORY BODIES

You must have complete knowledge of what publication misconduct comprises of, as well as the consequences of indulging in it. Most universities have their own set of rules and/or protocols which employ various strategies to discourage publication misconduct. It is always prudent to become acquainted with them before submitting your thesis/paper.

University Grants Commission (Promotion of Academic Integrity and Prevention of Plagiarism in Higher Educational Institutions) Regulation 2018

The Gazette notification states *"Every higher educational institute (HEI) should establish mechanisms as to enhance awareness about responsible conduct of research and academic activities, to promote academic integrity and to prevent plagiarism"*. Some of the salient points relevant to your thesis are as follows:

- Every student submitting a thesis shall submit an undertaking indicating that the document has been prepared by him/her, is original and free of any plagiarism.
- The undertaking shall include the fact that specific sections (Abstract, Summary, Hypothesis, Observations, Results, Conclusions, and Recommendations) have been duly checked through an approved Plagiarism detection tool which will not have any similarities. It can exclude a common knowledge or coincidental terms (up to 14 consecutive words).
- Each supervisor shall submit a certificate indicating that the work done by the researcher under him/her is plagiarism free.
- If any faculty member suspects plagiarism, it should be reported to the Departmental Academic Integrity Panel (DAIP) which will investigate and submit recommendations to the Institutional Academic Integrity Panel (IAIP).
- Students will be penalized according to quantity of plagiarism (**Table 23.2**).

Delhi University: Guidelines

The UGC guidelines are followed by Delhi University (DU) with relation to PhD thesis or dissertation (**Box 23.6**). With respect to MD/MS degrees, the Faculty of Medical Sciences, DU follows the Post Graduate Ordinance. The salient points regarding MD/MS theses include:

- A similar topic cannot be repeated within 5 years.

TABLE 23.2: Levels of plagiarism with corresponding penalty (UGC Guidelines).

Level	Extent of similarity	Penalty
0	≤10%	No penalty
1	10–40%	Submission of revised script within 6 months
2	40–60%	Debarment from submitting revised script for 1 year
3	≥60%	Cancellation of student registration program

Publication Misconduct and How to Avoid It | 173

> **Box 23.6: Guidelines for plagiarism check for PhD thesis (Delhi University).**
> - The PhD thesis must undergo a Plagiarism Check by either Turnitin or Ithenticate software
> - The exclusion at the time of performing the check should be limited to the following: Quotes, bibliography, phrases, small matches up to 10 words, small similarity less than 1%, mathematical formula, and name of institutions, departments, etc.
> - The Central library will issue the final certificate of plagiarism check called the Plagiarism Verification Certificate, certifying and authenticating the check performed by the student/department. This certificate has to be submitted to the exam branch at the time of submission of the thesis

- A declaration has to be given that the work has been done by the student and under the supervisor with the stipulated duration.
- The ordinance states, "*A student may be debarred from appearing in the examination and his/her registration cancelled on the recommendations of the Board of Research Studies (BRS) if he/she fails to submit...date, and his/her work or conduct is reported to be "Not Satisfactory" by the Supervisor/Head of Department/Head of the institution. Such students shall be debarred from joining any PG/Post-doctoral course for a period of 5 years from the date of cancellation of registration.*"

As you can see, the rules toward publication are not defined and fall under the realms of work and conduct. However, if a complaint is made to the BRS by the supervisor or reviewer regarding this, there is no doubt that it will be considered to be "not satisfactory" and the corresponding penalty will be carried out.

CONCLUSION

Do not regard your thesis as a necessary evil or a noose around your neck. Be proud and take ownership of your work. Do your research sincerely and you will actually start to enjoy your study as it grows into a robust body of scientific evidence. Who knows what kind of impact it may have in the future on scientific world? Do not get tempted by the easy ways out or swayed when you see your peers apparently getting away with acting unethically. Remember the age-old proverb "Honesty is the best policy".

> **KEY MESSAGES**
> - Accept ownership and responsibility of your thesis. It is your research.
> - Do not give into the temptation of copying from original articles, falsifying, and/or fabricating data.
> - Make notes of the important points when you are reading an article and make sure that you include the reference accurately.
> - While synthesizing a concept, keep the original texts out of sight and write your thoughts in your own words.
> - Be mindful while writing and do not fail to include citations of all the references that you use.
> - There are many ways by which publication misconduct can be detected. There are heavy penalties to pay if one is caught.

FURTHER READING

1. American Association of University Professors. Statement on plagiarism 2013. [online] Available from http://www.aaup.org/report/statement-plagiarism. [Last accessed 30 April, 2020].
2. Executive Council of the Rutgers Graduate School-New Brunswick. Guidelines on Using Previously Published Work in Theses and Dissertations. [online] Available from https://www.libraries.rutgers.edu/sites/default/files/copyright/Guidelines-on-Using-Previously-Published-Work-in-Theses-and-Dissertations.pdf. [Last accessed 30 April, 2020].
3. Institute of Medicine. On Being a Scientist: A Guide to Responsible Conduct in Research, 3rd edition. Washington, DC: The National Academies Press; 2009.
4. Kolin FC. Ethical Writing in the Workplace. In: Successful writing at work, Concise, 2nd edition. New York: Houghton Mifflin Harcourt Publication Company; 2009. pp. 17-26.
5. Kolin FC. Successful writing at work, 6th edition. Boston: Houghton Mifflin; 2002.
6. Roig M. Avoiding plagiarism, self-plagiarism, and other questionable writing practices: A guide to ethical writing. [online] Available from https://ori.hhs.gov/sites/default/files/plagiarism.pdf. [Last accessed April, 2020].
7. Mandal M, Bagchi D, Basu SR. Scientific misconducts and authorship conflicts: Indian perspective. Indian J Anaesth. 2015;59:400-5.
8. Dhingra D, Mishra D. Publication misconduct among medical professionals in India. Indian J Med Ethics. 2014;11(2):104-7.
9. White C. Suspected research fraud: difficulties of getting at the truth. BMJ. 2005;331:281-8.
10. Heitman E, Litewka S. International perspectives on plagiarism and considerations for teaching international trainees. Urol Oncol. 2011;29:104-8.
11. International Committee for Medical Journal Editors. Recommendations for the Conduct, Reporting, Editing, and Publication of Scholarly Work in Medical Journals. Updated December, 2013. [online] Available from http://www.icmje.org/recommendations/archives/2013_dec_urm.pdf. [Last accessed 30 April, 2020].
12. Singh S. Earlier version. Avoiding Academic Dishonesty: It Can be Detected! In: Gupta P. Singh N (Eds). How to write the thesis and thesis protocol: A primer for Medical, Dental and Nursing Courses, 1st edition. New Delhi: Jaypee Brothers Medical Publishers Pvt. Ltd.; 2014. pp. 153-7.
13. Mondal S, Mondal H. Google Search: A simple and free tool to detect plagiarism. Indian J Vasc Endovasc Surg. 2018;5(4):271-3.
14. Office of Research Integrity. [online] Available from https://ori.hhs.gov/content/case. [Last accessed 30 April, 2020].
15. Society for Scientific Values. [online] Available from: http://www.scientificvalues.org. [Last accessed 30 April, 2020.
16. University Grants Commission (Promotion of academic integrity and prevention of plagiarism in higher educational institutions) Regulation 2018. The Gazette of India. 2018:7-12.
17. Faculty of Medical Sciences. PG ordinance-Schedule of submission of protocol, thesis and annual Fees. [online] Available from https://www.fmsc.ac.in. [Last accessed 30 April, 2020].

CHAPTER 24

Elements of Writing Better English

Navjeevan Singh

■ INTRODUCTION

This chapter offers an overview of writing scientific English, and emphasizing particular problems and conventions. Many flaws are camouflaged in spoken language, but when the same person writes—errors of spelling, syntax, and punctuation are magnified. We expect that after reading through the chapter, you will be able to avoid common writing errors when you write your thesis.

It is imperative to be able to write well because examiners may equate shoddy English with shoddy Science. Poor language must not detract from the Science. In a sense, your language must be invisible to the reader so that the emphasis is firmly on the Science.

The examples used in this chapter, taken from actual manuscripts, illustrate common errors that should be corrected before the thesis is submitted. The following text comprises of examples of appropriate and inappropriate use of 10 basic elements of writing better English.

> *Note*: In the text boxes, the example appears in *italics*, regular font indicates the author's comments, and **bold**, the correct version. Many examples have multiple errors. Careful comparison of the text in *italics* and **bold** letters will help to identify them.

■ ABBREVIATIONS AND ACRONYMS

The function of abbreviations and acronyms is to aid readability by avoiding reading the same long phrase again and again.

Abbreviations are short forms of words that are used in text. "Standard abbreviations" are those that are widely understood and accepted by certain organizations such as Medline. Examples are: HBV, HPV, EBV, DNA, RNA, and PhD. When spoken, they are either spelt out, or said in full.

Acronyms are names formed from the first letters of consecutive words in a phrase. When spoken, they are pronounced as names, for example: for *E*nzyme *L*inked *I*mmuno *S*orbant *A*ssay (ELISA), and for *A*cquired *I*mmuno *D*eficiency *S*yndrome (AIDS).

- Avoid using abbreviations and acronyms in the Summary section, except for generally accepted ones like DNA, or ELISA, or standard units of measurement such as s (seconds), mg (milligram), mL (milliliter), and kg (kilogram).
- If you need to use an abbreviation or acronym in the main text, write it in full the first time with the abbreviation in brackets afterward, for example, human

papillomavirus (HPV). Subsequently use only the abbreviation.
- Never use abbreviations and acronyms in the Title of your thesis. Use standard abbreviations wherever possible.
- Avoid inventing or making new abbreviations. If you do make your own abbreviation, ensure that it does not sound like some other standard abbreviation. For example, do not use BP, the standard abbreviation for blood pressure, for balanoposthitis!
- Plurals of some standard abbreviations can be tricky. Species is abbreviated as sp. (singular). The plural form is spp. For example: *Klebsiella* sp. is singular while *Klebsiella* spp. is plural. Similarly, the abbreviation for a single page is p.; the plural is pp.
- Units of measurement are not pluralized. It is 1 mL, 100 mL, 10 L; and *not* 100 mLs or 10 Ls.

■ SPELLING AND TYPOGRAPHICAL ERRORS

A single misplaced alphabet can change the meaning of a word. If both versions form a correctly spelled word, the error will not be detected by computer software. Typographical errors commonly occur when the interchanged keys are adjacent to each other on the keyboard; for example, "worker" may inadvertently be typed as "worked".

The prostrate gland.
The prostate gland.

Twenty-five patients had intermittent claudification.
Twenty-five patients had intermittent claudication.

As easy and accepted way of curriculum planning is to follow the "systems approach".
The error is a single letter of the alphabet. Spell-check will not pick up the error if the wrong word is correctly spelt.

An easy and accepted way of curriculum planning is to follow the "systems approach".

The standard KOH mount lacks color contrast. Various dyes are available for contrast enhancement; these are Chicago Blue Stain (CBS), Chlorazole Black E (CBE), Parker stain and Calcofluor White (fluorescent dye), which stain different fungal elements.

These errors may be difficult to detect unless the reader is well-versed with the subject. When she is, she quickly concludes that the writer may not be. Here "Calcoflour" refers to a fluorescent dye. The discerning reader will notice the spelling error.

The standard KOH mount lacks color contrast. Various dyes are available for contrast enhancement; these are: Chicago Blue Stain (CBS), Chlorazole Black E (CBE), Parker Stain, and Calcofluor White (fluorescent dye), which stain different fungal elements.

■ COMMA, SEMICOLON, AND LISTS

Comma (,)

Missing commas are the most common writing errors. Misplaced commas and excess commas are also frequent. Commas separate the clauses in a sentence and indicate a pause in reading. One way to decide where a comma belongs is to read the sentence aloud. Where you pause is where a comma should be.

Nine out of 16 (56%) cases of pleomorphic adenoma showed intracytoplasmic PAS-D positive globules which were usually single and occasionally causing nuclear indentation.

Missing comma. Commas should separate the clauses in the sentence.

Nine out of 16 (56%) cases of pleomorphic adenoma showed intracytoplasmic PAS-D positive globules, which were usually single, and occasionally caused nuclear indentation.

This sentence is even better when split into two, with an appropriately placed comma in the second.

> Nine out of 16 (56%) pleomorphic adenomas had intracytoplasmic PAS-D positive globules. These were usually single, occasionally causing nuclear indentation.

> *Problem solving approach emphasizes the ability of the learner to solve a given problem and thus takes into account, both the above approaches.*
>
> Misplaced comma.
>
> **A problem-solving approach emphasizes the ability of the learner to solve a given problem and thus takes into account both the above approaches.**

> *Patients admitted to a hospital with no history of drug intake harbor gut flora less resistance to antibiotics (usually single, around 10%) than the patients taking antibiotics have gut flora with >50% of antibiotic resistance.*
>
> Multiple errors are often a problem. Missing commas are not the only reason that this sentence is difficult to comprehend, "less" is the wrong word to use, and sentence construction is flawed.
>
> **Around 10% of patients admitted to hospital with no history of drug intake harbor gut flora with low resistance, usually to a single antibiotic, compared to patients taking antibiotics, 50% of whom have high resistance gut flora.**

Semicolon (;)

> Semicolons are used to link two independent clauses when the thought is extended. Each clause could be a complete sentence that could have been separated by a full stop.
>
> *Infections by dermatophytes induce a specific immune response. However, the intensity of immune response that is raised varies by dermatophyte species.*
>
> A semicolon should precede "however".
>
> **Infections by dermatophytes induce a specific immune response; however, the intensity of the immune response varies by dermatophyte species.**

Lists

Use a list when the information you wish to convey has several related items. When there are more than six items, and two or more categories of information, prefer a table. When making lists, be careful to avoid some of the common errors shown in the examples below.

Comma-separated Lists

In a comma-separated list, individual items are separated by commas. This is the simplest and most commonly used method. The preposition must be repeated before each item in a list.

> *The slides were stained by May-Grunwald-Giemsa, Papanicolaou, Ziehl-Neelsen and Immunoperoxidase methods.*
>
> Repeating the preposition "by" emphasizes the items making up the list.
>
> **The slides were stained by May-Grunwald-Giemsa, by Papanicolaou, by Ziehl-Neelsen, and by Immunoperoxidase methods.**

> *The cellularity, cell type, cell distribution and diagnosis were recorded.*
>
> **The cellularity, the cell type, the cell distribution, and the diagnosis were recorded.**

> *Sera were tested for typhoid, malaria, tuberculosis, hepatitis and syphilis.*
>
> **Sera were tested for typhoid, for malaria, for tuberculosis, for hepatitis, and for syphilis.**

Always use a comma after the penultimate item in a list.

> *The patient had jaundice, pedal edema, a protuberant abdomen with ascites and a red eye.*
>
> It is never wrong to use a comma after the penultimate item in a list. Note that doing so in this example takes the eye out of the abdomen.
>
> **The patient had jaundice, pedal edema, a protuberant abdomen with ascites, and a red eye.**

Colon Lists

When the list is long, and there are short phrases in it, a colon (:) list is preferable.

> The inclusion criteria were: Age between 1 and 5 years, bilaterally symmetrically distributed skin lesions, and a negative Lepromin test.

Bullet Lists

Bullet lists have dots, or bullets, to identify and separate the clauses and sentences.

> Exclusion criteria:
> - Azoospermia
> - Liver enlargement
> - Fever

Avoid using bullet lists in your text.

■ PLURALS (COLLECTIVE NOUNS AND MULTIPLE SUBJECTS) AND NUMBERS

Some commonly used terms have less well-known singular forms:

Plural	Singular
Agenda	Agendum
Bacteria	Bacterium
Criteria	Criterion
Phenomena	Phenomenon
Memoranda	Memorandum
Media	Medium
Sera	Serum

"Data", the collective noun for a group of results, does have the singular "datum"; however, the usage has changed. The singular is seldom used. Both, "the data was collected" and "the data were collected" are correct.

Certain words end with "s" but are not plurals. Some false plurals are: Measles, Mumps, Mathematics, Politics, and Genetics.

> *The relationship between different levels can now be discussed in more details.*
> **The relationship between different levels can now be discussed in more detail.**
> Or better:
> **The relationship between different levels can now be discussed in greater detail.**

> *Serum of positive patients and healthy controls will be collected.*
> The plural of "serum" is "sera".
> **Sera of positive patients and healthy controls will be collected.**

> *These infections also limits occupational livelihood.*
> **These infections also limit occupational livelihood.**

Correct contextual use of collective nouns.

> *A pair of animals was housed in a cage.*
> **A pair of animals were studied.**

> *The number of patients studied was thirty-five.*
> **Thirty-five patients were studied.**

With neither/nor, the verb should take the number of the closest noun.

> *Neither the mice nor the rat were in the cage.*
> The singular "rat" should be followed by "was".
> **Neither the mice nor the rat was in the cage.**
> This is grammatically correct, but reads poorly.
> Note the effect of switching the nouns, with the plural following the singular.
> **Neither the rat nor the mice were in the cage.**
> Correct, and reads well.

- Conventions: Numbers
  - In the text of a thesis, some numbers are conventionally written as numerals:
    - Statistical or mathematical functions — 5.5 multiplied by 5, 3rd quartile.
    - Decimals, fractions including a whole number — 55.68 cm, 6½ minutes.

- All numbers above 10–50 patients.
- All numbers preceding a unit of measurement — 10 cm.
- Numbers that are exact quantities– IQ of 125, ₹ 25.
- When numbers below ten group with numbers above ten — 5 of 20 patients.
- Numbers that indicate part of a series — Figure 5, Chapter 1.

 o Numbers are conventionally written in full when:
- The measurements are not precise—a two-way interaction, repeated four times.
- Numbers below ten group with other numbers below ten—five out of six times.
- Any number that begins a sentence—25 patients met the inclusion criteria.
- Fractions without a whole number—increased by a quarter.
- "Zero" and "one" in most places when not with another number—and one culture was positive. The count remained zero.

■ MISPLACED MODIFIERS

Placement of modifiers can change the meaning of a sentence. Cultural and linguistic conditioning of the writer often influences the position of the modifier. In the following examples, "only" is the modifier. Note how the meaning changes with the position of the modifier.

a. Medication can ease the pain.
b. **Only medication can ease the pain.**
c. Medication only can ease the pain.
d. **Medication can only ease the pain.**
e. **Medication can ease only the pain.**
f. **Medication can ease the pain only.**

Note that c and f above are "Indianisms". "We are like that only." is a phrase I love to use in conversation, but would prefer to avoid in scientific writing.

The patient was referred to a psychiatrist with a severe emotional problem.
Real meaning: The psychiatrist had a severe emotional problem.
What was intended:
The patient with a severe emotional problem was referred to a psychiatrist.

ABC software has its own disadvantages like its inability to be used in pediatric patients.
What it means: The software is unable.
What is intended:
The inherent disadvantage of ABC software is that it cannot be used for pediatric patients.

Migraines strike twice as many women than men.
What was intended:
Migraines are twice as common in women as in men.

Women are more likely to take vitamins than men.
What was intended:
Women are more likely than men to take vitamins.

"Amniocentesis", written by a group of prenatal experts.
Real meaning: "Amniocentesis", a book written by people who were experts in the field before they were born.
What was intended:
"Amniocentesis", a book written by experts in the field of prenatal child care.

Lipoma forearm left side.
Real meaning: The patient has one forearm; the lipoma is on the left side of that forearm.
What was intended: The lipoma is on the left forearm.
Lipoma, left forearm.

Tuberculous abscess left chest.
Real meaning: The patient has two chests; a left, and a right. The abscess is on the left chest.
What was intended: The abscess is on the left side of the chest.
Tuberculous abscess, left side of chest.

> The administration should provide directions and limits to the staff's efforts.
>
> In this sentence "provide" is the modifier for both "directions" and "limits". It is appropriate for the first, but not for the second.
>
> **The administration should provide directions, and prescribe limits to the staff's efforts.**

> Nail infections may act as reservoir and may spread to adjacent area or may precipitate secondary bacterial infections.
>
> Misplaced/incorrect "and".
>
> **Nail infections may be reservoirs of infection, facilitating spread to adjacent areas; or precipitate secondary bacterial infections.**
>
> Or better:
>
> **Nail infections may act as reservoirs from where spread to adjacent areas may occur. They may also precipitate secondary bacterial infections.**

■ UNNECESSARY WORDS

In an effort to sound knowledgeable, scientists have developed their own specialized word use (jargon). Unnecessary words, or phrases (redundancy), and expressions that have lost their original meaning through pointless overuse (clichés) should be deleted. The resulting text will be crisp and focused. Some common examples of unnecessary words, jargon, and clichés are:

- *As a consequence of...*
- *Based on the fact that...*
- *Because of the fact that...*
- *Due to the fact that...*
- *In light of the fact that...*
- *In view of the fact that...*
- *On account of...*
- *On the grounds that...*
- *Owing to the fact that...*
- *The reason is because...*

All these mean the same, and can be replaced by one word: "Because".

Some more commonly used redundant phrases and clichés are:

- *As far as the... (methods/results) are concerned...*
- *Coming to the... (results/discussion)...*
- *As a matter of fact...*
- *In a very real sense...*
- *In a sense...*
- *It is interesting to note that...*
- *It should be noted that...*
- *You will appreciate that...*
- *Let us make it clear that...*
- *Needless to say...*
- *First and foremost...*
- *All said and done...*
- *Along with...*
- *Let us make it very explicit that...*
- *"Crystal" as in: Crystal clear.*
- *"Down" as in: Dropped down.*

Unnecessary words irritate the reader, add nothing to scientific writing, and must be ruthlessly deleted. Also, avoid clichés like the plague!

Some examples of inappropriate word use:

> *Much interest has been gained in mucosubstances produced in tumors.*
>
> Inappropriate use of "gained".
>
> A better alternative:
>
> **Much interest has been generated in mucosubstances produced in tumors.**

> *PAS positivity of all lesions along with grading of breast carcinoma is shown in **Table 2**.*
>
> "Along with" can easily be replaced by the simpler, shorter, and sweeter "and".
>
> **PAS positivity and grading of breast carcinoma are shown in Table 2.**

> *Let us illustrate it by an example.*
>
> The "it" is unnecessary.
>
> **Let us illustrate with an example.**

> *You will appreciate that none of the approaches outlined above are entirely satisfactory.*
>
> The phrase "You will appreciate that" is unnecessary.
>
> **None of the approaches outlined above are entirely satisfactory.**

Elements of Writing Better English | 181

> Or:
> **Notice that none of the approaches outlined above are satisfactory.**

> *The immunology of dermatophytosis is currently poorly understood.*
> The present tense adequately conveys the "current" trend.
> **The immunology of dermatophytosis is poorly understood.**

> *We shall discuss about that a little later.*
> "About" is implied in "discuss".
> **We shall discuss that a little later.**
> Or:
> **We shall discuss that later.**
> Or:
> **That will be discussed later.**

■ QUESTIONS AND STATEMENTS

> *Why a subject is being taught? How a subject is being taught?*
> Statements disguised as questions, or poorly constructed questions?
> **Why a subject is being taught. How a subject is being taught. (statements)**
> Or:
> **Why is a subject being taught? How is a subject being taught? (Questions)**

> *In this study, we would like to evaluate the macrophages on Pap smears in cervical epithelial lesions and assess whether they can aid in the diagnosis and grading of cervical neoplasms on Pap smears?*
> This is a statement; it should be punctuated with a semicolon and end with a full stop (and NOT a question mark).
> **In this study we wish to evaluate macrophages in Papanicolaou smears in cervical epithelial lesions, and assess if they can aid in the diagnosis and grading of cervical neoplasms.**

■ THE SENTENCE (CONSTRUCTION, FRAGMENTS)

> *The cases of pleomorphic adenoma showed stromal positivity which was not seen in basal cell adenoma on smears.*
> Use simple sentences.
> **Smears were examined for stromal positivity; it was present in pleomorphic adenoma but not in basal cell adenomas.**

> *Regular screening of Papanicolaou smears has decreased the incidence and mortality of cervical neoplasms. But the sensitivity of Papanicolaou smear is low and variable.*
> "But the sensitivity of Papanicolaou smear is low and variable." is a fragment. In this instance, it is intended to be the dependent clause of a longer sentence; replacing the full stop with a comma corrects the error.
> **Regular screening of Papanicolaou smears has decreased the incidence and mortality of cervical neoplasms, but the sensitivity of Papanicolaou smear is low and variable.**

Make simple, short sentences.

> *Before we close this discussion, we will like to re-emphasize that the outcome of a given curriculum is the result of interaction of various curricular components and our frustration with the present system of education is often the result of our inability to understand the interdependence of these components.*
> Eliminate unnecessary words and phrases. Use appropriate words. Make two sentences.
> **The components of a curriculum are interdependent.**
> **A curriculum that ignores this tenet will be frustrating to implement.**

> *Out of the 50 cases of breast lump, 29 (58%) were fibroadenoma, 19 (36%) were carcinoma and one case was (3%) of benign and malignant phylloides tumor each.*
> Sentence construction: Placement of (3%).

> Out of the 50 cases of breast lump, 29 (58%) were fibroadenoma, 19 (36%) were carcinoma and one case (3%) each was of benign, and malignant phyllodes tumor.
>
> Or:
>
> Of the 50 patients with breast lumps, 29 (58%) had fibroadenoma, 19 (36%) carcinoma, and one each (3%) benign, and malignant phyllodes tumor.
>
> Or:
>
> **There were 50 patients with breast lumps: Fibroadenoma 29 (58%), carcinoma 19 (36%), and one each (3%) benign, and malignant phyllodes tumor.**

■ THE PARAGRAPH

The paragraph is a unit of thought.

A simple paragraph will have three or four, sentences. The topic sentence comes at or near the beginning. The succeeding sentences explain, or establish, or develop the statement made in the topic sentence. The final sentence either emphasizes the thought of the topic sentence, or states some important consequence, and links it to the next paragraph.

> **Our data shows that food and education influence gender equality in India.** We must ensure that no mother should have to choose to feed her boy, and not her girl child, because there is food only for one. Likewise, no parent should have to choose to send the boy to school, and not the girl child, because there is money only to educate one. Two decades after we begin to feed and educate all our children, our nation can anticipate the dawn of an era of gender equality.

> Topic sentence:
>
> *Our data shows that food and education influence gender equality in India.*
>
> Development of the statement:
>
> *We must ensure that no mother should have to choose to feed her boy, and not her girl child, because there is food only for one. Likewise, no parent should have to choose to send the boy to school, and not the girl child, because there is money only to educate one.*

> Conclusion:
>
> *Two decades after we begin to feed and educate all our children, our nation can anticipate the dawn of an era of gender equality.*

■ COMMON PROBLEMS IN WRITING SCIENTIFIC ENGLISH

> *Cervical biopsy of lesional area would be taken for histopathological confirmation. Papanicolaou smears will be destained and immunostaining would be done by Streptavidin Biotin method.*
>
> In the "methods" of the thesis protocol, use the future tense "will be". Do not alternate between "will be" and "would be".
>
> **Cervical biopsy of the lesional area will be taken for histopathological confirmation of diagnosis. Papanicolaou smears will be de-stained for immunostaining by the Streptavidin Biotin method.**

> *Seventy-eight cases were diagnosed as tumors on fine needle aspiration cytology (FNAC).*
>
> Or worse:
>
> *FNAC diagnosed tumors in 78 cases.*
>
> Prefer "patients" to "cases", wherever possible. It conveys empathy. FNAC does not diagnose tumors, doctors do.
>
> **Tumors were diagnosed in 78 patients by FNAC.**

> *Alcian blue staining was performed by method proposed by Bancroft at a pH of 2.5.*
>
> "pH 2.5" is a modifier of "staining", and belongs with it.
>
> **Alcian blue staining was performed at pH 2.5 by the method proposed by Bancroft.**

"Since" and "for"
- Use "since" when referring to a fixed time in the past.
    - The patient had been sick since 12 September.
    - She had been having a cardiac arrhythmia since 2 AM.
- Use "for" when a time period is specified.
    - The patient had been sick for 12 years.

o The slides will be covered with 4% hydrogen peroxide for 30 minutes.

> *All patients with diarrhea and vomiting since 24 hours will be included.*
> For, not since:
> **All patients with diarrhea and vomiting for 24 hours will be included.**

- Use a colon, when introducing a word or phrase.

> *Take a simple example you are going on a vacation to Nainital.*
> When introducing a word, or phrase, use a colon(:).
> **Take a simple example: You are going on a vacation to Nainital.**

- Use of "that"

> *To comment that under what circumstances this happened.*
> Unnecessary "that", misplaced modifier.
> **To comment on the circumstances in which this happened.**

- Missing "article"

> *Affective domain includes ethical aspect also.*
> Missing "the".
> **The effective domain includes the ethical aspects also.**

> *Onychomycosis affects approximately 5% of population worldwide.*
> Missing article "the"
> **Onychomycosis affects approximately 5% of the world population.**

> *Onychomycosis usually develops in presence of predisposing factors.*
> Missing "the".
> **Onychomycosis usually develops in the presence of predisposing factors.**

- Miscellaneous

> *Till date, no study has been done on immunological response of Indian population in onychomycosis.*
> "Till date" is unnecessary. The sentence can be simplified to:
> **The immunological response to onychomycosis has not been studied in Indians.**

> *Onychomycosis is difficult to treat because of slower growth of nails.*
> Slower compared to what?
> **Onychomycosis is difficult to treat because of slow growth of nails.**

> *Secondary syphilis: Some newer observations.*
> Newer compared to what?
> **Secondary syphilis: Some new observations.**

> *The number of patients in this study is very less.*
> "Less" is not the right word to use here.
> **The number of patients in this study is very small.**

> *The histopathological report came out to be carcinoma.*
> Avoid literal translations.
> **The histopathology report was carcinoma.**

Attention to language will ensure that the thesis is readable, and conveys what is intended.

> **KEY MESSAGES**
> - Avoid using abbreviations and acronyms in the title and summary.
> - Stay vigilant; avoid spelling and typographical errors, especially ones that might convey a lack of scientific or technical knowledge.
> - Use commas appropriately; use them in places where you would normally pause while reading a sentence.
> - Use semicolons to link two independent clauses.
> - Prefer tables for longer lists; other options include comma-separated lists or colon lists. Avoid bullet lists.
> - Statistical functions, decimals and fragments with a whole number, numbers greater than 10, numbers followed by units of measurement, numbers <10 grouped with numbers >10, and numbers indicating the members of a series should be written out as numerals (i.e., the digit form).
> - Avoid jargon and clichés.
> - Make simple, short sentences. Longer sentences do not necessarily convey more information or exhibit your erudition.
> - Use a paragraph to work as a unit of thought. It should have a topic sentence at or near the beginning, followed by explanatory sentences, and end with explanatory sentences, and end with a sentence that either closes or emphasizes the thought, or helps it to flow smoothly into the next paragraph. Paragraphs, like sentences, should be kept short.
> - The language in your thesis should be "invisible" so that the focus is on the context (the Science) and not on the text (the English, or the lack of it).

FURTHER READING

1. Burnham NA, Hutson FL. Scientific English as a foreign language. [online] Available from https://users.wpi.edu/~nab/sci_eng/ScientificEnglish.pdf. [Last accessed 30 April, 2020].
2. John BK. Entry from backside only: Hazaar fundas of Indian-english. New Delhi: Penguin Books; 2007.
3. Strunk W Jr, White EB. The elements of style. [online] Available from https://faculty.washington.edu/heagerty/Courses/b572/public/StrunkWhite.pdf. [Last accessed 30 April, 2020.
4. The Economist: Style guide. London: The Economist Newspaper Limited; 2014.
5. Truss L. Eats, shoots and leaves: the zero tolerance approach to punctuation. London: Profile Books; 2003.

CHAPTER 25

Showcasing Thesis Through an Effective PowerPoint Presentation

Pooja Dewan, Piyush Gupta

■ POWERPOINT AND THESIS

PowerPoint, a virtual presentation software, was developed jointly by Robert Gaskins and Dennis Austin at an American software startup company named Forethought, Inc between 1984 and 1987. It was first developed for McIntosh computers but was soon acquired by Microsoft and became a component of Microsoft Office suite starting 1990. Since then, over a dozen improved versions of PowerPoint have emerged, incorporating several new features, the latest version being PowerPoint 16 launched in 2016 and updated in 2019. It uses slides incorporating multimedia to display information whilst including word, excel, and other office tools. It is now virtually impossible to imagine a visually interactive presentation for a large audience in any other mode.

During the pursuit of your thesis, you will be required to present the protocol of your thesis in the college, mid-term results of your thesis work in your department, your thesis work at a scientific conference, etc. It is here that you will need a skillful presentation of your thesis to generate an impact; PowerPoint is a very handy tool for the same. In this chapter, we help you to prepare yourself to make a good PowerPoint presentation, though the act of delivering an effective presentation can only be mastered by practice.

■ WHY USE THE POWERPOINT?

Microsoft PowerPoint is a visual presentation software program which combines text, images, drawing features, animations, and other objects to create self-running or interactive displays to aid oral presentations. Each file created by PowerPoint is called a *presentation* and each presentation is made up of *slides*.

A PowerPoint presentation has several advantages over the conventional modes of presentation like overhead projections using transparencies or chalk and talk (blackboard).

- Using slides with a mix of text, images, photos, and drawings, you can make your presentation more vivid which aid a better retention.
- Images are brighter, sharper and larger, with no keystone effect (where the image narrows toward the bottom) and the entire image is in focus.
- It enables interplay of sound, animation, and graphics.
- It allows use of the web or software programs.

- You can use various keys on the keyboard to interact with your audience during presentation such as by pressing the key B you can hide the screen, by pressing W you can blank out the screen, by pressing Ctrl + P you can transform the mouse to a pointer/pen, Ctrl + E can be used to erase the drawings made using pen/pointer during slideshow, etc.
- If you use the remote control, you can move around the stage or room interacting with your audience, as you deliver your presentation.
- The slide sorter function can be used to find a particular slide easily.
- A PowerPoint file can be easily edited, copied, maintained, transferred and printed, making it a durable and economical mode of presentation.
- Instant transition from slide to slide saves time and helps to maintain the flow during presentation.
- The newer versions of PowerPoint are not only compatible with computers (windows and Macintosh) but also mobile phones (android and iOS) and laptops and tablets (windows and iPad).
- The version PowerPoint 16.0 offers the option for display of real-time translation of a presenter's spoken words to on-screen captions in one of the over 60 languages using inbuilt software "Presentation translator."

HOW TO PREPARE AN EFFECTIVE POWERPOINT PRESENTATION?

To make an effective PowerPoint presentation, a stepwise approach is needed. These include:
- Defining the session contents.
- Creating a good presentation.

Defining the Contents of your Presentation

This involves the following four components:
a. Decide the topic.
b. Outline the goals and objectives of the presentation.
c. Accumulate appropriate reference material.
d. Subdivide the content.

The first step is to identify the topic and outline the learning goals and specific learning objectives of your topic. Identify the expectations of your presentation, such as "the intent of this presentation"—is it to inform, influence, analyze, teach, or motivate? The contents of your presentation would be dictated by the aim of your presentation. If you need to convince a biased audience, the contents of your presentation should include compelling evidence. You should modulate your tone and body language to reassure your skeptical audience that you are a responsible expert.

Since you would be presenting your protocol or thesis, the flow of the content material should be systematic. Start from the title and proceed along to the Introduction (or background) including the need (or rationale) for your study, research question and hypothesis of your study, Aims and objectives, the body of presentation (materials and methods, outcome measures, and sample size), Results (or observations), and finally the Conclusions and recommendations. The contents of your presentation should be chosen keeping in mind five elements: (1) Utility, (2) Novelty, (3) Emotional value, (4) Entertainment, and (5) Conversational value. You also need to decide if your presentation will include text only, text plus images, graphs, figures and/or tables or in addition would have some video or audioclips.

Creating a PowerPoint Presentation

Once you are ready with the contents of your presentation, you can start making the presentation using the PowerPoint software. Click "Start," go to "Programs," and then click on "Microsoft PowerPoint." It will open a file tentatively named "Presentation 1" (which may later be renamed as per your choice). All PowerPoint files have the suffix "*.ppt*" or "*.pptx*" after the filename. The "X" in the file format stands for "XML." It is possible for you to save your file in either format. However, if your computer has only older office software, it may not be possible to open the *pptx* format.

Choosing a Slide Layout

When you create a PowerPoint presentation, you would be asked about the type of presentation to be made through an Opening Dialog Box, which shows three options: (1) "Auto Content Wizard"(automatically guides the user through pre designed background and placeholder settings and content suggestions), (2) "Design Template"(providing a selection of predesigned backgrounds and placeholder settings without content suggestions), and (3) "Blank Presentation"(which allows total freedom to the user to choose various parameters). Placeholders are the dotted-line containers on slide layouts that hold content such as titles, body text, tables, charts, SmartArt graphics, pictures, clip art, videos, and sounds.

In case you opt for a blank presentation, you can choose the layout of your slide by clicking on the "new slide" option or selecting the appropriate layout using a dropdown menu as shown in **Figure 25.1**. There are 24 inbuilt slide layouts. The layouts will appear as either "Text layouts," "Content layouts", "Text and content layouts," or "Other layouts" (blank, title slide, title only, bulleted list, two-column text, text with table/chart/clipart, flowchart)." Depending if your current slide is a mix of figures, texts, tables or diagrams, choose an appropriate layout for that slide. The slide layout may be selected by using the autocontent wizard, particularly if you are a beginner.

Few of the available slide layouts are listed below:
- *Blank*: It does not contain any placeholders. Text and/or picture can be added according to one's own specifications.
- *Title slide*: There are two boxes to insert text for creating heading/title and subheadings; for example, the title of your thesis protocol can be put in the upper box and your name and affiliation in the lower box.
- *Title and content*: Allows insertion of a heading followed by the relevant content enlisted in the content box (*bulleted list*).
- *Two-content*: A title bar with two columns of text used for showing contrasting text or comparative text.
- *Text with table/chart/clipart*: Allows insertion of these along with text on one side.
- *Flowcharts*

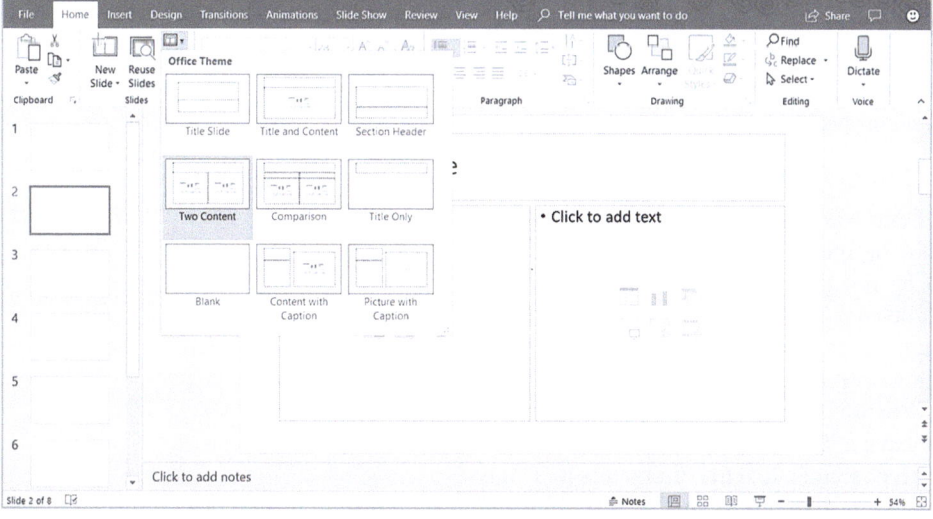

Fig. 25.1: Choosing a slide layout. *(For color version, see Plate 3)*

Adding Text

Text can be typed in the slide if there is a layout for inserting text. However, to add text to a blank slide, click on the "Text Box" option.

Follow the 6 × 6 rule for inserting textual content in any slide, not more than 6 rows in a slide and not more than 6 words per dot point. If a slide is too verbose and is not written in a point form, it will make it difficult for you to present each point. Your audience too will spend too much time and effort trying to read this paragraph. Use telegraphic language incorporating key words. Remember the "*three-word challenge*," i.e., most statements can be summarized in three simple and crisp words. The statement "Vitamin D is important for the body as it boosts the immune system of the body" should be replaced with "Vitamin D boosts immunity."

Show one point at a time (by appropriate use of animation): This will focus attention of the audience on one point, prevent reading ahead, and help keep your presentation focused. Use bullet points as default text format and use assertion-evidence structure in your presentation, wherever feasible.

While typing text, remember to leave generous margins on all sides. An extra wide margin at the bottom is better as the backbenchers in your audience may not be able to actually read the lower part of the slides as their line of vision to the lower half of the screen may be blocked.

Best Fonts for Presentation Slides

The fonts you use in your PowerPoint slides should be readable and large enough to be read by the people seated at the back. You must be consistent in the use of the same font throughout your presentation. Do not use more than two complementary fonts (e.g., Arial and Arial Narrow). The letters or symbols in some fonts have a little line at the end of the stroke in each character, like the characters in Times New Roman. These fonts are "Serif fonts." Fonts that do not have these lines are called "Sans serif fonts" (**Fig. 25.2**). Examples of a "Sans serif" font are Arial, Calibri, Cambria, Geneva, Helvetica, Lucida Sans, Trebuchet, and Verdana. The fonts you use in a PowerPoint presentation must preferably be of "Sans serif type." "Serif fonts" are preferred for printed text. Serif fonts are to be avoided in visual presentation as these are more difficult to read at small font sizes. Do not use a complicated font.

Choosing Point Size of the Font

The font size is a very important factor in using the PowerPoint effectively. Use different size fonts for heading (title) and text to show hierarchy (**Fig. 25.3**). The title font size is 44 points, the main text is 32 points, and the secondary text is usually 24 and 28 points (default settings). You may use 36–44-point size for titles. **Never use a font size smaller than 18 points**. You may use different font sizes to emphasize the main points or key words in the presentation, but use this as sparingly as possible. To check the appropriateness of your

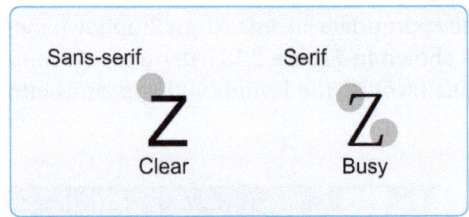

Fig. 25.2: Fonts: Serif and sans serif.

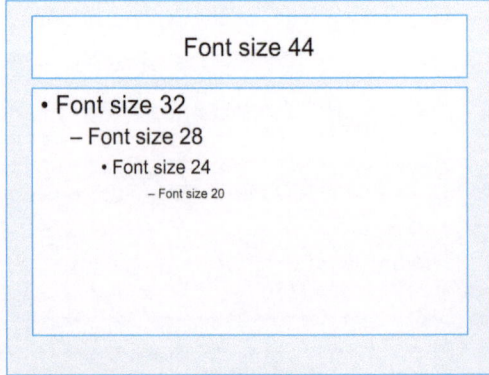

Fig. 25.3: Appropriate font size.

font size, stand at a distance of 7 feet from the screen of your computer and assess if you can read the slides without difficulty.

Font Color and Slide Background

The color of font should be in contrast with the background color. Never use yellow on white or black color fonts on a blue background. We should prefer to use dark fonts (black, blue) on a light background (white, pastel shades) to bring out a contrast. You may use black or blue color on a white background or vice versa. Stick to one or two font colors throughout your presentation. Avoid using exotic colors or color for decoration as it can put off your audience. Avoid using a different color for each point. Writing each character/word in a point with a different color in your zeal to be creative can also look particularly bad and foolish.

Choose an appropriate and contrasting background color (**Fig. 25.4**). Use backgrounds that are attractive but simple and be consistent throughout your presentation. We would prefer a light-colored background. Avoid using gaudy colors such as red or bright orange or canary yellow as the slide background color as it can make your slides look jarring (**Fig. 25.5**).

Inserting Charts, Graphs, Tables, and Flowcharts

Microsoft PowerPoint can be used to insert different types of data charts and graphs including column charts, line graphs, pie charts, bar charts, area graphs, scatter graphs, stock charts, surface charts, doughnut charts, bubble graphs, and radar graphs in your presentation. Try to incorporate graphs instead

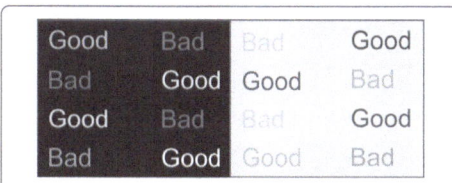

Fig. 25.4: Use of appropriate font color and background color to enhance contrast. *(For color version, see Plate 3)*

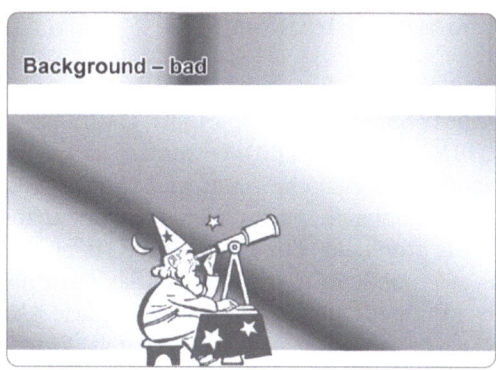

Fig. 25.5: Bad background for slides. *(For color version, see Plate 3)*

of tables/raw data as trends in a graph are easier to comprehend and retain than raw data.

- To insert a chart or table, choose an appropriate layout. Alternately, you can create charts and tables on the blank slide layout using these options from the Formatting toolbar.
- To create a chart, simply click on Insert>Chart and select the type of chart you want to insert. Once you decide the type of chart, you will be prompted to enter the relevant data in an Excel sheet and the resultant chart will be displayed. You can also update the data in the Excel sheet as and when needed and the associated chart will be modified.
- Tables can be created by using either of the two options, the first one being "Insert Table," which creates tables with a preset number of columns and rows, and the second one using the "Draw Table" feature, which requires manual creation of the tables.
- Always remember to title your graphs. Avoid making your graphs too complicated by inserting minor gridlines or by using too many bright colors, or excessive shading, or very small fonts.
- You can create a Flowchart using the "SmartArt Graphics." Click on "Insert," go to "SmartArt," and then select the appropriate format for the flowchart.

Choosing Attributes

Attributes such as bold font, underline, or italics should be used sparingly. CAPITALIZE ONLY WHEN NEEDED. Lowercase letters are easier to read and have a greater visual appeal for the audience. When a word is in capital, the eye is presented with a rectangular shape that is more difficult to read. Even titles must not be in upper case (capitals); use title case. Use of italics should be avoided as the italic form is hard to read. However, you may use italics for attribution of a quote or statistics. In case you are using italics for emphasizing a point, use animation instead. Underlining is usually not acceptable in a PowerPoint slide except for the hyperlinks to websites/URLs.

Animation, Pictures, Clip Art, and Special Effects

Animations

To animate your slides, select the appropriate text on the slide and then click on the "Custom Animation" in the formatting toolbar and choose the appropriate animation. See **Figure 25.6**. You can now choose the entry and exit paths, motion effects, or emphasis. For text use, you may use the following animation effects, namely: appear, wipe (left to right, very fast), or fade (very fast). For graphics, acceptable animation effects include wipe, fade, or dissolve in.

- Do not use distracting animation such as transitions and sound effects.
- Do not use too many animations.
- Use consistent animation.
- Animate quickly and simply.

Pictures

You can insert pictures into presentations to make the presentation engrossing. To add a picture onto a slide, click on the "Insert" button on the main toolbar and go to pictures menu to specify the source (from either downloads, drop box, pictures in your library, files on your computer, scanner, or a digital camera). Pictures can be saved in different formats such as JPEG, PNG, GIF, TIFF, and BMP. JPEG stands for Joint Photographic Expert Group, PNG denotes Portable Network Graphic, GIF stands for Graphics Interchange Format, TIFF stands for Tagged Image File Format, and BMP denotes Bitmap Image File. While adding pictures, it is prudent to use the format that takes less disk space (e.g., .jpeg and .gif) and avoid those taking more space (e.g., .bmp, .tiff, .png) so that the presentations could be easily copied on to a pendrive. The size, magnification, and contrast of the image can

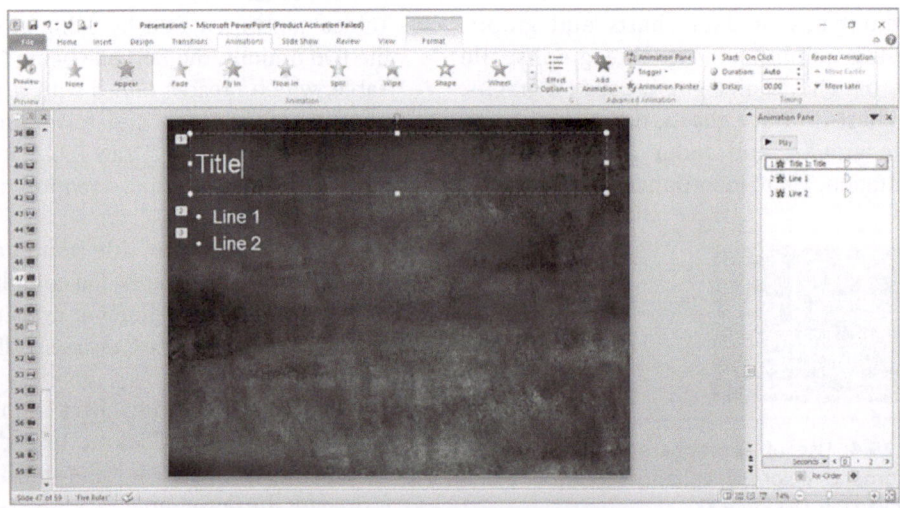

Fig. 25.6: Customizing animation. *(For color version, see Plate 4)*

be edited by clicking on the picture and then selecting the "format" option from the toolbar. Ensure that the picture is clearly visible even to the backbenchers. Refrain from trite clipart as it can look unscientific compared to a color photograph specific to your presentation. Avoid using images for decoration.

Headers and Footers

Other things that may be added to the slides include Headers and Footers (in the toolbar at the top).

Inserting Date, Time, or Slide Numbers

The toolbar also allows you to insert the date, time, or slide number in your presentation.

Notes/Comments

It is possible for you to add notes or comments on a slide which may remind you of the key message or relevant additional information to the text matter on the slide. The panel below the slide will allow you to add notes (**Fig. 25.7**). These may be hidden during a presentation.

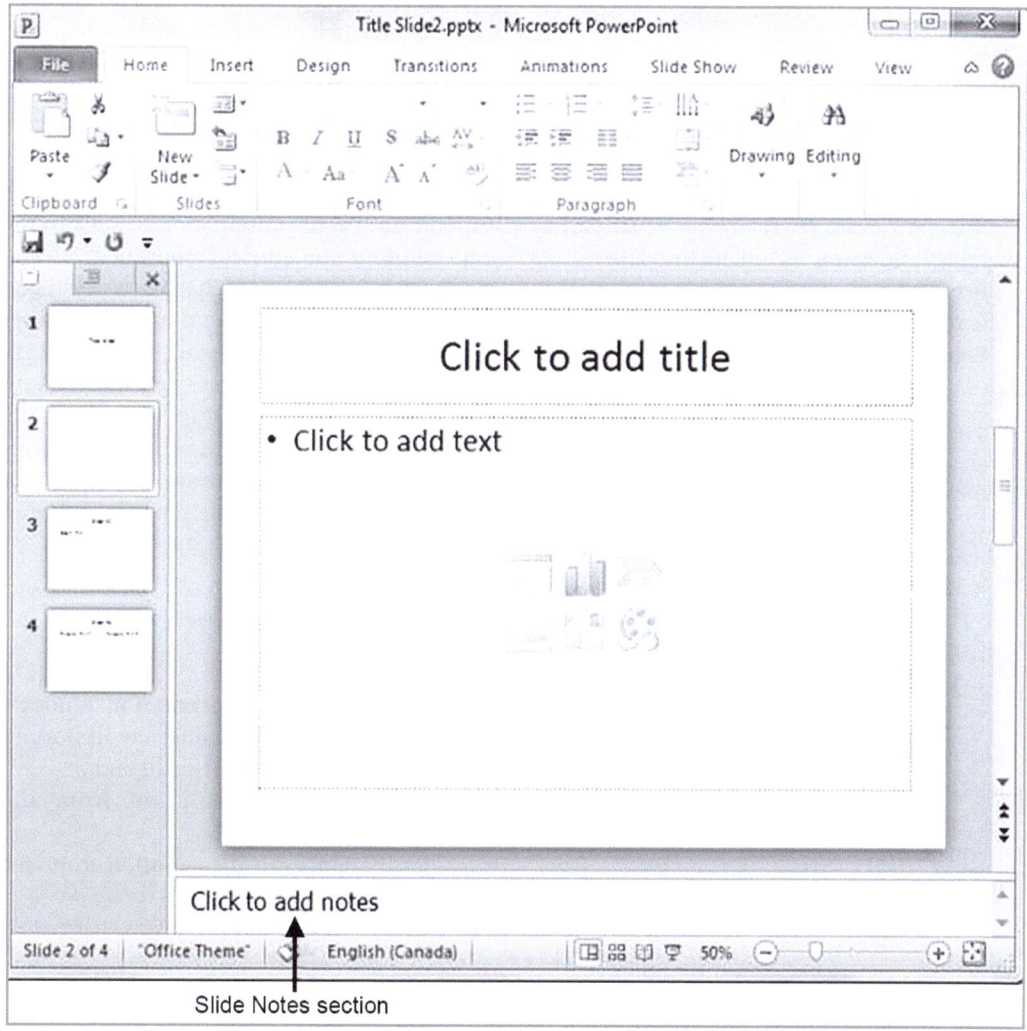

Fig. 25.7: Inserting notes in presentation. *(For color version, see Plate 4)*

Editing the Slides: Making a Global Change

Slide Master is a useful tool which allows you to make a global change to all the slides, except the title slide. Click on the "View" option toolbar and now select the Master option. You will be presented with a slide with an option to make a global change by changing just one slide. For example, if you wish to insert your name or your institution's logo in all slides, or wish to change the background, or font size/style, you could change that in just one slide which would then be applied to all slides.

Change the Order of the Slides

Slide Sorter shows all the slides lined up on the screen as thumbnails. In case you want to change the order of the slides, you have to drag the slide number up or down the list in the Outline view to do so. However, be careful as dragging it sideways will delete the slide.

Box 25.1 enlists ten key points to remember while making good slides.

Figure 25.8 shows some examples of bad slides.

> **Box 25.1: Ten points for making good slides.**
> 1. Keep the template structured and concise
> 2. Add text judiciously (use point form, follow 6 × 6 rule, avoid wordiness)
> 3. Fonts: Reasonably big, simple, and clear
> 4. Use text to support your communication
> 5. Use pictures to simplify complex concepts
> 6. Use animations for complex relationships
> 7. Use visuals to support, not to distract
> 8. Use sounds only when absolutely necessary
> 9. Limit the number of slides: Three slides per minute is the maximum
> 10. Proofread your slides

■ PREPARING FOR A GOOD PRESENTATION

Checking and Rechecking

Once you are ready with your slides, always proofread your slides for any spelling or grammatical errors, or repetition of words. When checking, it is always good to take a break before you come back to your slides. You will be amazed at the mistakes you are able to pick up on the second reading. You do not want your mistakes magnified and projected onto a wall for all to see. You could also ask a friend or colleague to go through them in case you are too exhausted in the process of making of your slides.

Timing

Always practice reading your slides and have a friend time your presentation to stick to the time allotted for your presentation. If you stick to the 6 × 6 rule, each slide would need about 20–30 seconds. So, adjust the number of slides accordingly. For your thesis protocol presentation, you would need to make about 18–20 slides, assuming that you would be allotted about 7–8 minutes to make your presentation. In case you are allotted more time, you are at liberty to increase the number of slides.

Useful Keyboard Shortcuts for Presentation

You can make your presentation smooth, quick, and seamless by using few important keys during the PowerPoint presentation.
- *F5*: Start the presentation from the beginning.
- *Shift+F5*: Start the presentation from the current slide.

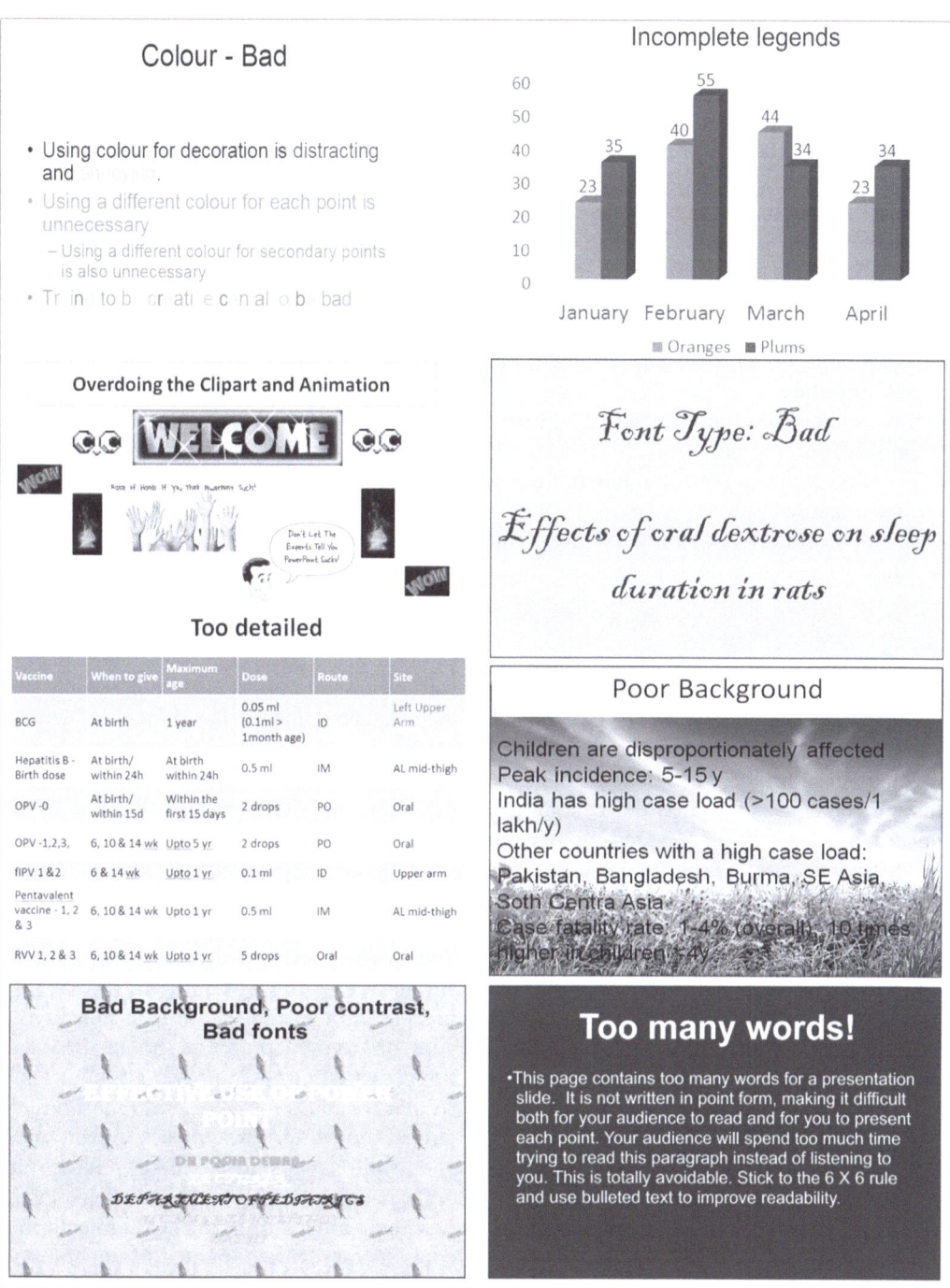

Fig. 25.8: Some bad slides in PowerPoint presentation. *(For color version, see Plate 5)*

- *Ctrl+P*: Activate the pen tool during a slideshow.
- *Ctrl+A*: Convert the pen to a pointer during presentation.
- *Ctrl+H*: Hide the pen or pointer during the show.
- *Home*: Go to the first slide, or from within a text box, go to the beginning of the line.
- *End/Esc*: Go to the last slide.
- *PgDn or → or ↓ (arrow key) or N*: Go to the next slide.
- *PgUp or ← or ↑ (arrow key) or P*: Go the previous slide.
- *W*: Makes the screen white during presentation.
- *B*: Makes the screen go black during presentation.
- *S*: Stop or restart an automatic PowerPoint show.

Carry all Accessories

You may manually advance the slides using the mouse or arrow keys on the keyboard. Alternately, you could carry a wireless mouse or a wireless remote (**Fig. 25.9**) to navigate through your slides; the latter device may also function as a laser pointer. There is no need to install any software in order to use these. You just need to plug the receiver into a USB port and you are ready to go. In case you wish to use a pointer, you should carry your own to the venue.

Rehearsing

Remember that a good presenter can do without multimedia techniques but not vice versa. Practice your speech several times before the actual presentation as stage fright is extremely common. Rehearse your speech in front of your good friends to decrease nervousness. A survey of more than 2,500 Americans revealed that 41% of the people feared public speaking; in contrast, only 19% feared death (Stephen E. Lucas, *The Art of Public Speaking*).

Do not read directly from the slides; keep a notes handout and prepare the script of your talk well in advance. Keeping a printout of the slides at hand is useful so that you can refer to them while speaking. You should rehearse your presentation preferably at the venue itself to make sure that all the things are working seamlessly. Make sure that the venue has the provision for LCD display and the systems at the venue support the version (like PowerPoint 2016) used by you.

Backup

You never know when technology can fail, so be ready for alternatives. Carry your presentation to the venue in a pendrive in addition to your laptop. You should also e-mail the presentation to your own e-mail account so that it can be retrieved any time from any part of the world. Always carry a print-out of your slide set which could be photocopied on transparencies for overhead projection, in case there is a failure of the LCD projector. You could also provide handouts to the audience in case there are major technical difficulties at the venue like electricity failure. PowerPoint Viewer is the name for a series of small free

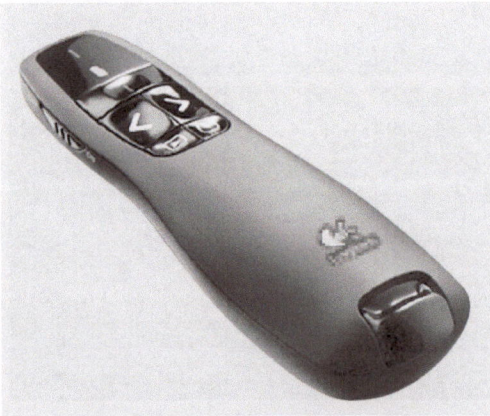

Fig. 25.9: A wireless digital presenter/remote for navigating through the slides.

application programs to be used on computers without PowerPoint installed. Alternately, use PowerPoint for the web or PowerPoint mobile on your mobile device.

MAKING THE FINAL PRESENTATION

- A good communication is the key to successful presentation. Remember that making an oral presentation is very different from writing a paper. Hook the audience by striking a common note and build credibility.
- Make the audience travel with your presentation in a flow. You could do so by numbering your points and making old-to-new transitions.
- Help the audience follow your ideas by using some tricks of the trade such as repeat key words or ideas, group a set of ideas together under a single heading, and always explain to the audience exactly *why* you are telling them a particular piece of information.
- Do not minify your own results or understate your expertise on the topic. Speak with conviction.
- If you need a specific slide more than once in your presentation, it is better to reproduce it at the appropriate places rather than going back to it.
- Keep the momentum of your presentation. To keep the audience engrossed, you may sometimes be doing the unexpected (use humor, change your tone or volume, present an attention-grabbing visual). Modulate your voice and tone effectively. Do not speak too quickly or end your sentences on a high note. Use appropriate pauses when you are stating a major result, raising a question or showing a complicated figure. However, do not dramatize or gesticulate excessively during your presentation.
- Control any nervousness. Do not pace, rock, slouch, tap your feet, adjust your hair or clothes and avoid eye contact. Avoid using stalling words such as: Um, er, uh, and, basically, you know.
- Always summarize your main results to improve clarity and use an effective and strong closing/concluding statement as it usually leaves an impact on the audience.
- Be prepared to answer questions related to your presentation. Do not use "sorry" to excuse incompetence or lack of preparation. Be humble but firm. You should apologize if you are late or shown to be incorrect. You should appear confident, but not overconfident and foolish.

ALTERNATIVES TO POWERPOINT

In the current age of digital technology, several new software programs have emerged which offer useful alternatives to PowerPoint. These include the following:

- *Visme:* Cloud-based, drag-and-drop presentation software which offers several high-definition backgrounds and layouts with a variety of fonts, free images, and graph tools. Since it is HTML5-based, it can be run on any browser and device.
- *Haiku Deck:* This cloud-based presentation solution with an inbuilt Artificial intelligence helper called "Zuru" is a mobile alternative to Prezi and PowerPoint. It offers great visuals and uses large fonts.
- *Emaze:* Like Visme, it uses HTML5-based technology and hence is compatible with any browser and all kinds of computers, tablets, and laptops.
- *Prezi:* One of the most popular cloud-based software characterized by nonlinear presentations. The features of Zoom and motion may be useful for some kinds of presentations. It is compatible with

Windows as well as Mac. It has been found to have a greater aesthetic appeal.
- *Keynote:* This is the Apple's version of PowerPoint. It also uses a cloud-based platform and is free for all Mac computers. Another useful feature is its compatibility with PowerPoint.
- *Google slides:* It is free with a Google account and is emerging as a powerful competitor to PowerPoint. When logged into Google account, you can access Slides at any time, from anywhere. The templates are neat and crisp. One can open the Slides, prepare the presentation, and export as PowerPoint presentation.
- *Sway:* This is Microsoft's own alternative to PowerPoint and can be accessed by anyone with Hotmail or Outlook account for free.

CONCLUSION

PowerPoint is a useful tool for allow for a lucid presentation of your thesis. A PowerPoint presentation should be made using appropriate slide layout, font (color, style, and sizes), content, with minimum use of animations and graphics. The presentation must be in a logical sequence with emphasis on your results. Remember to summarize your work before you conclude. Additionally, good oratory skills are the key to a successful presentation.

KEY MESSAGES

- In the current age of digital technology, several software programs including the PowerPoint, Prezi, Keynote, and Google slides serve as useful media to present your research work.
- An appropriate intermix of text, figures, tables, and graphs in your presentation, along with correct background, colors, and fonts can help you to make an impactful presentation.
- Always prepare your presentation in advance and rehearse it before the final date.
- Remember to have a backup just in case technology falters on the day of presentation.

FURTHER READING

1. Evans ML. Polished, professional presentation: unlocking the design elements. J Contin Educ Nurs. 2000;31(5):213-8; quiz 238-9.
2. Gunderman RB, McCammack KC 4th. PowerPoint: know your medium. J Am Coll Radiol. 2010;7(9):711-4.
3. Gupta P, Guglani L, Shah D. Exploring the power of PowerPoint. Indian Pediatr. 2002;39(6):539-48.
4. James C, Linte CA. Tips on effective presentation design and delivery. Conf Proc IEEE Eng Med Biol Soc. 2010;2010:1108.
5. Mormer E. What's in Your Teaching Toolbox? Semin Hear. 2018;39(1):107-14.
6. Moulton ST, Türkay S, Kosslyn SM. Does a presentation's medium affect its message? PowerPoint, Prezi, and oral presentations. PLoS One. 2017;12(7):e0178774.
7. Norvig P. PowerPoint: shot with its own bullets. Lancet. 2003;362(9381):343-4.

CHAPTER 26

Writing the Thesis Protocol

Dheeraj Shah, Navjeevan Singh

■ INTRODUCTION

The thesis protocol is a plan of your research proposal. It is reviewed by a committee of experts in the institute, and amendments suggested by the committee need to be incorporated before it is sent for approval to the university. The protocol is an official document to which your proposed research must conform. You need to write your protocol very carefully as once approved, changes cannot be made to the research work without approval of the university, which may be a tedious job. To simplify writing an acceptable research protocol without omitting essential information, a structured format is useful. The following format has been devised with detailed instructions to guide you in writing a complete protocol.

■ A MODEL PROTOCOL FORMAT

This document contains sections "A" to "K" and amplifies them for ease of use; however, some sections will not be needed in every study. When you identify such a section, e.g., the one on interventional studies, and if your study does not have an intervention, you should delete it.

Instructions, or sample text, are provided in each section to generate ideas of what should be included therein. The text should be substituted with information that pertains to your study. Do not rearrange the sections of the protocol. The format for writing the protocol (in the order in which they appear in text) is given below:

Cover Page

(*Centered alignment*)

> **Title of Thesis**
> **Protocol of Thesis to be Submitted to the**
> [Insert Name of University/Board]
> **Toward Partial Fulfillment of the Requirement for the Degree of**
> [Insert Degree and Subject (e.g., MD Microbiology)]
> **Session/Batch** [Insert time of postgraduate training (e.g., 2018–2021)]
> **Name of Student**
> **Name of Primary Department**
> **Name of Institution**

Title Page

(*Start on a fresh page*)

> **Protocol of thesis to be submitted to the** (Name of University/Board) **toward partial fulfillment of the requirement for the**
> **Degree of** MD/MS (Discipline)
> **Session/Batch:** *from "Year" to "Year"*
> **Title of Thesis:** *(Write in Title Case)*
> **Name of student: Signature:**
> **Name and designation of Supervisor: Signature:**
> **Name and designation of Co-supervisor(s): Signature(s):**
>
> **Place of work: Department(s)**
> *(Name of the Institution)*

Summary of Protocol

(*Start on a fresh page, maximum 1 page*)

The summary must provide the reader with a rapid assessment of the research proposal. It also serves as a format for a PowerPoint presentation of the protocol using each subheading as the title of each slide. A good presentation can, thus, be managed using a maximum of 12 slides in approximately 7 minutes.

- The protocol summary should be no more than 300 words and, at the most, a page long (Follow the guidelines of your university if they differ from those mentioned here).
- The summary should be able to stand on its own.
- Fragments/phrases can be used instead of complete sentences.

All the central elements of the protocol should be summarized (preferably in a structured manner) as given here:

Study title: Enter the full title.
Rationale: Specify the reason for conducting this research in light of current knowledge, i.e., why the research needs to be done, and its relevance.
Aim and objective(s): State what you want to find out (aim) and how you are going to do it (objectives). Align them to your research question/hypothesis/title.
Setting: Place (e.g., community, hospital) and department(s) where the study will be conducted.
Study design: Descriptive or analytical. If descriptive, whether case series, survey, cross-sectional, diagnostic accuracy study, etc. If analytical, whether observational (cohort, case-control or cross-sectional) or interventional (randomized control trial, crossover).
Time frame: Time during which the study will be conducted (from inception to submission).
Population/participants: List the nature (age, gender, sociodemographic characteristics), inclusion and exclusion criteria, and method of enrollment.
Sample size: State the total number of patients to be recruited to the study.
Methods: List of procedures/intervention.
Outcome measures: List primary and secondary outcome measures [pertaining to primary and secondary objective(s) respectively].
Statistical analysis: Statistical methods proposed to be used for data analysis.

Introduction

(*Start on a fresh page, maximum 2 pages*)

The introduction should be focused on the research question and should be directly relevant to the objectives of your study. Organize the information in paragraphs, presenting the more general aspects of the topic early in the introduction (background), then narrowing to specific information that states the problem and rationale, and end with the research question/hypothesis. The introduction should answer the question of why and what: Why the research needs to be done and what its relevance will be.

See Chapter 10 for a guide to writing an Introduction. It is vital to frame a crisp and concise introduction while writing the protocol, which can be used again when writing the thesis.

Review of Literature

(*Start on a fresh page, maximum 4 pages*)
It should start with the brief statement of the problem including magnitude, affected geographical areas, considerations, etc. This should be followed by a brief analysis of the most relevant studies published on the subject as they apply to your research question. This section should answer the questions: What is the current knowledge about the subject of study? In what ways has the problem been approached by others and what are the results? Are the reported studies contradictory? What are the lacunae in the existing knowledge?

Move from what is known to what is unknown, ending with a compelling rationale of how your study will fulfill the lacunae in the literature.

Do not merely list the findings of the studies one after the other. Analyze the findings that affect your study and report them theme-wise. For example, you may write about studies that suggest drug A is better than drug B, the next thematic paragraph could be studies that contradict this finding, another paragraph could mention lacunae in the study designs that resulted in these differences, and so on.

See Chapter 11 for a guide to writing the Review of Literature. Take care to be brief while writing the Review of Literature for your protocol. Later, when you are writing the full thesis report, a detailed Review of Literature is desired.

Aim and Objectives

(*Start on a fresh page; 1 page*)
Aim is a broad statement of what the research study hopes to accomplish. The steps taken to achieve the aim are the "objectives" of the study; they must be linked to the research question/hypothesis. Objectives should be SMART: Specific (not vague), Measurable, Achievable, Relevant, and Timebound. Mention the primary and secondary objectives. Primary objectives directly contribute to answering the research question. Secondary objectives may not directly contribute to answering the research question but are important to the study. Aim and objectives must be aligned to the title of the thesis.

Material and Methods

(*Start on a fresh page; 4–5 pages approximately*)
This section is the most important part of the protocol as it exactly describes the work you will be carrying out.

Checklist for "Material and Methods"

Study design: Descriptive or analytical. If descriptive, whether case-series, survey, cross-sectional, or diagnostic study. If analytical, whether observational (cohort, case–control, or cross-sectional), or interventional (randomized control trial, crossover) study.

Study setting: Place where subjects will be recruited from.

Study duration: When and where the study will be carried out.

Ethical aspects: Name of ethics committee from where ethical clearance is sought. Mention about written informed consent. Mention issues about confidentiality.

Participants: Target population (age group, sex).

Inclusion criteria: Define ages, criteria for defining disease condition/normalcy, including for controls (if any).

Exclusion criteria: Subjects who fulfill inclusion criteria but would be excluded because of other conditions that could possibly introduce bias.

Describe basis for assignment of participants into case or control group, or for receiving one or other intervention. Provide details related to sequence generation, allocation concealment, and blinding in randomized controlled studies.

Intervention/procedure: Detail if using a new method or else quote standard reference if the

method you are going to use has already been described. Describe the following:
- Modifications you have made to a standard or published method.
- *Quantitative aspects*: Masses, volumes, incubation times, concentrations, and machine specifications (include manufacturer's name and address).
- Who will make the assessments, and the tools that will be used.
- Frequency and duration of intervention.
- Procedures and schedules of examination/investigations/treatment, and observation of outcome measures.
- Dosage, formulations, schedules, duration of drug treatments, if any.

Outcome measures:
Primary: These are the outcomes which are based on the research question/hypothesis. The main thrust of interest in the protocol pertains to the primary objective(s).

Secondary: These are other outcomes of possible interest; they pertain to the secondary objective(s), if any.

Study flow chart: A graphic outline of the study design using a flow diagram should be provided. This should include the timing of intervention (if any) and assessments/monitoring in various groups of participants. This should be named as a figure (e.g., Fig. 1), and must be cited in the text of Material and Methods section.

Sample size: You should mention the basis for sample size calculation. Provide the reference(s) for data used to calculate the sample size. Mention calculated sample size, and the number you plan to enroll accounting for feasibility/attrition.

Data management and statistical analysis: The protocol should provide information on how the data will be managed including data handling, and coding for computer analysis, monitoring, and verification/cleaning of data. The statistical methods proposed to be used for the analysis of data including reasons for the sample size selected, power of the study, level of significance to be used, and procedures for accounting for any missing or spurious data should be clearly outlined.

For projects involving qualitative approaches, specify in sufficient detail how the data will be analyzed.

References

(*Start on a fresh page; limit to 20–30 most pertinent and recent references*)
References that have been cited in the text of the protocol should be listed in this section in the chronological order of their appearance in the text. Standard and uniform Vancouver method should be used to cite references (See Chapter 22).

Case Record Form

(*Clinical data sheet, Start on a fresh page*)
The data sheet must capture the required, relevant, accurate, and analyzable data about the participants (patients); the procedures carried out; outcome measure(s) at predefined intervals; and observations about each case.

A sample case record form is provided in *Annexure* 1.

Informed Consent Form

(*Including patient information sheet*)
The form should have two parts: (1) Patient/parent information sheet, and (2) certificate of consent. Before requesting consent to participate in research, the investigator must provide the individual with information about the purpose of the study, the expectations from the participant, the responsibility of the investigators, risks, and benefits of the intervention, the alternatives available (if interventional study), and the options to withdraw from the study. These should be part of patient/parent information sheet. The second part should include statements by patients/parents about their willingness to participate in the study, along with their

signatures. Both parts of the informed consent form should be in English as well as in local language, and title of the study should be clearly mentioned in the beginning.

A sample of informed consent form in English has been provided in Chapter 14. Informed consent form templates of the World Health Organization are available with their own detailed instructions from https://www.who.int/ethics/review-committee/informed_consent/en/ or Indian Council of Medical Research. Choose the template suitable for your study. Many institutions also provide sample consent forms, which should be used by student of that institute for the sake of uniformity.

Informed consent must be obtained in a language known to the patient; therefore, a translation of the informed consent form may be necessary. Translation into a local language should be performed by somebody knowing both languages and then it should be typed in local language. Online automated translation facilities should not be used as it often results in major errors.

Annexures

Any other annexure (e.g., validated questionnaires, marking sheets, forms) can be appended if it is a part of research methods. Any annexure used must be cited in the text at appropriate place.

Other Technicalities

- *Pages*: Generally, should not exceed 12-14 (excluding title page, summary, forms, and annexures). Number the pages consecutively starting from the title page. It should be printed, preferably at the bottom of the page.
- *Font size*: 12 minimum
- A4 size paper
- *Line spacing*: Double space
- *Margins*: At least 2.5 cm on all four sides. Justified

CONCLUSION

Thesis protocol is the backbone of the future work to be done. A well-written protocol goes a long way in ensuring quality of the research work and uniformity in data collection. You should refer to the protocol whenever you face any problem in deciding whether to include or exclude a potential research participant, how to assess, and how to manage his/her condition. Your protocol should always be available with you while carrying out any part of the research so that it can be readily referred to.

KEY MESSAGES

- Initial pages of a protocol are: Cover page, Title page (with signatures), and Summary.
- Main body of protocol should be written under headings of Introduction (1–2 pages), Review of Literature (3–4 pages), Aim and Objectives (1 page), Material and Methods (4–5 pages), and References (1–2 pages).
- End pages of protocol are constituted by Case Record Form, Informed Consent Form (including patient/parent information sheet), and any other Annexure.
- Protocol should be typed neatly ensuring uniformity of font type and size, heading/subheading style, spacing, and page margins.

FURTHER READING

1. Al-Jundi A, Sakka S. Protocol writing in clinical research. J Clin Diagn Res. 2016;10:ZE10-3.
2. Cameli M, Novo G, Tusa M, Mandoli GE, Corrado G, Benedetto F, et al. How to write a research protocol: Tips and tricks. J Cardiovasc Echogr. 2018;28:151-3.
3. Indian Council of Medical Research. (2017). National Ethical Guidelines for Biomedical and Health Research Involving Human Participants. [online] Available from https://www.icmr.nic.in/sites/default/files/guidelines/ICMR_Ethical_Guidelines_2017.pdf. [Last accessed April, 2020].
4. World Health Organization. Recommended Format for a Research Protocol. [online] Available from https://www.who.int/ethics/review-committee/format-research-protocol/en/. [Last Accessed April,2020].
5. World Health Organization. Templates for Informed Consent Forms. [online] Available from https://www.who.int/ethics/review-committee/informed_consent/en/. [Last accessed April,2020].

CHAPTER 27

Converting Thesis into a Scientific Paper

Dheeraj Shah

■ INTRODUCTION

The objectives of a research work, thesis in this case, remain unfulfilled unless it is published in form of a scientific paper that is available to researchers and policy makers all over the world. However, a thesis report cannot be simply "converted" into a scientific paper publishable in a good journal. It involves lot of effort and perseverance on part of the student and the supervisors, but the effort is worth it as publication in form of a scientific paper not only results in dissemination of the work to the scientific community but also brings credit and career advancement opportunities, especially for those aspiring for a career in academics or research.

Converting a thesis report into a journal article involves many steps because there are important differences between a full thesis report and a journal article (**Table 27.1**). The first and foremost difference is that a journal article is much shorter. However, it is not possible to make a journal article out of thesis report by using cut-and-paste. Remember that the journal article (paper) is not a miniature version of the full thesis. The format of thesis report and a journal article also differs substantially. The scientific paper thus needs to be written afresh using information from

TABLE 27.1: Important differences between thesis and scientific paper.

Characteristic	Thesis	Scientific paper
Length	~100 pages	5–6 printed pages
Elements/Sections		
• Summary/Abstract	Summary, usually at the end	Abstract, in the beginning
• Introduction	2–3 pages	1–2 paragraphs
• Aim and Objectives	Presented as a separate section	Presented within the Introduction
• Review of Literature	Present and detailed	Absent
Tables and Figures	No restrictions	Usually not more than three each
Language/Format	As per University guidelines	As per Journal guidelines
Number of references	~100	20–30 maximum

the thesis report, and simultaneously topping it up with additional information that may be available by the time you write a journal article from your thesis report.

■ WHEN SHOULD YOU WRITE A PAPER FROM THESIS?

You can consider writing a paper from thesis report at many stages. For PhD theses, some university guidelines mandate publication of a journal article before thesis submission/acceptance. However, University Grants Commission (UGC) of India is reconsidering this policy of mandatory publication during PhD courses as it is considered to be one of the reasons for flourishing of poor-quality predatory journals and unethical publication practices. Irrespective of mandatory policy, you should consider writing a scientific paper out of your thesis as early as possible, and preferably during your postgraduate training itself.

A manuscript-based thesis (see Chapter 28) is a format where thesis report is written in a format that facilitates publication in form of a scientific paper. However, it is still only a concept in India, which has not been adopted by universities. This also carries a risk of loss of complete data collected during thesis because of the inherent brevity of a scientific manuscript.

You may write a scientific paper either simultaneously with thesis report or follow it over next few months. However, it is easier said than done as most students will get busy with preparation of examinations and find no time (and also inclination) to write and submit a paper for publication in a journal. As there is no incentive involved, the job is often left for afterwards and after examinations your priorities will again change to finding further career or training opportunities. By the time one is "settled" it may be too late and the research work may become outdated. As a result, most theses never get published in form of scientific papers.

Overall, it is important that you write a scientific paper from your thesis early, preferably during postgraduate training. A good way to ensure that you write a scientific paper from your thesis during your postgraduate training itself is to submit it as a full paper for presentation at a conference or for an award. In case you were not able to do so, do it as early as possible after examinations are over; otherwise, there is a real risk that thesis will never be published as a journal article. Supervisors have an important role to play in motivating and guiding the students to write a paper.

■ SELECTING A JOURNAL

The first step in writing a journal article from thesis is to select the most appropriate journal. This is important at early stage as you need to write and format the manuscript as per instructions to the authors of that particular journal. The important factors for choosing the journal are its scope and priorities, indexing status, accessibility, publication fee, and time to publication. While publication of scientific paper from a thesis paper is important, you should not fall prey to poor quality predatory journals, which make bogus claims regarding their indexing status and cite fake impact factors. Predatory journals are poor quality journals that publish almost everything submitted to them in exchange of money in name of article processing charges and display low levels of transparency and integrity. These journals usually have fancy prefixes to their titles such as "Global", "International," but have poor quality practices of peer review and journal operations. The exact designations and location of their editors and publishers cannot be verified easily, and the language of their communication is deceptive. Publishing your paper in such journals with questionable integrity may bring disrepute to you and your supervisor rather than providing the joy of seeing one's name in print. You may refer to an article by Dewan and Shah for more tips on choosing a journal (Dewan P, Shah D. A writer's dilemma: where to publish and where not to? Indian Pediatr. 2016;53:141-5).

WRITING THE CONTENT

As emphasized earlier, the paper is to be written afresh using the data in thesis as a starting point. You will need to write a paper in various sections such as Introduction, Methods, Results, and Discussion. An abstract will also be required. While nomenclature of many of these sections is similar to that in thesis, there are important differences while you write them in a scientific paper.

Title

It is not necessary to retain the title of the research work that you used in your thesis.

The title of a journal article should be clear and concise, and should include the key ingredients such as population, condition, intervention (if any), outcome, and study design. Though all these principles also hold true for title of a thesis, you might not have given enough importance to them at the stage of writing thesis protocol. Moreover, the journal guidelines also sometimes dictate the type of title to be used for scientific paper. For example, some journals may want declarative title (where key result is declared in title itself) or query title, but most journals will prefer descriptive or neutral title. In case you are presenting only a part of the thesis work in form of a scientific paper, the title will have to be modified accordingly.

Abstract

Your thesis report may not have this section but will have a section of "Summary" which is somewhat similar to Abstract. You need to write all major elements of your paper in abstract and format it as per journal's guidelines. Some journals will ask you to write structured abstract (4-point, 8-point, 10-point, etc.) under various subheadings, (e.g., Objectives, Methods, Results, Conclusion), while others may want an unstructured abstract. You also need to check recommended word limit of abstract for the journal you wish to prepare your paper for. A good abstract should be a complete, stand-alone document that provides all important elements of a paper including data on key outcomes in a concise manner. For a journal article, you also need to include few keywords for the purpose of indexing of article.

Introduction

This section will be much shorter in a research paper in comparison to that written in thesis report. This should be no >1–2 paragraphs that should clearly outline the lacunae in existing literature, need for the current study, and the study objectives. Remember that the journal article (in contrast to thesis report) does not have a separate subsection of "Aim and Objectives," and thus, objectives should be presented in Introduction itself as the last statement.

Methods

This section in a research paper will be much similar to that of thesis or protocol but will avoid detailed descriptions of procedures which have been already described in literature. Just a reference to the procedure with detail of any modification will suffice. In thesis report, you might have included few pictures of instruments/materials used in research, but you must avoid including them in a journal article. If you are presenting only a part of the research work carried out during thesis project in a scientific paper, you need to write only relevant part of methodology. However, while doing so, you must clearly mention it in the research article and the justification for doing so. In any case, you cannot change the broad description of methodology of a paper as the research has already been completed.

Results

You will be utilizing data in your thesis report for writing this section in a scientific paper but it will not be possible for you to directly replicate tables and figures from your thesis. The number of tables and figures will be guided by the requirements of the publishing journal and no >2-3 tables and 1-2 figures will be allowed by most journals. Thus, you will need to reorganize results by omitting unnecessary tables and figures, combining tables with similar content, (e.g., continuous and categorical outcomes, primary and secondary outcomes), and omitting data that has little or no relevance to the proposed objectives. Description of statistics is also to be guided by the journal's policy. The presentation of results in a scientific paper will have to broadly adhere to the prescribed guidelines for that study design, (e.g., CONSORT for interventional studies, STARD for diagnostic accuracy studies, and STROBE for observational studies). While presenting results, you have to ensure that they are in synchrony with the proposed objectives and outlined methodology, and no part described in methods is omitted from results.

Discussion

This section will substantially differ between thesis and scientific paper. Apart from being shorter and crisper, it needs to be unstructured and tailored as per journal's policy. Most importantly, by the time you prepare an article for submission to the journal, new evidence might have emerged. Thus, you need to carry out a revised search of literature to find any important research that has been carried out on the similar topic and use it to build this section. This section in a research article must be coherent and requires several rounds of editing, rewriting and reorganization. You should avoid discussing results piecemeal—the style often followed in writing a thesis report. Focus on important/primary outcomes while preparing discussion for a scientific paper.

Broadly, the discussion should be organized in following sequence using paragraphs: Summary of study findings (without repeating data), comparison with existing literature and reasons for differences if any, strengths and limitations of the study, implications of study for practice, policy or research, and conclusions. Few journals may ask for a separate section on conclusions; for others, these need to be presented along with discussion.

References

Include only relevant and recent references in the article to be submitted for publication. Check the journal's guidelines for the number limit and adhere to the same while preparing the article. You also need to format the style of writing the references to match the journal's recommendations.

OTHER FACETS

Authorship

There are other important issues to be considered while preparing a scientific article. The authors' name and sequence need to be decided in consultation with your supervisor and co-supervisors. It is unethical to not include name of any person who has substantially contributed to the work and fulfills the following authorship criteria for a scientific manuscript.
- Substantial contributions to the conception or design of the work; or the acquisition, analysis, or interpretation of data for the work; and
- Drafting the work or revising it critically for important intellectual content; and
- Final approval of the version to be published; and
- Agreement to be accountable for all aspects of the work in ensuring that questions related to the accuracy or integrity of any part of the work are appropriately investigated and resolved.

All supervisors and co-supervisors should be involved in manuscript writing or its critical assessment even if they have seen and approved the thesis report earlier. Sometimes, other persons who might not have been supervisors or co-supervisors of thesis might qualify for authorship by virtue of their contribution in various capacities. It is important to include them as authors, simultaneously avoiding gift authorship to those who do not qualify above authorship criteria. Other people, who have contributed to the project but do not qualify to be an author, should be acknowledged in title page of scientific paper.

Publication Ethics

- Write various components of research paper in your own language and plagiarism must be avoided (see Chapter 23). Plagiarism becomes a stronger misconduct if replicated in a scientific paper rather than when confined to thesis alone.
- Falsification of data and omitting/manipulating outcomes to make your results more attractive and "publishable" are gross misconducts, which editors/reviewers of good journals will easily recognize, and it will bring disrepute not only to you and your supervisors but also to the institute and country.
- Submit the paper to only one journal at a time. You are not allowed to submit the paper simultaneously to different journals; you can submit to the next journal only if the manuscript is rejected or formally withdrawn from the first journal.
- Avoid slicing data of your thesis into different scientific papers just to increase number of publications. All important results of a focused research should be presented in one scientific paper. For example, if you have collected data on clinical and radiological features of pulmonary tuberculosis over 1 year, publishing clinical data in a Pediatric journal and publishing radiological features in a Radiology journal amounts to slicing of data (also called salami publication). If there are strong reasons to present some results separately, you need to clearly mention the same in the Methods section of manuscript with citation to the other paper published/submitted for publication from the same data.

Revision

Same in case the journal editors ask you to revise the submission after or before peer review, you need to do accordingly. In case the manuscript is rejected by one journal, submit to the next target journal, but modify the manuscript as per instructions to authors of the next journal. This will involve much less effort than writing a paper afresh as only some aspects need to be changed, (e.g., reference style, word count, abstract structure). Do not get disheartened by rejection of manuscript as it is often a rule than exception and submit to the next journal in consultation with your supervisor. Most manuscripts will need to undergo few rounds of revision and submission before they are finally accepted.

■ CONCLUSION

The objective of a thesis project remains incomplete unless the work is presented to scientific word in the form of an article (paper) in a scientific journal. As there are important differences between a thesis and a journal article, the latter is to be written afresh using information from the thesis report intelligently, rather than by cut-and-paste. Writing a journal article requires scientific temperament and writing skills, and it is important to seek training and supervision from people well versed with writing and publishing scientific papers. While it is important to write a paper out of thesis, you need to keep in mind the ethics of publication, and not fall prey to unethical practices and journals following such practices.

KEY MESSAGES

- Choose a suitable journal for your research work. Avoid predatory journals.
- Read carefully all instructions to authors of the chosen journal.
- Write manuscript afresh, utilizing data from the thesis work. Avoid copy paste.
- Reorganize results; reconstruct tables, keeping in mind the instructions of the target journal.
- Search and read relevant recent literature again, and prepare a focused discussion after inclusion of recent studies.
- Format and organize your manuscript including references as per the style recommended by target journal.
- Follow publication ethics by strictly avoiding plagiarism and falsification of data. Avoid writing many papers out of one thesis.
- Do not get disheartened by rejection. Use comments to improve the manuscript and submit to another journal.

FURTHER READING

1. Arora SK, Shah D. Writing methods: How to write what you did? Indian Pediatr. 2016;53:335-40.
2. Bagga A. Discussion: The heart of the paper. Indian Pediatr. 2016;53:901-4.
3. Cobey KD, Lalu MM, Skidmore B, Ahmadzai N, Grudniewicz A, Moher D. What is a predatory journal? A scoping review. F1000Res. 2018;7:1001.
4. Dewan P, Gupta P. Writing the title, abstract and introduction: Looks matter! Indian Pediatr. 2016;53:235-41.
5. Dewan P, Shah D. A Writers Dilemma: Where to publish and where not to? Indian Pediatr. 2016;53:141-5.
6. Equator Network. Reporting guidelines for main study types. [online] Available from https://www.equator-network.org/reporting-guidelines/. [Last accessed April 30, 2020].
7. International Committee of Medical Journal Editors. Defining the role of authors and contributors. [online] Available from: http://www.icmje.org/recommendations/browse/roles-and-responsibilities/defining-the-role-of-authors-and-contributors.html. [Last accessed April 30, 2020].
8. International Committee of Medical Journal Editors. Manuscript preparation and submission. [online] Available from http://www.icmje.org/recommendations/browse/manuscript-preparation/. [Last accessed April 30, 2020.
9. Mishra D, Shah D (Eds). The Art and Science of Writing a Scientific Paper. New Delhi: CBS Publishers; 2020.
10. Mukherjee A, Lodha R. Writing the results. Indian Pediatr. 2016;53:409-15.

CHAPTER 28

Manuscript-based Thesis: A New Paradigm

Somashekhar Nimbalkar

■ INTRODUCTION

The most common method of publication followed in India is publishing a manuscript derived from the dissertation of a master's degree or a doctoral degree. In this manner, a thesis may result in publication of a scientific paper in a journal. However, as most students and supervisors know, often due to other pressing needs, a thesis may never get published and precious work is lost to the academic world. To circumvent this and to ensure that a high degree of peer review is already met when the thesis is submitted, few universities across the world have shifted to a new paradigm of a manuscript-based thesis.

■ WHAT IS A MANUSCRIPT-BASED THESIS?

A thesis that incorporates published manuscripts/accepted manuscripts (or manuscripts in publishable form) from the research work undertaken by the student for his/her master's or doctoral thesis would meet the definition of a manuscript-based thesis. The manuscripts need to be derived from the research work done and there needs to be a cohesive body of work that shows its unitary character. The manuscripts can be of various types and range from narrative reviews, systematic reviews, protocol manuscripts, methodology papers, original articles, or even animal research as long as it stems from a single body of research. The student would need to be the first author signifying that he/she has done the major work on writing the manuscript and thus fulfill the criteria for authorship.

How Many Manuscripts are there in a Manuscript-based Thesis?

University academics, rigor, and standards determine the number of manuscripts required for a thesis. While two manuscripts are the minimum usually required in Indian DM/MCH programs for a master's or doctoral thesis, some programs may require up to four manuscripts for a doctoral thesis and just one manuscript for a master's thesis. It is a requirement that at least one manuscript be based on data that is obtained during the conduct of the research by the student.

Should the Manuscripts be Published/Accepted/Submitted?

There is no standard guideline and this falls under the purview of the university. Most renowned universities would want the

TABLE 28.1: Differences between manuscript-based thesis and traditional thesis.

Manuscript-based thesis	Traditional thesis
Advantages	
Published articles based on the research done have more value than a thesis that is less accessible to the academic community	Allows the student to have freedom to structure the thesis based on guidelines that are broad
It is likely to have more citations for a published paper than a thesis	Often journals are wary of publishing radical new ideas and these will find more acceptance in a traditional thesis and thus allow the student to complete his course in time
A published article in a high impact factor journal with a high number of citations will be viewed with greater respect and increases the chances of the student getting a better academic position in universities	A student who has limited availability of time may find a traditional thesis easier to complete as he/she needs to navigate fewer guidelines and peer reviewers
The student can develop a flair for writing manuscripts that are suitable to be published in journals	The traditional thesis allows a beginner to develop his/her writing skills and not to be overawed by stringent requirements of journals
The student needs the support of his supervisors/guides who have experience in publishing manuscripts, have the time to guide, and the patience to go through the peer review process of journals	A relatively inexperienced guide/supervisor may be more amenable to a traditional thesis and would be able to do a better handholding of the student
Disadvantages	
The process can be unnecessarily prolonged, as the guide and student have to depend on an external factor such as the editors to achieve their goals	If there is poor oversight and supervision, the quality of the traditional thesis drops over time and good research work may not get published

manuscripts to be accepted before they can be incorporated in the thesis. However, it is acceptable to have manuscripts that have been submitted or ready for submission incorporated in this form of thesis.

Should I Choose a Manuscript-based Thesis or a Traditional Thesis?

Some universities may offer a choice between the two types of thesis and the student would need to consider the options before selecting between either of them. **Table 28.1** outlines the important differences between a manuscript-based thesis and traditional thesis.

Thus, choice depends on various factors and it should be a joint decision of the supervisor and the student. There also needs to be guidance from the academic committee of the university that oversees dissertations. It may also depend on research work that will be undertaken and whether the design and execution of research will lend itself to the publication of manuscripts.

■ SUGGESTED FORMAT

It should ideally encompass all the items that are present in a traditional thesis. However, it also depends on what articles are published and the extent of details included there. If three articles have been prepared/published in the form of a systematic review, methodology paper, and an original article, very little additional information may be needed in the final

> **Box 28.1: Suggested components of a manuscript-based thesis.**
> 1. Title Page
> 2. Abstract/Summary
> 3. Introduction
> 4. Aim and Objectives
> 5. Review of Literature (Manuscript on systematic review or desk review can also be included here)
> 6. Methodology (Any methodology paper/published protocol can be included here)
> 7. Manuscript 1 (original article)
> 8. Manuscript 2 (if any)
> 9. Manuscript 3 (if any)
> 10. Results (if any remaining)
> 11. Discussion
> 12. Conclusion
> 13. Bibliography
> 14. Appendices

thesis. However, if three original articles have been prepared/published, adding additional information in the thesis of the methodology and review of literature would be needed as the original articles may not have enough details for these parts of the research work.

Suggested components and their sequence of a manuscript-based thesis are listed in **Box 28.1**.

Introduction

The Introduction needs to be written separately. The manuscripts have word limits for the introduction and hence what could not be incorporated in the manuscripts can be used in the thesis so as to give a better idea of the need for doing the research work. This section should have the conceptual framework of the research work and also show that the manuscripts published form an integral part of this work. It should cite the manuscripts published or give details of where they have been sent for publication. The contributions of the authors may be detailed in this section.

Aim and Objectives

The manuscripts by themselves will have the research questions incorporated in them. However, if there are 2–4 original articles, there may be a different research component being evaluated in them. In this section of the thesis, the aim and objectives pertaining to all the manuscripts can be detailed at a single place, so that an impression of the complete research work is provided at one place. If there is only a single original paper-based manuscript in the thesis, this section may become superfluous.

Review of Literature

This section of the manuscript-based thesis allows the student to detail more studies as many cannot be incorporated into the manuscripts themselves. It allows for greater latitude in the number of papers that can be cited as some journals have a cap on the number of papers that can be cited. The review also tends to be more focused than what can be seen in a traditional thesis. If a systematic review has been published, that manuscript can replace this section.

Methodology

Manuscripts do not have the space for detailed methodology unless a methods paper has been published. Therefore, the student can add more details of the methods in this section, including various photographs that may not find space in a manuscript. If a methods/protocol paper has been published, that manuscript can replace this section.

Data-based Manuscripts

The manuscripts based on various objectives of the research work and those based on secondary data/projections should be listed next in sequence. This section is essential in a manuscript-based thesis.

Results

This section complements the manuscript, and tables and graphs that could not be included in the manuscripts can be utilized in this section. Many journals allow supplementary web tables where detailed results can be published. If this is the case, this section may not be necessary and the supplementary web tables or supplementary files can be used along with the manuscript.

Discussion

This section can utilize additional details that are not shared in the manuscripts. If 3–4 original articles have been written, this section may not be extensive or refer to the discussions in the manuscripts.

Conclusions

This section can contain the conclusions as well as recommendations and the contribution of the thesis to the improvement in knowledge of the research area that was addressed.

Bibliography

The references in the thesis need to be arranged as a single comprehensive alphabetical list including all references cited in the entire thesis (i.e., those cited both in manuscripts and in chapters, which are not included in the manuscripts). It is expected that the in-text referencing is consistent throughout the thesis.

WHY A PARADIGM SHIFT?

Academics need to ensure that research work is made available to the larger scientific community. Moving to a manuscript-based thesis may be one way for academia to increase the value of scholarship in society as shared information helps build newer concepts and advances in all spheres of education whether science, humanities, or business.

CONCLUSION

A manuscript-based thesis is encouraged by many universities and should be an option that is available to all students of a university. It provides a unique opportunity within the training period to publish one's work (or prepare a manuscript that is ready to submit) and thus gives the student a stronger footing for an academic career. The university also benefits from having more published literature in the public domain, which can enhance its academic standing and rating. However, this approach requires a more experienced guide and a supportive administration.

KEY MESSAGES

- The student needs to have a flair for academic writing and a supervisor who has some publishing experience for a manuscript-based thesis to be successful.
- The decision to choose between a manuscript-based thesis and a traditional thesis should be a joint one between the supervisor and the student and should have approval of the academic committee of the university.
- A traditional thesis is a better choice if the topic is unlikely to get traction with journals, especially when it is a new topic or the research work is replicating previous work.

FURTHER READING

1. Ryerson University. Guidelines for manuscript-based dissertations/theses 2019. [online] Available from https://www.ryerson.ca/Content/Dam/Graduate/Programs/Ensciman/Documents/EnSciMan-Manuscript-Thesis-and-Dissertation-Guidelines.pdf. Ryerson University. [Last accessed April 30, 2020].
2. University of Calgary. Guidelines for manuscript-based thesis 2019. [online] Available from nursing.ucalgary.ca/sites/default/files/teams/4/2019_01%20Guidelines%20for%20Manuscript%20Based%20Thesis.pdf. [Last accessed April 30, 2020]
3. University of Uottawa. Manuscript-based thesis 2016. [online] Available from health.uottawa.ca/nursing/sites/health.uottawa.ca.nursing/files/manuscript-basedthesis2016.pdf. [Last accessed April 30, 2020].

Annexure: Case-Record Form
Title: Clinical and Biochemical Profile of Neonatal and Infantile Cholestasis

Basic Information

CR No.: ....

Date of Admission: ....

Telephone (Mobile) No.: ....

Name: ....

Birth Weight: ....

Date of Birth: ....

Address: ....

....

Age: .... Gender: ....

Gestational Age: ....

Clinical Details

Past history of jaundice:	Yes/No	Edema:	Yes/No
Family history of liver disorder:	Yes/No	Skin bleeds:	Yes/No
Acholic stools:	Never/Persistent/Intermittent	Vitamin deficiency signs:	Yes/No
		Palmar erythema:	
Bleeding from any site:	Yes/No	Liver size (BCM):	Yes/No
Nature:		Spleen size (BCM):	
Duration:		Ascites:	
Itching or scratch marks:	Yes/No		Yes/No

Investigation	Date	Result	Date	Result	Date	Result
S. bilirubin: Total/direct						
AST						
ALT						
ALT/AST						
Alkaline phosphatase						
PT						
APTT						

Treatment Given

Antibiotics: ....

Blood and blood products: ....

Vitamins and supplements: ....

Final Diagnosis

Outcome

Discharged/Died/LAMA   Cause of death   Condition at discharge

Index

A

Abbreviations 175
  glossary of 21
  in the title 47
Acknowledgments 20
Acronyms 175
Accountability 98
Aim 13, 60
  vs. objectives 60, 61t
Aim and objectives 13, 60-65
  aligning with title 62
  in a manuscript-based thesis 210
  in protocol 199
  steps to formulate 64t
  translating research question to 61
Allocation concealment 40, 80
Alpha error 87
Alternate hypothesis 28
Analytical studies 36
Ancillary data 128, 129
Animations 190
Annexure 16
  in protocol 201
Appendices 16, 21
Applied research 26
Area under the curve 38
Assent 99
Authorship 169b, 205
Axis
  in a graph 135

B

Bar chart 136f
Baseline data 80, 124
Basic research 26
Beneficence 97
Beta error 87
Bibliography 154
  in a manuscript-based thesis 211
Binary logistic regression analysis 115
Binding 22
Blinding 40, 80
Block randomization 40
Boolean operators 55, 56
Boxplot 135f

C

Captions
  of a graph 135
Case record form 22, 106-108, 200, 212
Case studies 44t
Case-control study 36, 37f, 44t
  objective of 63
Categorical data 110
Central tendency
  measures of 111
Certificate
  of consent 102b
  of participation 99
  of thesis 20f
Charts 189
Citing 154
Clinical informatics 58
Clinical Trials Registry India (CTRI)
ClipArt 190
Clipboard 55
Cluster randomization 40
Cochrane collaboration 41
Cochrane database of systematic reviews 57
Cochrane library 57
Cohen's d 89
Cohort 36

Cohort study 36, 37f, 44t
  objective of 63
Collective nouns 178
Columns 134
Comma 176
Comma separated lists 177
Comparison group 79
Complete plagiarism 167t
Conclusion 15, 143-147
  do's and don'ts 144
  errors in writing 145
  essential elements of 143
  sample 144
  styles of 146t
  using tense in 145t
  in a manuscript-based thesis 211
Confidence interval 86, 120
Confidence level 120
Confidence limits
  for calculating sample size 92
Confidentiality 101b
Confounder 37
Consent form 22
CONSORT 44, 77
  flow diagram 126f
Consortium for academic and research ethics (CARE) 58
Continuous data 110
Control group 79
Controls
  selection of 37
Convenience sampling 79
Correlation 113
  and regression 115b
Correlation coefficient 113, 114b
Cover design 19f, 22
Cover page 197
Crossover study design 42
Cross-reference 154

Cross-sectional study 36, 37, 37f, 44t
Cryptomnesia 166

D

Data
  acquisition of 103
  categorical *vs.* numerical 110
  collection 81
  fabrication 168
  falsification 168
  management 200
  monitoring 81
  ownership 103
  paired *vs.* unpaired 110
  type of 124
Data Safety Monitoring Board (DSMB) 104
Data sheet 22
Data slicing 206
Data-based manuscripts 210
Databases 53t
Decimal 129
Declaration 19, 20f
Declaration of Helsinki 104
Demographic data 125
Descriptive research question 28
Descriptive studies 35
Diagnostic studies 37, 43t, 77
Diagnostic test 121
Digital presenter 194f
Direct plagiarism 167t
Discussion 138-142
  checklist 141
  components of 15
  contents of 138
  elements of 139
  how to organize 140
  in a manuscript-based thesis 211
  of thesis paper 205
  purpose of 138
Dispersion
  about mean 88
  measures of 111
Dissertation 2
Distributive justice 98
Dropout rates 90

E

Effect size 43t, 88, 89
Efficacy studies 43t
Electronic case record form 108
Embase 53t
Environmental protection 98
English
  elements of writing 175-184
  problems in writing 182
Epi Info 91, 91f
Essentiality 98
Ethics 97-105
  in methods 78
  in patient care and research 103
Ethics committee 104
Ethical writing 166
Evidence
  levels of 42
Exclusion criteria 79
Expected frequency
  for calculating sample size 91
Experimental studies 34, 44t
Experimental study design 39
Exposure 36

F

Fabrication 168
False negative 38t, 121
False positive 38t, 121
Falsification 168
  examples of 169b
Feasibility sampling 79
Filters 54
Fonts
  serif *vs.* sans-serif 188f
  size, for slides 188
Footnote
  of table 134
Forest plot 42

G

Gaussian distribution 112f
Ghost authorship 169
Glossary 21
Good clinical practice guidelines 104

Google 51
Google Scholar 52, 53t, 57
Google slides 196
Grab bag conclusion 146t
Graph 132f, 134
  components of 135
  considerations for 134
  in PowerPoint 189
  selecting appropriate 135
Guru 5

H

Haiku deck 195
Harvard style 157
Headers and footers 191
Heading
  and subheadings 23
  of table 134
Health informatics 58
Hypothesis 26, 28
  elements of 28
  framing of 29
  studies to test 86
  types of 28b
Hypothesis testing
  concept of 116
  steps of 117

I

ICMJE style 157, 158
Inclusion criteria 78
Index 21
Index test 38
IndMED 58
Inferential research question 28
Informed consent 98
Informed consent document 99
Informed consent form 100b
  in protocol 200
Institutional arrangements 98
Institutional Ethics Committee (IEC) 104
Intellectual theft 167t
International conference on harmonization (ICH) 104
Internet
  as source of literature 51
  citation 159

Interquartile range (IQR) 111
Intervention 48, 80
Interventional studies 77
Introduction
  components of 13
  funnel approach 67
  in a manuscript-based thesis 210
  in summary 149
  of protocol 198
  of thesis paper 204
  purpose of 66
  structure of 67
  what not to include in 67
  when to write 66

J

Journal
  name, abbreviating 159
  selection of 203

K

Keyboard shortcuts 192
Keynote 196

L

Law 97
Legally acceptable/authorized representative (LAR) 99
Legends
  of graph 135
Levels of evidence (LOE) 42
  for different research questions 43t
  hierarchy of 43f
Linear correlation 113
Lists 177
Literature
  critical analysis of 73
  primary, secondary, tertiary 51, 69
  scholarly *vs.* nonscholarly 51
  sorting and prioritizing 72
  sources of 51
Literature review. Also *See* Review of literature
  chronological 71
  conceptual 71
  goal of 71
  methodological 71
  organization of 71
  writing the 73
Literature search 51-59
Logistic regression 115

M

Manipulation 166
Manuscript based thesis 203, 208-211
  components of 210b
  format of 209
  traditional thesis *vs.* 209t
Margin of error 87
Master chart 22
Matched control 110
Material and methods 14, 76-84
  checklist for 83b
  components of 76
  in a manuscript-based thesis 210
  in protocol 199
  in summary 149
  of thesis paper 204
  tips for writing 14, 82
  what not be include in 84
Mathew effect 52
Maximization of benefit 98
Mean 111
Measures of dispersion 88
Median 111
Medical information 52f
Medical informatics 58
Medline 53
Mendeley 160-162
Mentee 7
Mentor 7
Mentoring 5, 6t,
Mentor–Mentee relationship 2-9
  do's and don'ts of 7
Mentorship program 7
MeSH 56
MeSH database 56
MeSH-based search 54f, 56
Meta-analysis 41, 77
Methodology oriented literature review 70
Misattribution 167t
Misquotation 166
Misrepresentation 166
Mixed-methods study 42
Mode 111
Model protocol 197
Modifiers 179
Morals 97
Multinomial logistic regression analysis 115
Multiple regression 115
My bibliography 55

N

National Center for Biotechnology Information (NCBI) 54
National guidelines for biomedical and health research in 2017 104
National institute of health (NIH) 54
National library of medicine (NLM) 54
Negative predictive value (NPV) 38t, 122
Nested case–control study 42
NLM catalog 57
Non-linear correlation 113
Nonexploitation 98
Nonmaleficence 97
Nonrandomized study 39
Nonresponse rate 90
Null hypothesis 28, 117
Numbers 178
Nuremberg code of 1947 103

O

Objectives 60
  essential elements of 63
  primary and secondary 61
  SMART 13, 63
Observational studies 33, 35, 77
Odds ratio (OR) 115
Optional thesis 24
Outcome 36
Outcome data 126, 129
  of a single group 126
  of categorical variables 127
  of more than one group 127

Outcome measures 81
   in protocol 200
   estimated value of 87
Outcome oriented literature
   review 70

P

P value 117, 128
Pagination 23
Paired data 110
Paragraph 182
Paraphrasing 165, 171
   appropriate and
      inappropriate 171b
Parenthesis 55
Participant 78
Participant data 124, 129
Participant flow 125, 126f
Patient information sheet 22, 99
Patient information sheet,
   additional elements 102
   essential elements of 101
Photographs 136
Photomicrographs 136
PICO 28
   comparison in 29f
   in conclusion 143
   in objectives 63
   intervention on 29f
   outcome in 29f
   population in 29f
Picture 190
Pilson's law 12
Plagiarism 166
   Delhi University Guidelines
      173b
   how to avoid 170
   types of 167
   UGC guidelines 172t
Plagiarism check software 171
Plurals 178
Population 48, 78, 109
   for calculating sample size 91
Positive predictive value (PPV)
   38t, 122
Post-hoc analysis 128
Power 88, 120
PowerPoint 185-196
   alternatives to 195
Predictive value 122

Presentation
   defining contents of 186
   finalization of 195
   preparing 192
Prevalence study 43t
Prezi 195
Primary literature 51, 69
Primary outcome 81
   and sample size 87
Primum non nocere 97
Privacy 98
PRISMA 77
Professional competence 98
Protocol. *See* Thesis Protocol
PS2 software 92, 93f
Publication ethics 206
Publication misconduct 165-174
   reasons for 170b
   types of 166
PubMed 53
   clipboard in 55
   filters in 54
   my bibliography in 55
   opening page 54f
   other features of 57
   parentheses in 55
   quotation marks in 55
   search 53, 55f
   truncation in 55
PubMed mobile 57

Q

Qualitative research 26
Qualitative studies 33
Quantitative data 110
Quantitative studies 33
Quotation marks 55

R

Randomization 39, 80
Randomized controlled trial 40
   objectives of 63
   parallel group 41f
Receiver operating
   characteristic (RoC) curve
   38, 39f
References 15, 154-164
   for a book chapter 159
   for a journal article 158

Harvard style 157
   how to write 156
   ICMJE style
   importance of 154
   in protocol 200
   key-terms for 154
   numbering of 158
   of thesis paper 205
   selection of 156
   sources of 155
   styles for writing 157
   Vancouver style 157
Reference list 154
Reference managers 160
Referencing software 58
Regression analysis 114
Rehearsing 194
Relative risk (RR) 116
Reporting guidelines 43
Research
   categories of 27t
   fields of 27
   for the practicing physician 1
   importance of 1
   in postgraduate courses 1-4
   opportunities for 2
   planning and conducting 103
   reporting of 103
   responsible conduct of 103
   types of 26
Research question 11, 26-32
   characteristics of 30b
   descriptive *vs.* inferential 28
   developing a 31f
   elements of 28
   framing 29
   good *vs.* bad 30
Respect for autonomy 97
Results 124-130
   components of 14
   in a manuscript-based thesis
      211
   in discussion 139
   in summary 149
   of thesis paper 205
   presentation of 129f
   sequence of presentation 128
   structure of 132
   what to include in 131
Review of literature 69-75
   components of 70

in a manuscript-based thesis 210
in protocol 199
mistakes in writing 74
process of 72
tips for writing 13
Right to refuse or withdraw 101b
Risk minimization 98
ROC curve 38
Rows 134

S

Salami publication 206
Sample 109
Sample size 81, 82, 85-96
 adjusting the 89
 Epi Info for calculating 94
 for a case-control study 93f
 for a randomized trial 94f
 for prevalence study 86
 for studies involving hypothesis testing 88
 formulae for 90
 how to calculate 86
 PS2 software for calculating 93
 software for calculating 90, 90b
 why to calculate 85
Sampling 79
Scales
 in graph 135
Scatter plot 136f
Scholarly literature 51
Secondary literature 51
Secondary outcome measures 81
Self-plagiarism 167t
Semicolon 177
Sensitivity 38t, 121
Sentence 181
Sequence generation 80
Sequential sampling 79
Setting 48
Sherlock Holmes conclusion 146t
Shishya 5
Simple randomization 39, 79
Simple regression 114
Six by six rule 188

Skewed data 112
Slides 185
 10 points for making 192b
 background of 189
 bad 193f
 editing of 192
 layout 187
SMART 13
Smart art graphic 190
Social data 125
Social responsibility 98
Software
 for literature search 53
 for plagiarism check 171
 for sample size 90, 93, 94
Source-based plagiarism 167t
Specificity 38t, 121
Spelling 176
SPICED 48
Standard deviation (SD) 111
 for calculating sample size 88
Standard test 38
STARD 43, 77
Statistical analysis 82, 109-123
 in the text 133
 in protocol 200
Statistical tests 118, 119f
 significance of 128
Stop words 56
Stratified randomization 39
Stratified sampling 79
STROBE 43, 77
Structured summary 148
Studies of diagnostic accuracy 37
Study design 33-44, 76
 additional 41
 case–control vs. cohort 35t
 choosing the 34
 limitations and strengths 44t
 outline of 34f
 qualitative vs. quantitative 33
 reporting guidelines for 77
Study period 78
Study setting 78
Summary 148-153
 4-point checklist 149t
 10-point checklist 149t
 attributes of a good 152
 do's and don'ts of 152
 elements of 149

format for writing 148
 in the thesis 152
 of protocol 198
 structured vs. unstructured
Supervisor
 and supervisee 6
 as a mentor 6
 expectations from 6,8
 expectations of 8
Swag 196
Systematic random sampling 79
Systematic reviews 41, 77

T

Table,
 2 × 2 38t
 components of 134
 considerations for 134
 in PowerPoint 189
 presentation of 134
Table of contents 21
 sample of 21f
Tertiary literature 51, 70
Text 132
Text-based search 54f, 55, 56
Thesis protocol 12, 197-201
 elements of 198
 summary of 198
Thesis 10-25
 10 essential components of 18
 advantages and disadvantages of 3
 author names in 158
 content of 13
 converting into a scientific paper 3, 16, 202-207
 in postgraduate courses 3
 margins of 23
 optional 24
 paper quality of 22
 preparing final 23
 rationale for 1-4
 rectification in 24
 role of 3
 spine of 22f
 submission of 23
 time guidelines for submission 24
 timetable for 12

typing and formatting 22
vs. dissertation 2
vs. scientific paper 202*t*
Three-word challenge 188
Title 45-50
   abbreviations in 47
   elements of 47, 48
   importance of 45
   of thesis paper 204
   what all to include 48
   when to write 49
Title page 19, 198
   sample of 19*f*
Topic
   selection of 11
Totality of responsibility 98
Translation plagiarism 167*t*
Transparency 98
Trial registration 104
True negative 38*t*, 121
True positive 38*t*, 121
Truncation 55
Type I error 87, 118, 119*t*, 119*f*
Type II error 88, 118, 119*t*, 119*f*
Typographical errors 176

U

UGC guidelines on academic integrity 172
UGC guidelines on prevention of plagiarism 172
Universal declaration on bioethics and human rights (2005) 104
University grants commission regulation 2018 172

Unpaired data 110
Unstructured summary 148

V

Values
   of conducting research 103
Vancouver style 157, 158
Variables
   and data 110
   dependent *vs.* independent 111
Visme 195
Voluntariness 98

W

Writing malpractice 166

Plate 1

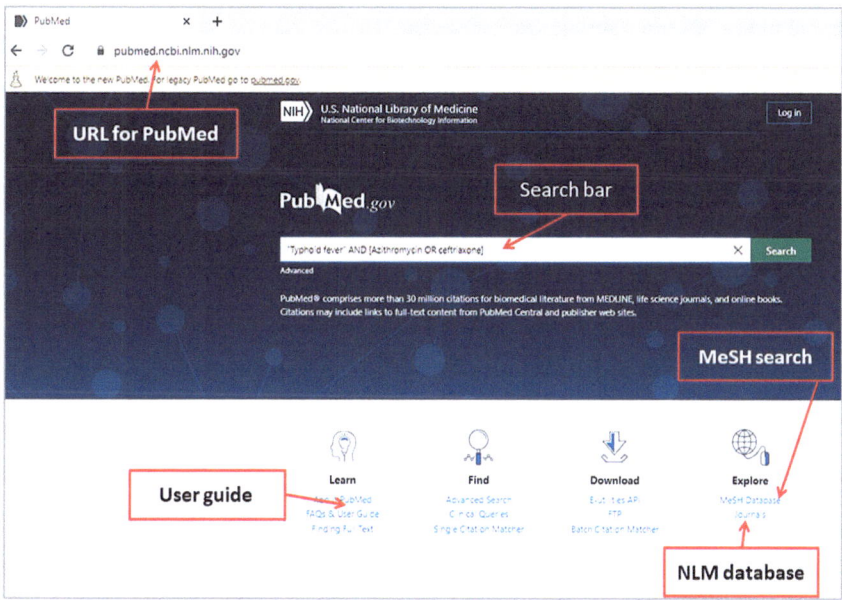

Fig. 8.1: Opening page of NCBI–PubMed revealing the search bar for text-based search, MeSH database for MeSH-based search, NLM database for searching journal, and user guide for troubleshoot. *(Chapter 8)*

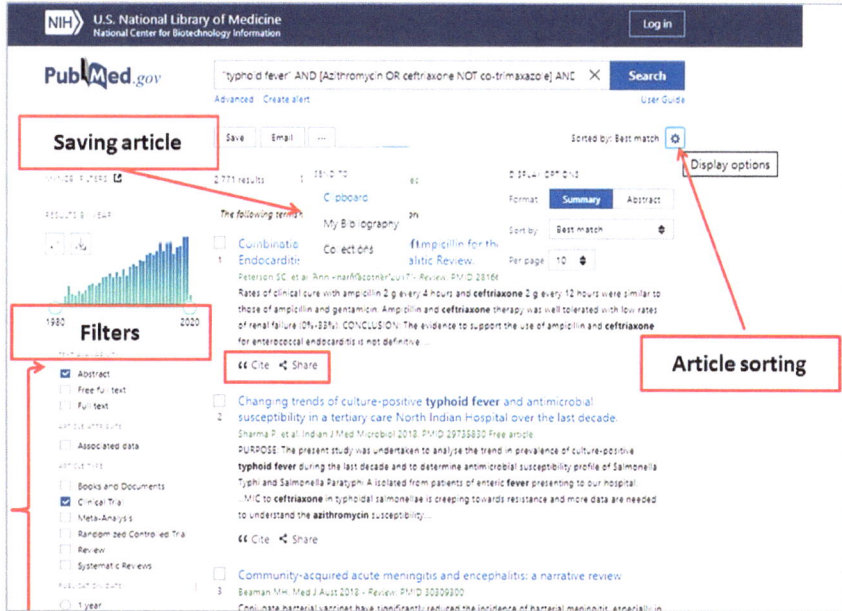

Fig. 8.2: PubMed search on typhoid fever depicting method to sort the articles, save the articles, cite and share them using appropriate filters. *(Chapter 8)*

Plate 2

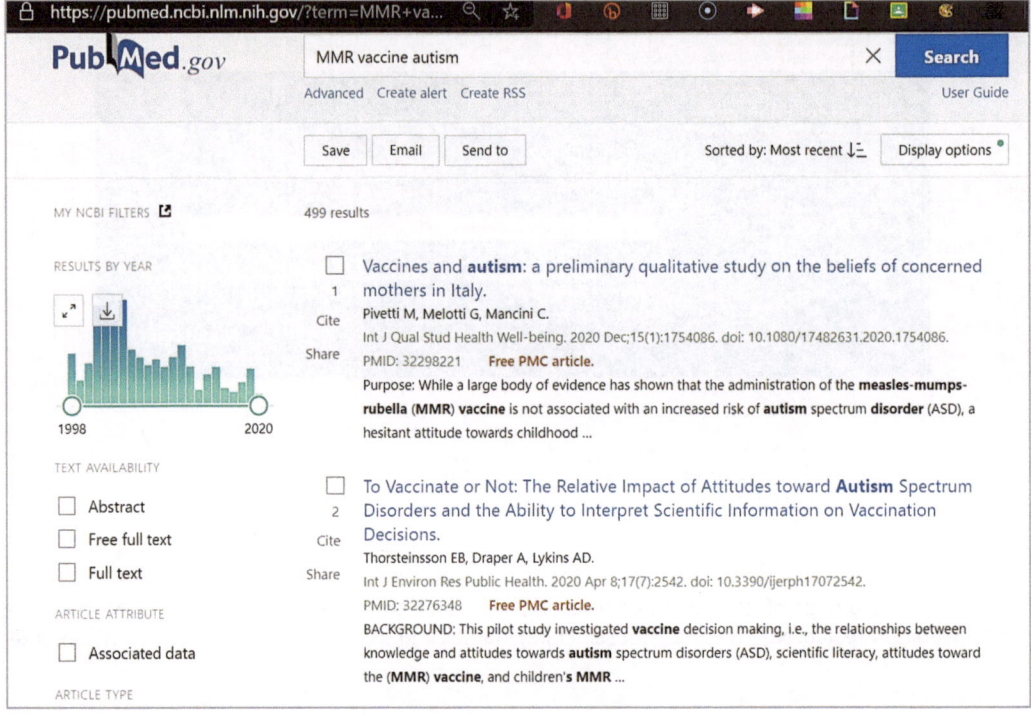

Fig 22. 1: Searching for literature on measles, mumps, and rubella (MMR) vaccine and autism. *(Chapter 22)*

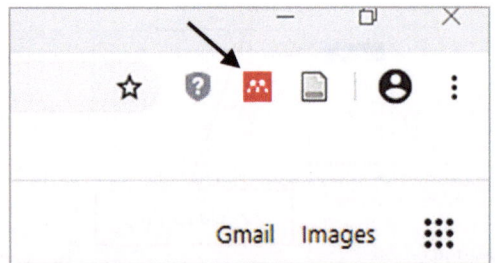

Fig. 22.3: Mendeley web importer icon (indicated by an arrow) as displayed in Google Chrome browser. *(Chapter 22)*

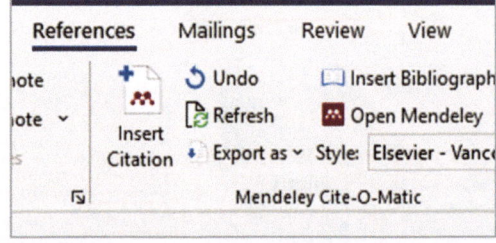

Fig. 22.4: Mendeley section displayed in the references tab of Microsoft Word document. *(Chapter 22)*

Plate 3

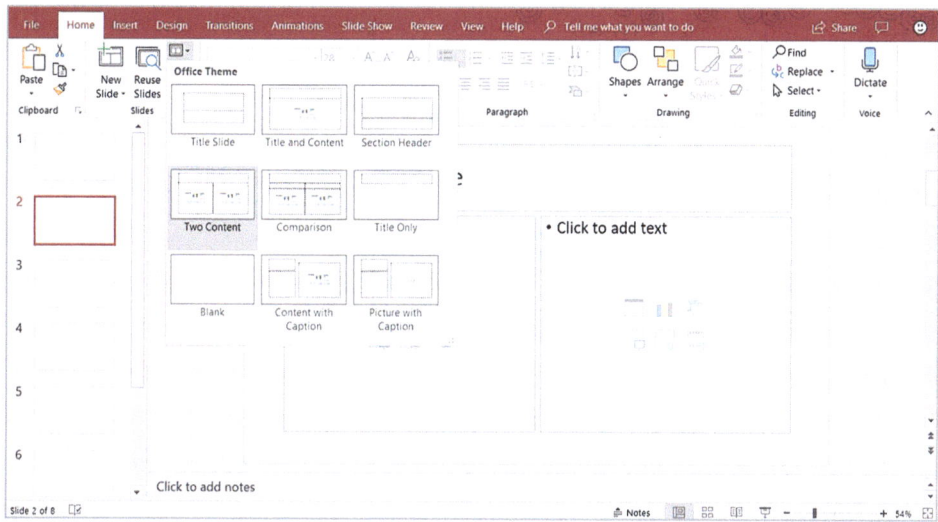

Fig. 25.1: Choosing a slide layout. *(Chapter 25)*

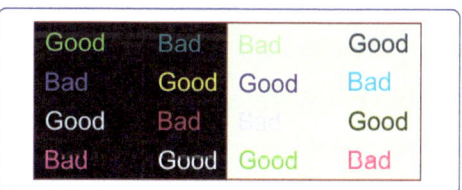

Fig. 25.4: Use of appropriate font color and background color to enhance contrast. *(Chapter 25)*

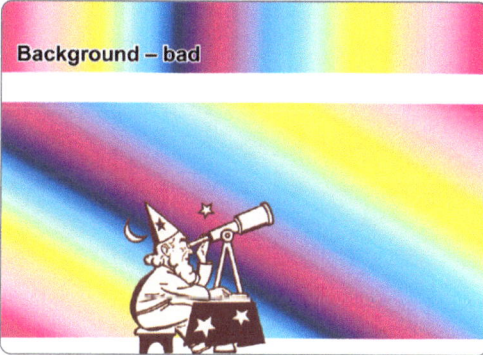

Fig. 25.5: Bad background for slides. *(Chapter 25)*

Plate 4

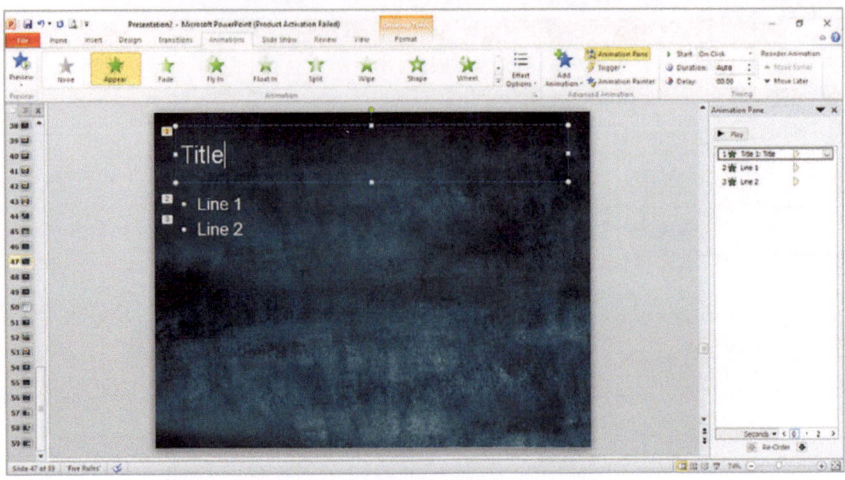

Fig. 25.6: Customizing animation. *(Chapter 25)*

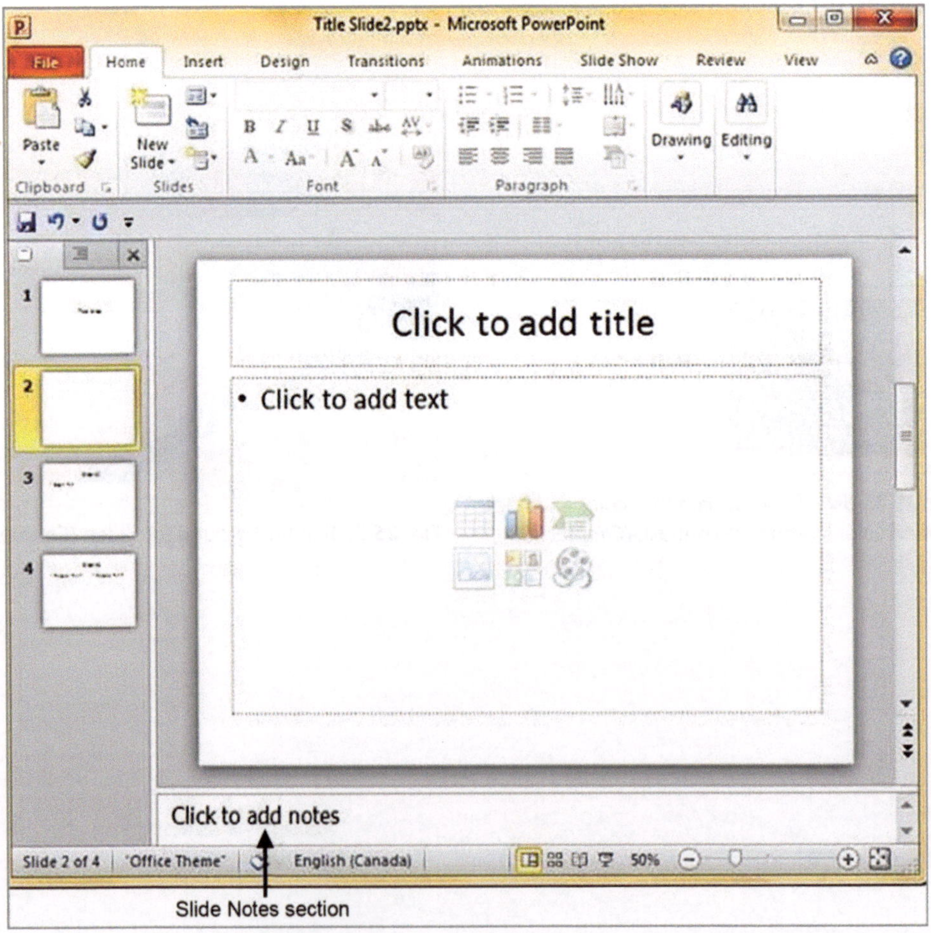

Fig. 25.7: Inserting notes in presentation. *(Chapter 25)*

Plate 5

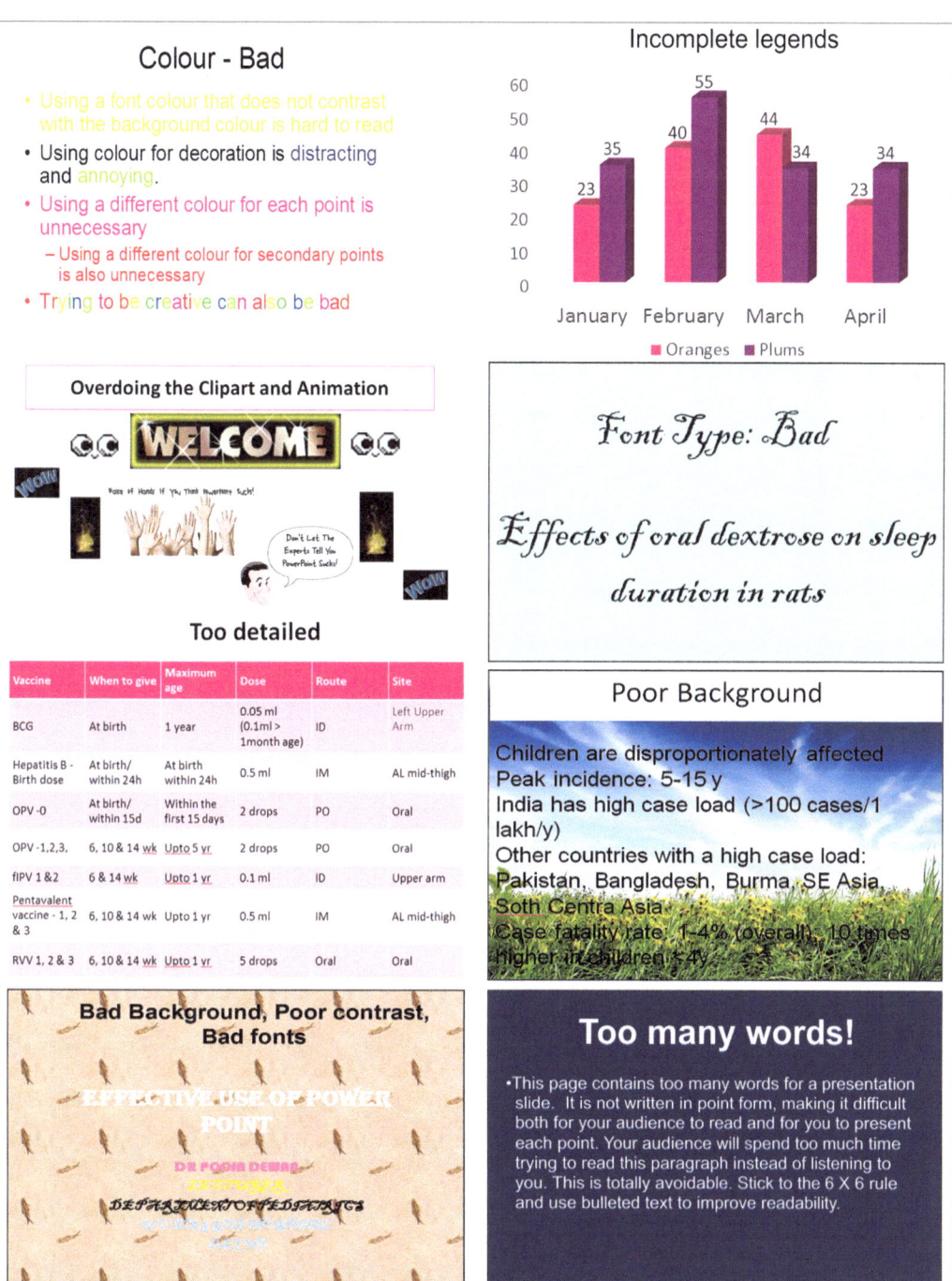

Fig. 25.8: Some bad slides in PowerPoint presentation. *(Chapter 25)*